ESSENTIALS OF

MEDICAL GENETICS

for Nursing and Health Professionals

An Interprofessional Approach

Laura M. Gunder McClary, DHSc, MHE, PA-C

Professor
Physician Assistant Department
Medical College of Georgia School of Allied
   Health Sciences
Augusta, Georgia

Professor
Nova Southeastern University
Fort Lauderdale, Florida

JONES & BARTLETT
LEARNING

World Headquarters
Jones & Bartlett Learning
5 Wall Street
Burlington, MA 01803
978-443-5000
info@jblearning.com
www.jblearning.com

Jones & Bartlett Learning books and products are available through most bookstores and online booksellers. To contact Jones & Bartlett Learning directly, call 800-832-0034, fax 978-443-8000, or visit our website, www.jblearning.com.

Production Credits

VP, Product Management: David D. Cella
Director of Product Management: Amanda Martin
Product Manager: Rebecca Stephenson
Product Assistant: Christina Freitas
Production Editor: Kelly Sylvester
Senior Marketing Manager: Jennifer Scherzay
Product Fulfillment Manager: Wendy Kilborn
Composition: S4Carlisle Publishing Services
Cover Design: Kristin E. Parker
Text Design: Michael O'Donnell
Rights & Media Specialist: John Rusk

Media Development Editor: Troy Liston
Cover Image: © Science Photo Library/ Getty Images (Genetics research and Genetic research conceptual image), © nicolas_/ E+/ Getty Images (Scientist looking at a DNA sequence), © D3Damon/ iStock/ Getty Images (Pills with DNA structure), © BSIP/ Getty Images (Biological specimen), © monsitj/ iStock/ Getty Images (DNA molecules on abstract technology background), © Natali_Mis/ iStock/ Getty Images (DNA shows doctor on a blue background concept design)
Printing and Binding: LSC Communications Kendallville
Cover Printing: LSC Communications Kendallville

Library of Congress Cataloging-in-Publication Data

Names: Gunder McClary, Laura M., author.
Title: Essentials of medical genetics for nursing and health professionals / Laura M. Gunder McClary.
Description: Burlington, Massachusetts : Jones & Bartlett Learning, [2019] | Includes bibliographical references.
Identifiers: LCCN 2018028651 | ISBN 9781284154245 (paperback)
Subjects: | MESH: Genetics, Medical | Genetic Diseases, Inborn--diagnosis | Genetic Diseases, Inborn--therapy
Classification: LCC RB155 | NLM QZ 50 | DDC 616/.042--dc23
LC record available at https://lccn.loc.gov/2018028651

6048

Printed in the United States of America
22 21 20 19 18   10 9 8 7 6 5 4 3 2 1

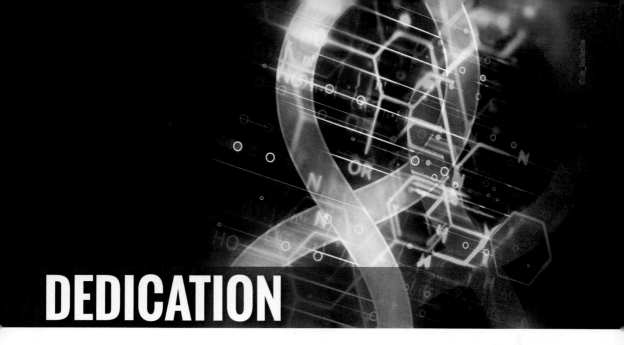

DEDICATION

The profound privilege of being a healthcare provider revolves around our dedication to improving the human condition through our service to others. With the exception of our own families, we find our greatest joy in serving patients and their families as well as in mentoring and teaching students in our charge. This text is for the students, teachers, patients, colleagues, and families who seek to know more and serve better. May your knowledge and skills always be tempered by compassion, integrity, and humility—these virtues are essential to the character of a true Servant.

SPECIAL ACKNOWLEDGMENTS

Most often in one's career, it is the person's family who make the greatest sacrifices. Families are unseen contributors in even our smallest accomplishments. This is certainly the case of those persons engaged in clinical practice, research, and academia, as working during many weekends, holidays, and evenings is required of us. Thank you all for your love, encouragement, and prayers and for making that sacrifice.

It is also important to note the collaborative efforts of numerous disciplines that culminated in a truly interprofessional approach to this curriculum. This is a reflection of how we work in everyday practice to achieve the best outcomes for our patients.

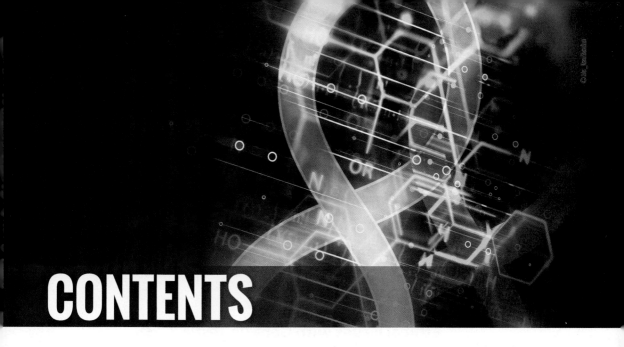

CONTENTS

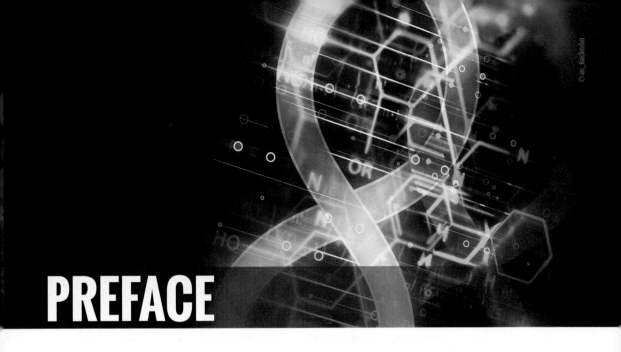

PREFACE

Learners enrolled in every healthcare training program need to have a basic understanding of medical genetics so that they can successfully transition from students to clinicians. The field of medical genetics is advancing at a fast pace and is becoming increasingly integral to all aspects of medicine. This fact emphasizes the need for every practicing clinician and faculty member to develop an in-depth knowledge of the principles of human genetics, given that they are applicable to such a wide variety of clinical presentations. Underscoring that importance, multiple accrediting bodies now require that medical genetics be included in the various curriculums, including the Liaison Committee for Medical Education (LCME), Accreditation Review Commission on Education for Physician Assistants (ARC-PA), Accreditation Commission for Education in Nursing (ACEN), Commission on Accreditation for Physical Therapy Accreditation (CAPTA), National Accrediting Agency for Clinical Laboratory Science (NAACLS), and the American Bar Association (ABA).

Likewise, there is a need to train primary care providers and related health professionals to meet the growing demand for genetic intervention. Although genetic counselors typically address most questions asked by the patient and family when a genetic test result is received, it falls to the primary care clinician and those involved in the direct patient care to address the same issues recurrently over the patient's lifetime. With the Human Genome Project's rapid progress and sequencing of the human genome completed ahead of schedule, genetic conditions and their multifactorial nature are increasingly requiring that treatment and prevention measures become highly individualized. The primary care provider in particular stands at the frontline of this interface and will play an integral role in intervention and prevention of genetically based diseases.

The incorporation of medical genetics into medical education and residency training programs has long since begun. However, because the understanding of genomics is relatively new, a gap exists between the education and training of those practicing clinicians, the existing curriculum, and the integration of the principles into clinical practice. Curriculum guidelines exist to assist developers and educators in integrating medical genetics into the existing curricula for most disciplines.

Because the concepts and principles of medical genetics are multidisciplinary and complex, it is especially important to consider the most efficient and effective methods of delivery of genetics-related education during the program planning. In addition to genetic diseases and disorders, the program should include an appreciation of the rapid advances in genetics, the need for lifelong learning, the need for referral, and the role of genetic counselors and medical geneticists. On a practical level, it should ensure that students develop the ability to construct and analyze a three-generation pedigree.

This text is intended to serve as the basis for a medical genetics curriculum that provides an opportunity for students to integrate genetic knowledge, skills, and attitudes early in their medical education and training. Other benefits of the text include improved student understanding of genetic concepts in clinical medicine and improved clinical skills, which will ultimately translate into improved patient outcomes. It is further recommended that faculty and other medical educators receive formal instruction in medical genetics education.

This text is designed to introduce the discipline of clinical genetics to physician assistant students, medical students, and other healthcare providers. Although many other genetics texts are available, most are inappropriate for the accelerated curriculum associated with medical education programs. Students have commented that many of these texts are very cumbersome and too detailed, requiring too much time to extract the most important clinical information. Accordingly, the overarching goal of this book is to assist the reader in making the transition from knowledge-based learning in the didactic curriculum to competency-based practice in the clinical training period and beyond. Moreover, it aims to encourage all practicing providers to integrate their new knowledge, skills, and attitudes related to the latest medical genetics into their everyday clinical practice.

To achieve these ends, the approach taken toward the specific disorders profiled in this text includes an explanation of the genetics involved, signs and symptoms of the disease, treatment and management options, and disease surveillance. A brief review of chromosomes, DNA, RNA, protein synthesis, inheritance patterns, diagnostic techniques, embryonic development, and teratogens is also provided. Finally, the roles of genetic counseling and prenatal testing and screening and an introduction to some ethical and legal issues related to medical genetics are included. Keeping in mind that many faculty will seek out this text as the foundation for a course in clinically relevant medical genetics, this book covers selected topics encountered in a primary care setting that may be ameliorated by early diagnosis and intervention and that cover every organ system.

This book is written in a simple-to-read format that avoids excessive use of genetics jargon. Chapters cover disease topics in all organ systems, ensuring that the text can be used in a variety of curricular formats—either as the sole text in a stand-alone course or as a supplemental resource for teaching clinical medicine in an organ system format across the curriculum. *Please realize that this book is not meant to be an all-inclusive textbook on genetics, as many such books are readily available today.* You will find that this text not only has application in the classroom setting for allied health students and medical students but is also clinically useful and timely for practicing clinicians (i.e., physician assistants, nurse practitioners, physicians, nurses) who want to learn more and stay abreast of new information in the area of genetics.

Many of the chapters offer a list of resources, including many website addresses, given that most students and providers today are likely to access a peer-reviewed website to obtain the most up-to-date medical information. Tables, figures, chapter summaries, and chapter review questions assist the reader in extracting the most pertinent information in a timely manner.

We hope that students, educators, and clinicians will find this text to be a concise, user-friendly, and clinically relevant read.

L. M. Gunder McClary

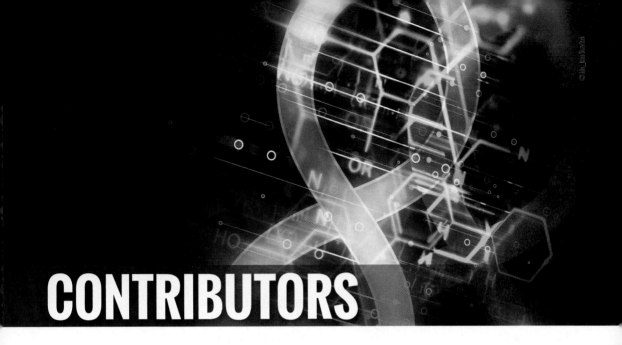

CONTRIBUTORS

Jay Amrien, PA-C
Program Director
Assistant Professor
Bryant University
Smithfield, Rhode Island

Belinda Worley Baron, DHSc, MHA, CLS (ASCP)
Exact Sciences Laboratory
Madison, Wisconsin

Cecelia A. Bellcross, PhD, MS, CGC
Associate Professor
Director, Genetic Counseling Training Program
Emory University School of Medicine
Atlanta, Georgia

Lorilee Butler, DHSc, MPAS, MEd, PA-C
Program Director
Assistant Professor
NOVA Southeastern University, Orlando
Orlando, Florida

Lisa Daitch, MPAS, PA-C
Associate Professor
Augusta University
Augusta, Georgia

Kelly Dayhoff, BSN, RN, MMSc, PA-C
Emory University Hospital
Atlanta, Georgia

Lisa Dickerson, MD
Mercer University
Atlanta, Georgia

Taylor Frering, MMSc, PA-C

Shawn Gunder, JD, MPAS, PA-C
University Hospital
Augusta, Georgia

Laura M. Gunder McClary, DHSc, MHE, PA-C, CLS (ASCP)
Professor
Augusta University
Augusta, Georgia
Professor
NOVA Southeastern University
Fort Lauderdale, Florida

Liz Hayes, MMSc, PA-C
Crestwood Medical Center Emergency
    Department
Huntsville, Alabama

Michael Kehoe, PhD, MMS, PA-C
Sound Clinic
Denver, Colorado

Maha Lund, DHSc, PA-C
Program Director
Associate Professor
Emory University School of Medicine
Atlanta, Georgia

Ingrid Pichardo Murray, DPT, MPAS, PA-C
Academic Director
Associate Professor
Adventist University of Health Sciences
Orlando, Florida

Tansyla Nicholson, MD
Assistant Professor
NOVA Southeastern University
Fort Lauderdale, Florida

Lisa Oakes, MS, CGC
Associate Director, Genetic Counseling Training
    Program
Emory University School of Medicine
Atlanta, Georgia

Melba Ovalle, MD
Professor
NOVA Southeastern University
Orlando, Florida

Chris Roman, PA-C
Assistant Professor
Butler University
Indianapolis, Indiana

Betsy Schmidt, PA-C
Assistant Professor
Butler University
Indianapolis, Indiana

Kristen Smethurst, MPAS, PA-C

Tori Smith, MSN, FNP-C
Florida Hospital
Orlando, Florida

Tia Sohl, MPAS, PA-C
Assistant Professor
Mercer University
Macon, Georgia

Michelle Sousa, MMS, PA-C
Assistant Professor
Gannon University
Ruskin, Florida

Ami Robinson Steele, MMSc, PA-C
Chair and Program Director
Associate Professor
Gardner Webb University
Boiling Springs, North Carolina

Ben Taylor, PhD, PA-C
Clinical Professor
Augusta University
Augusta, Georgia

Adam Wood, PharmD, DABAT
Assistant Professor
NOVA Southeastern University
Nemours Children's Hospital
Fort Lauderdale, Florida

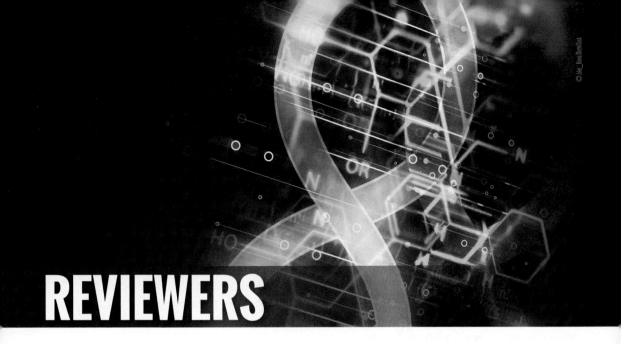

REVIEWERS

Joe Bethle, PA-C
Assistant Professor
Francis Marion University
Florence, South Carolina

James R. Cacchillo, DO
Ohio University
Dublin, Ohio
Medical Director
Capital City Hospice
Westerville, Ohio

Damon B. Cottrell, DNP, APRN, FNP-C, CCNS, ACNS-BC
Assistant Dean & Clinical Professor
Texas Woman's University
Denton, Texas

Ann Crickard, DO
Medical Director and Clinical
    Assistant Professor
Ohio University
Dublin, Ohio

Bonnie Dadiq, EdD, PA-C
Chair and Professor
Augusta University
Augusta, Georgia

Alicia Ela, PharmD
Associate Professor
Augusta University
Augusta, Georgia

Rachel Fink, MPAS, PA-C
Assistant Professor
Augusta University
Augusta, Georgia

Jeffrey Fisher, MPAS, PA-C
Assistant Professor
Ohio University
Dublin, Ohio

Amanda J. Flagg, PhD, RN, EdD/MSN, ACNS, CNE
Associate Professor
Middle Tennessee State University School of Nursing
Murfreesboro, Tennessee

Cheryl Geng, MS, PA-C
Assistant Clinical Professor
Ohio University
Dublin, Ohio

Tracy George, DNP, APRN-BC, CNE
Assistant Professor of Nursing
Francis Marion University
Florence, South Carolina

Sara Haddow-Liebel, MSA, PA-C
Associate Professor
Augusta University
Augusta, Georgia

Cevette M. Hall, DNP, DHSc, ANP-BC, CPHQ
Adjunct Professor
Maryville University
St. Louis, Missouri

Maggie Klusman, MMSc, PA-C
Winter Park Memorial Hospital
Orlando, Florida

Barbara Whitman Lancaster, DNP, APN, WHNP-BC, NCMP
Assistant Professor
Middle Tennessee State University
Murfreesboro, Tennessee

Lee Anne Martinelli, RPh, MMSc, PA-C
Assistant Professor
Emory University School of Medicine
Atlanta, Georgia

Augusto Montalvo, MD, MPH
Advanced Dermatology
Clermont, Florida

Kristen Lugo, PharmD
Assistant Clinical Professor
Director of Clinical Education
Ohio University
Dublin, Ohio

Allan Platt, PA-C, MMSc, DFAAPA
Assistant Professor
Physician Assistant Program
Emory University School of Medicine
Atlanta, Georgia

Mary Smania, DNP, FNP-BC, AGN-BC
Assistant Professor
MSU College of Nursing
East Lansing, Michigan

Mariya Tankimovich, DNP, MSN, RN, APRN, FNP-C, CNE
FNP Track Director for Clinical Education
UTHealth Cizik School of Nursing
Houston, Texas

CHAPTER OBJECTIVES

‹ Review molecular genetics and associated terminology.
‹ Review Mendelian genetic principles.
‹ Define mutation and give examples of different types of mutations.
‹ Describe different inheritance patterns.

KEY TERMS

Allele
Amniocentesis
Aneuploidy
Autosomal dominant
Autosomes
Chorionic villus sampling (CVS)
Chromosomal aberration
Chromosome
Codon
Consanguinity
Degenerate
Deletion
Deoxyribonucleic acid (DNA)
Dominant
Down syndrome

Gene
Genomics
Germinal mutation
Hemizygous
Heterozygous
Homozygous
Inborn errors of metabolism
Inversion
Klinefelter syndrome
Locus
Mendelian genetics
Messenger ribonucleic acid (mRNA)
Mitochondrial chromosome
Monogenic
Monosomy

Mutation
Nondisjunction
Pedigree analysis
Polygenic
Polysomy
Recessive
Ribosomal RNA (rRNA)
Sex chromosome
Somatic mutation
Transcription
Transfer ribonucleic acids (tRNA)
Translation
Translocation
Trisomy
Truncated protein
Turner syndrome

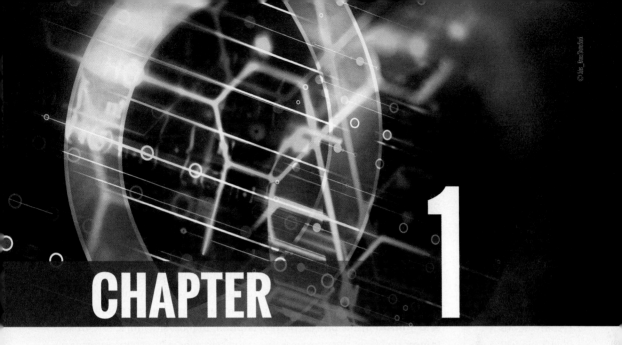

CHAPTER 1

Introduction

The goal of this chapter is not to go into exhaustive genetic detail, but to familiarize the reader with basic genetic concepts (e.g., meiosis and mitosis, haploid vs. diploid) by providing a basic overview of molecular genetics, simple inheritance patterns, chromosomal aberrations, and mutations. For more detailed information or to refresh your memory, the reader is referred to any one of a number of comprehensive genetics textbooks. The following texts are all recommended:

» Hartl, D. L., & Ruvolo, M. (2019). *Genetics: Analysis of genes and genomes* (9th ed.). Burlington, MA: Jones & Bartlett Learning.
» Jameson, J. L., & Kopp, P. (2012). Principles of human genetics. In A. S. Fauci, E. Braunwald, D. L. Kasper, S. L. Hauser, D. L. Longo, J. L. Jameson, & J. Loscalzo (Eds.), *Harrison's principles of internal medicine* (18th ed.). New York, NY: McGraw-Hill Medical.
» Jorde, L. B., Carey, J. C., Bamshad, M. J., & White, R. L. (2016). *Medical genetics* (5th ed.). Philadelphia, PA: Elsevier.
» Nussbuam, R. L., McInnes, R. R., & Willard, H. F. (2016). *Thompson & Thompson genetics in medicine* (8th ed.). Philadelphia, PA: Elsevier.

Basic Genetics

Genetics is the study of biologically inherited traits determined by elements of heredity that are transmitted from parents to offspring in reproduction. These inherited elements are called **genes**. Recent advances in the field of **genomics** have led to development of methods that can determine the complete

KEY TERMS

Gene: a region of DNA containing genetic information, which is usually transcribed into an RNA molecule that is processed and either functions directly or is translated into a polypeptide chain; the hereditary unit.

Genomics: systematic study of an organism's genome using large-scale DNA sequencing, gene-expression analysis, or computational methods.

Deoxyribonucleic acid (DNA): a macromolecule usually composed of two polynucleotide chains in a double helix that is the carrier of genetic information in all cells.

Messenger ribonucleic acid (mRNA): an RNA molecule that is transcribed from a DNA sequence and translated into the amino acid sequence of a polypeptide.

deoxyribonucleic acid (DNA) sequence of an organism. Genomics is the latest advance in the study of the chemical nature of genes and the ways that genes function to affect certain traits.

The work of Gregor Mendel, a monk and part-time biologist, with garden peas is regarded as the beginning of what would become the science of genetics. Mendel is credited with showing the existence of genes as well as illuminating the rules governing their transmission from generation to generation. The study of genetics through the analysis of offspring from mating is sometimes referred to as classical genetics.

The billions of nucleotides in the nucleus of a cell are organized linearly along the DNA double helix in functional units called genes. Each of the 20,000 to 25,000 human genes is accompanied by various regulatory elements that control when that gene is active in producing **messenger ribonucleic acid (mRNA)** by the process of **transcription**. In most situations, mRNA is transported from the nucleus to the cytoplasm, where its genetic information is used in the manufacture of proteins (a process called **translation**); these proteins perform the functions that ultimately determine phenotype. For example, proteins serve as enzymes that facilitate metabolism and cell synthesis; as DNA binding elements that regulate transcription of other genes; as structural elements of cells and the extracellular matrix; and as receptor molecules for intracellular and intercellular communication. DNA also encodes many small RNA molecules that serve functions that are not yet fully understood, including regulating gene transcription and interfering with the translational capacity of some mRNAs.

Chromosomes are the means by which the genes are transmitted from generation to generation. Each chromosome is a complex of protein and nucleic acid in which an unbroken double helix of DNA is tightly wound (**Figure 1-1**). Genes are found along the length of chromosomes. A variety of highly complicated and integrated processes occur within the chromosome, including DNA replication, recombination, and transcription. In the nucleus of each of their somatic cells, humans normally have 46 chromosomes, which are arranged in 23 pairs. One of these pairs, consisting of the **sex chromosomes** X and Y, determines the sex of the individual; females have the pair XX, and males have the pair XY. The remaining 22 pairs of chromosomes are called **autosomes**. In addition to these nuclear chromosomes, each mitochondrion (an organelle found in varying numbers in the cytoplasm of all cells) contains multiple copies of a small chromosome. This **mitochondrial chromosome** encodes a few of the proteins for oxidative metabolism and all of the **transfer ribonucleic acids (tRNA)** used in translation of proteins within this organelle. Mitochondrial chromosomes are inherited almost entirely from the cytoplasm of the fertilized ovum and, therefore, are maternal in origin.

FIGURE 1-1	Molecular structure of a DNA double helix. (A) A space-filling model in which each atom is depicted as a sphere. (B) A diagram highlighting the helical backbones on the outside of the molecule and stacked A-T and G-C pairs inside.

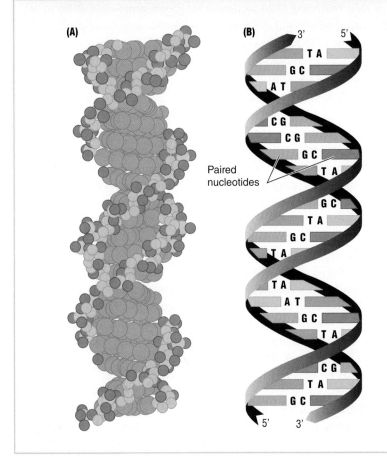

(A)

(B)

Paired nucleotides

KEY TERMS

Transcription: the process by which the information contained in a template strand of DNA is copied into a single-stranded RNA molecule of complementary base sequence.

Translation: the process by which the amino acid sequence of a polypeptide is synthesized on a ribosome according to the nucleotide sequence of an mRNA molecule.

Chromosome: a DNA molecule that contains genes in linear order to which numerous proteins are bound.

Sex chromosome: a chromosome, such as the human X or Y, that plays a role in the determination of sex.

Autosomes: all chromosomes other than the sex chromosomes.

The exact location of a gene on a chromosome is known as its **locus**, and the array of loci constitutes the human gene map. Currently, researchers have identified the chromosomal sites of more than 11,000 genes (i.e., those for which normal or abnormal function has been identified).

Homologous copies of a gene are termed **alleles**. In comparing alleles, it must be specified at which level of analysis the comparison is being made. For

KEY TERMS

Mitochondrial chromosome: a small circular chromosome found in each mitochondrion that encodes tRNA, rRNA, and proteins that are involved in oxidative phosphorylation and ATP generation.

Transfer ribonucleic acids (tRNA): a small RNA molecule that translates a codon into an amino acid in protein synthesis; it has a three-base sequence, called the anticodon, complementary to a specific codon in mRNA, and a site to which a specific amino acid is bound.

Locus: the site or position of a particular gene on a chromosome.

Allele: any of the alternative forms of a given gene.

Homozygous: having the same allele of a gene in homologous chromosomes.

Heterozygous: carrying dissimilar alleles of one or more genes; not homozygous.

example, if alleles are truly identical, their coding sequences and the number of copies do not vary, so the individual is **homozygous** at that specific locus. However, if the DNA is analyzed using either restriction enzyme examination or nucleotide sequencing, then, despite having the same functional identity, the alleles would be viewed as different, and the individual would be **heterozygous** for that locus. Heterozygosity based on differences in the protein products of alleles has been detectable for decades and represents the first hard evidence proving the high degree of human biologic variability. In the past decade, analysis of DNA sequences has shown genetic variability to be much more common, with differences in nucleotide sequence between individuals occurring about once every 1,200 nucleotides.

Mutation

A **mutation** is defined as a change in DNA that may adversely affect the host. A heterozygous allele frequently results when different alleles are inherited from the egg and the sperm, but it may also occur as a consequence of spontaneous alteration in nucleotide sequence that results in a mutation. A **germinal mutation** occurs during formation of an egg or a sperm. If the change occurs after conception, it is termed a **somatic mutation**. The role of somatic mutation is now increasingly recognized as a key factor in the etiology of human disease.

The most dramatic type of mutation is an alteration in the number or physical structure of chromosomes, a phenomenon called a **chromosomal aberration**. Not all aberrations cause problems in the affected individual, but some that do not may lead to problems in their offspring. Approximately 1 in every 200 live-born infants has a chromosomal aberration that is detected because of some effect on phenotype. The frequency of this finding increases markedly the earlier in fetal life that the chromosomes are examined. By the end of the first trimester of gestation, most fetuses with abnormal numbers of chromosomes have been lost through spontaneous abortion.

For example, during the reduction division of meiosis that leads to production of mature ova and sperm, failure of chromosome pairs to separate in the dividing cell (**nondisjunction**) causes the embryo to have too many or too few chromosomes. When this type of error occurs, it is called **aneuploidy**, and either more or fewer than 46 chromosomes are present. Three types of aneuploidy may occur: (1) **monosomy**, in which only one member of a pair of chromosomes is present; (2) **trisomy**, in which three chromosomes are present instead of two; and (3) **polysomy**, in which one chromosome is represented four or more times.

During **translocation** or **inversion**, there is a rearrangement of chromosome arms. This effect is considered a mutation even if breakage and reunion do not disrupt any coding sequence (**Figures 1-2** and **1-3**). In an inversion,

FIGURE 1-2

(A) Two pairs of nonhomologous chromosomes in a diploid organism. (B) Heterozygous reciprocal translocation in which two nonhomologous chromosomes (the two at the top) have interchanged terminal segments.

(A)   Homozygous normal (both pairs normal)

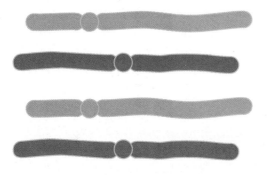

(B)   Heterozygous translocation (one pair interchanged, one pair normal)

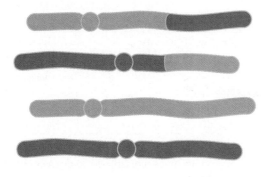

KEY TERMS

Mutation: heritable alteration in a gene or chromosome; also, the process by which such an alteration happens.

Germinal mutation: a mutation that takes place in a reproductive cell.

Somatic mutation: a mutation arising in a somatic cell.

Chromosomal aberration: alteration in the number or physical structure of chromosomes.

Nondisjunction: failure of chromosomes to separate (disjoin) and move to opposite poles of the division spindle; the result is loss or gain of a chromosome.

Aneuploidy: a condition in which extra or fewer copies of particular genes or chromosomal regions are present compared with the wild type.

Monosomy: a condition in an otherwise diploid organism in which one member of a pair of chromosomes is missing.

KEY TERMS

Trisomy: a disorder in which a normally diploid organism has an extra copy of one of the chromosomes.

Polysomy: condition of a diploid cell or organism that has three or more copies of a particular chromosome.

Translocation: a mutation that results from an exchange of parts of two chromosomes.

Inversion: a structural aberration in a chromosome in which the order of several genes is reversed from the normal order

Deletion: loss of chromosomal material.

Codon: a sequence of three adjacent nucleotides in an mRNA molecule, specifying either an amino acid or a stop signal in protein synthesis.

Degenerate: a feature of the genetic code in which an amino acid corresponds to more than one codon.

FIGURE 1-2 (C) Homozygous reciprocal translocation.

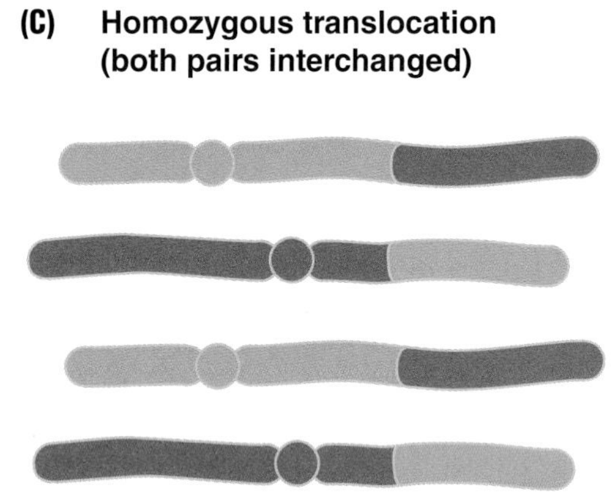

(C) Homozygous translocation
(both pairs interchanged)

FIGURE 1-3 Origin of an inversion by reversal of the region between two chromosomal break points.

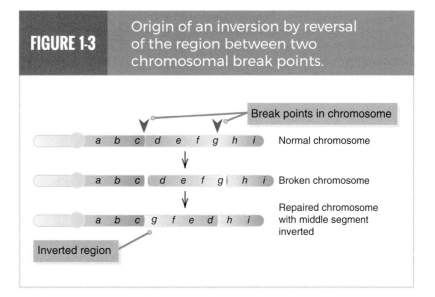

Break points in chromosome
a b c d e f g h i
Normal chromosome
a b c d e f g h i
Broken chromosome
a b c g f e d h i
Repaired chromosome with middle segment inverted
Inverted region

a chromosomal region becomes reoriented 180 degrees out of the ordinary phase. In each case, the same genetic material is present but appears in a different order. Consequently, the phenotypic effect of gross chromosomal mutations can range from profound (as in aneuploidy) to innocuous.

Less obvious, but still detectable cytologically, are **deletions** of part of a chromosome. These mutations almost always alter phenotype, because a number of genes are lost. However, a deletion may involve only a single nucleotide, whereas 1–2 million nucleotides (1–2 megabases) must be lost before the defect can be visualized by the most sensitive cytogenetic methods. More sensitive molecular biology techniques are needed to detect smaller losses.

Changes in one nucleotide can alter which amino acid is encoded. For example, if the amino acid is present in a critical region of the protein, normal protein function might be severely disrupted (e.g., sickle cell disease). In contrast, some other amino acid substitutions have no detectable effect on function, such that the phenotype is unaltered by the mutation. Also, within the genetic code, two or more different three-nucleotide sequences called **codons** may encode the same amino acids (**degenerate**), such that nucleotide substitution does not necessarily alter the amino acid sequence of the protein. Three specific codons signal termination of translation, so a nucleotide substitution that generates one of the stop codons prematurely usually causes a **truncated protein**, which is frequently abnormal.

Nondisjunction Syndromes

Mutations may occur spontaneously or may be induced by radiation, medication, viral infections, or other environmental factors. Both advanced maternal and paternal age are associated with different types of mutations. In women, meiosis is completed only when an egg ovulates, and chromosomal nondisjunction is increasingly common as the egg becomes older. An example is trisomy 21, also known as **Down syndrome**. The risk that an aneuploid egg will result increases exponentially and becomes a major clinical concern for women older than their early 30s who wish to conceive a child (**Figure 1-4**). In men, mutations affecting nucleotide sequences are more subtle and increase with age. Offspring of men older than 40 years of age are at an increased risk for having primarily **autosomal dominant** Mendelian conditions.

Down syndrome is one of the most common trisomies, with approximately 1 of every 800 babies born in the United States being affected by this condition, which includes a combination of birth defects. Affected individuals have some degree of intellectual disability, characteristic facial features, and, often, heart defects and other health problems. They are typically short with round, moonlike faces (**Figure 1-5**). Their tongues protrude forward, forcing their mouths open, and their eyes slant upward at the corners. The severity of these problems varies greatly among affected individuals.

Some of the health problems associated with Down syndrome are shown in **Table 1-1**. Fortunately, most are treatable. Thus, life expectancy for persons with trisomy 21 is now approximately 55 years. The degree of intellectual disability varies from mild to severe. Because severe intellectual disability is less likely, most affected individuals are able to go to school and participate in special work programs.

KEY TERMS

Truncated protein: a protein that does not achieve its full length or its proper form and thus is missing some of the amino acid residues that are present in a normal protein. A truncated protein generally cannot perform the function for which it was intended because its structure is incapable of doing so.

Down syndrome: a chromosomal dysgenesis syndrome consisting of a variable constellation of abnormalities caused by triplication or translocation of chromosome 21. Affected individuals have some degree of mental retardation, characteristic facial features, and, often, heart defects and other health problems.

FIGURE 1-4 Frequency of Down syndrome (number of cases per 100 live births) related to age of mother. The graph is based on 438 Down syndrome births (among 330,859 total births) in Sweden in the period 1968 to 1970.

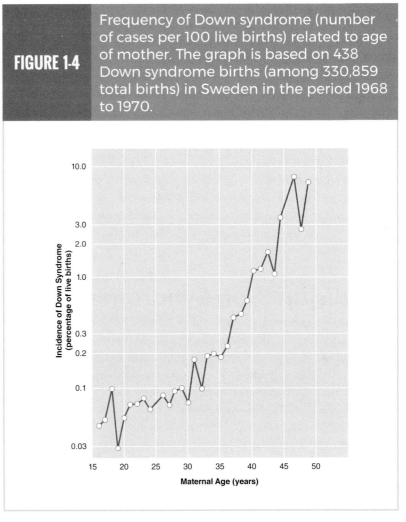

Data from Hook, E. B., & Lindsjö, A. (1978). *American Journal of Human Genetics, 30,* 19.

The American College of Obstetricians and Gynecologists recommends that all pregnant women be offered a screening test for Down syndrome, regardless of the woman's age. Screening may consist of a maternal blood test done in the first trimester (as early as 10 weeks of pregnancy) known as cell free DNA (cfDNA). This can be done with or without a special ultrasound examination of the back of the baby's neck (called nuchal translucency). Alternately, a maternal blood test can be done in the second trimester (at 15–20 weeks of pregnancy). These tests help to identify pregnancies that are at higher-than-average risk of Down syndrome and other trisomies, but cannot definitively diagnose Down syndrome or other birth defects.

| **FIGURE 1-5** | Down syndrome. (A) Karyotype of Down syndrome girl with trisomy of chromosome 21. (B) Distinguishing characteristics of Down syndrome. |

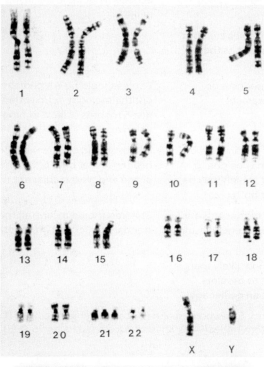

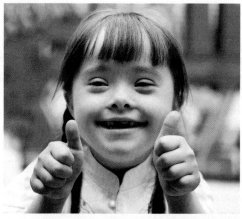

(A) © L. Willatt, East Anglian Regional Genetics Service/Science Source.
(B) © Denis Kuvaev/Shutterstock.

TABLE 1-1	Health Problems Associated with Down Syndrome	
Problem	**Specifics**	**Recommendation**
Heart defects	Almost half of babies have heart defects.	Babies should be examined by a pediatric cardiologist and have an echocardiogram in the first 2 months of life.
Intestinal defects	Approximately 12% of babies are born with intestinal malformations that require surgery.	
Vision problems	Crossed eyes, nearsightedness or farsightedness, and cataracts.	Babies should have a pediatric ophthalmologist exam within the first 6 months of life and have regular vision exams.
Hearing loss	Approximately 75% of children have some hearing loss. It may be due to fluid in the middle ear (which may be temporary), a nerve, or both.	Babies should be screened for hearing loss at birth or by 3 months of age and have regular exams.
Infections	Children tend to have many colds and ear infections as well as bronchitis and pneumonia.	Children should receive all the standard childhood immunizations.
Memory loss	Affected individuals more likely than unaffected individuals to develop Alzheimer's disease at an earlier age.	

Data from *Down syndrome*. Pregnancy & Newborn Health Education Center. March of Dimes website. http://www.marchofdimes.com/pnhec/4439_1214.asp. Accessed January 16, 2010.

Women who have an abnormal screening test result are offered a diagnostic test, such as **amniocentesis** or **chorionic villus sampling (CVS)**, that will either confirm or disprove the presence of Down syndrome in the fetus. Amniocentesis involves the removal and examination of a small sample of the amniotic fluid that surrounds the fetus. Chorionic villus sampling involves taking a tiny tissue sample from outside the sac where the fetus develops (chorionic villi) and is done earlier in pregnancy (usually between 10 and 12 weeks) than amniocentesis (usually 15–20 weeks). Both procedures pose a small risk of miscarriage, with CVS having a slightly higher risk than amniocentesis. These tests are highly accurate for diagnosing or ruling out Down syndrome.

Nondisjunction of the sex chromosomes can lead to a variety of nonlethal genetic disorders. One of the most common occurs when an ovum with an extra X chromosome is fertilized by a sperm with a Y chromosome. This process results in an XXY genotype, known as **Klinefelter syndrome**. Klinefelter syndrome occurs in approximately 1 out of every 700–1,000 newborn males. Even though these individuals are males, their masculinization is incomplete. Their external genitalia and testes are unusually small, and approximately 50% of these individuals develop breasts. Spermatogenesis is abnormal, and affected males are generally sterile. Klinefelter syndrome is the most common chromosomal disorder associated with male hypogonadism and infertility.

Another disorder associated with nondisjunction of sex chromosomes is **Turner syndrome**. This monosomy syndrome results when an ovum lacking the X chromosome is fertilized by a sperm that contains an X chromosome. It may also occur when a genetically normal ovum is fertilized by a sperm lacking an X or Y chromosome. The result is an offspring with 22 pairs of autosomes and a single, unmatched X chromosome (XO).

Turner syndrome occurs in only 1 out of every 10,000 female births, as the XO embryo is more likely to be spontaneously aborted. These individuals look like females and are characteristically short with wide chests and a prominent fold of skin on their necks. Because their ovaries fail to develop at puberty, they are sterile and have low levels of estrogen and small breasts. Mental retardation is not associated with this disorder, so individuals lead fairly normal lives.

Genes in Individuals

Most human characteristics and common diseases are **polygenic**, whereas many of the disordered phenotypes thought of as "genetic" are **monogenic** but still influenced by other loci in a person's genome. Phenotypes due to alterations at a single gene are frequently referred to as **Mendelian**, after Gregor Mendel, the monk/biologist who studied the reproducibility and recurrence of variation in garden peas. Mendel showed that some traits were **dominant** relative to other traits; he called the latter traits **recessive**. Dominant traits require only one copy of a "factor" to be expressed, regardless of what the other copy is, whereas recessive traits require two copies before expression occurs. We now recognize that the Mendelian factors are genes, and the alternative copies of the gene are alleles. For example, if *B* is the common (normal) allele and *b* is the mutant allele at a locus, then the phenotype is dominant regardless of whether the genotype is *BB* or *Bb*. Conversely, the phenotype is recessive when the genotype is *bb*.

Inheritance Patterns

As described earlier, phenotypes due to alterations at a single gene are characterized as Mendelian, and monogenic human diseases are frequently referred to as Mendelian disorders. The mode of inheritance for a given phenotypic

KEY TERMS

Chorionic villus sampling (CVS): a prenatal test that involves taking a tiny tissue sample from outside the sac where the fetus develops. It is performed between 10 and 12 weeks after a pregnant woman's last menstrual period.

Klinefelter syndrome: a disorder that occurs when an ovum with an extra X chromosome is fertilized by a sperm with a Y chromosome. This results in an XXY genotype male who is sterile.

Turner syndrome: a monosomy syndrome that results when an ovum lacking the X chromosome is fertilized by a sperm that contains an X chromosome. It may also occur when a genetically normal ovum is fertilized by a sperm lacking an X or Y chromosome. The result is an offspring with 22 pairs of autosomes and a single, unmatched X chromosome.

FIGURE 1-6   Conventional symbols used in depicting human pedigrees.

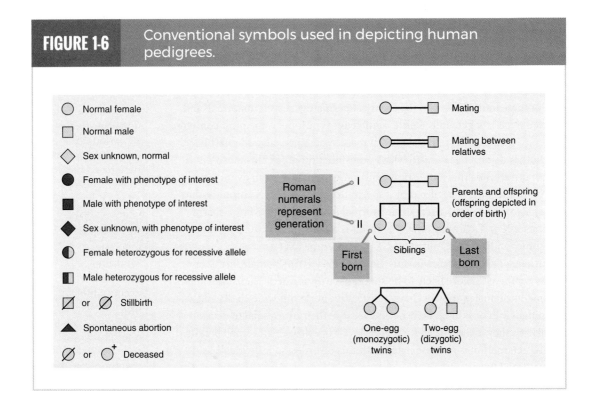

trait or disease is determined by **pedigree analysis**. All affected and unaffected individuals in the family are recorded in a pedigree using standard symbols (**Figure 1-6**). The principles of allelic segregation, and the transmission of alleles from parents to children, are illustrated in **Figure 1-7**. One dominant (A) allele and one recessive (a) allele can display any of three Mendelian modes of inheritance: autosomal dominant, autosomal recessive, or chromosome X-linked. Approximately 65% of human monogenic disorders are autosomal dominant, 25% are autosomal recessive, and 5% are X-linked. Genetic testing is now available for many of these disorders and plays an increasingly important role in clinical medicine.

Autosomal Dominant Inheritance

Autosomal dominant disorders are relevant because mutations in a single allele are sufficient to cause the disease (**Figure 1-8**). In contrast to recessive disorders, in which disease pathogenesis is relatively straightforward because

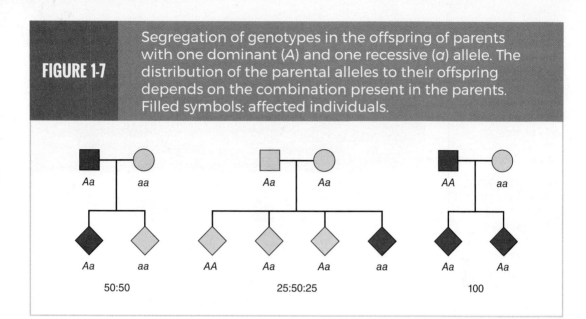

FIGURE 1-7 Segregation of genotypes in the offspring of parents with one dominant (*A*) and one recessive (*a*) allele. The distribution of the parental alleles to their offspring depends on the combination present in the parents. Filled symbols: affected individuals.

there is loss of gene function, dominant disorders can be caused by various disease mechanisms, many of which are unique to the function of the genetic pathway involved (**Box 1-1**).

Autosomal Recessive Inheritance

In the case of recessive disorders, mutated alleles result in a complete or partial loss of function. An example of a pedigree of autosomal recessive inheritance is shown in **Figure 1-9**. Recessive disorders frequently involve enzymes in metabolic pathways, receptors, or proteins in signaling cascades. The affected individual can be of either sex and either a homozygote or compound heterozygote for a single-gene defect. Fortunately, autosomal recessive diseases are, for the most part, rare and often occur in the context of parental **consanguinity**. The relatively high frequency of certain recessive disorders, such as sickle cell anemia, cystic fibrosis, and thalassemia, is partially explained by a selective biologic advantage for the heterozygous state. Heterozygous carriers of a defective allele are usually clinically normal, but they may display subtle differences in phenotype that become apparent only with more precise testing or in the context of certain environmental influences (i.e., sickle cell disease) (**Box 1-2**).

KEY TERM

Mendelian genetics: the mechanism of inheritance in which the statistical relations between the distribution of traits in successive generations result from three factors: (1) particulate hereditary determinants (genes), (2) random union of gametes, and (3) segregation of unchanged hereditary determinants in the reproductive cells.

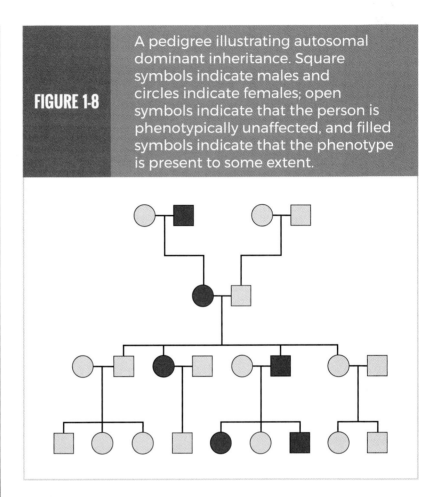

FIGURE 1-8 A pedigree illustrating autosomal dominant inheritance. Square symbols indicate males and circles indicate females; open symbols indicate that the person is phenotypically unaffected, and filled symbols indicate that the phenotype is present to some extent.

Autosomal recessive phenotypes are often associated with deficient activity of enzymes and are thus termed **inborn errors of metabolism**. Such disorders include phenylketonuria, Tay-Sachs disease, and the various glycogen storage diseases. They tend to be more severe, less variable, and less age dependent than dominant conditions. When an autosomal recessive condition is quite rare, the chance that the parents of affected offspring are consanguineous for the phenotype is increased. As a result, the prevalence of rare recessive conditions is high among inbred groups such as the Old Order Amish and Ashkenazi Jews.

X-Linked Inheritance

Because males have only one X chromosome, a daughter will always inherit her father's X chromosome in addition to one of her mother's two

| **BOX 1-1** | Characteristics of Autosomal Dominant Inheritance |

» A vertical pattern is observed in the pedigree, with multiple generations being affected.
» Heterozygotes for the mutant allele show an abnormal phenotype.
» Males and females are affected with equal frequency and severity.
» Only one parent must be affected for an offspring to be at risk for developing the phenotype.
» When an affected person mates with an unaffected one, each offspring has a 50% chance of inheriting the affected phenotype. This is true regardless of the sex of the affected parent—specifically, male-to-male transmission occurs.
» The frequency of sporadic cases is positively associated with the severity of the phenotype. Autosomal dominant phenotypes are often age dependent, less severe than autosomal recessive phenotypes, and associated with malformations or other physical features.

Data from Pyeritz, R. E. Medical genetics. In L. Tierney et al. *Current medical diagnosis & treatment,* 42nd ed. 2003.

| **FIGURE 1-9** | A pedigree illustrating autosomal recessive inheritance. |

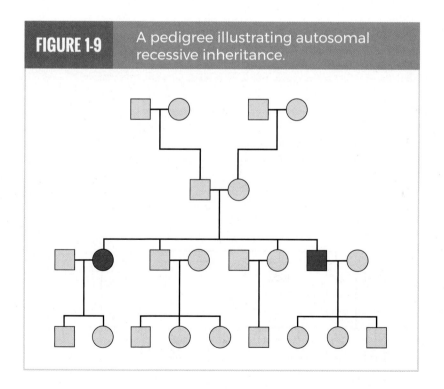

X chromosomes (**Figure 1-10**). Conversely, a son inherits the Y chromosome from his father and one maternal X chromosome, so the risk of developing disease due to a mutant X-chromosomal gene differs in the two sexes. Because of the presence of one X chromosome, males are said to be

BOX 1-2   Characteristics of Autosomal Recessive Inheritance

» A horizontal pattern is noted in the pedigree, with a single generation being affected.
» Males and females are affected with equal frequency and severity.
» Inheritance is from both parents, each of whom is a heterozygote (carrier) and each of whom is usually clinically unaffected by his or her carrier status.
» Each offspring of two carriers has a 25% chance of being affected, a 50% chance of being a carrier, and a 25% chance of inheriting neither mutant allele. Thus, two-thirds of all clinically unaffected offspring are carriers of the autosomal recessive phenotype.
» In matings between individuals, each with the same recessive phenotype, all offspring will be affected.
» Affected individuals who mate with unaffected individuals who are not carriers have only unaffected offspring.
» The rarer the recessive phenotype, the more likely it is that the parents are consanguineous (related).

Data from Pyeritz, R. E. Medical genetics. In L. Tierney et al. *Current medical diagnosis & treatment*, 42nd ed. 2003.

FIGURE 1-10   A pedigree illustrating X-linked inheritance.

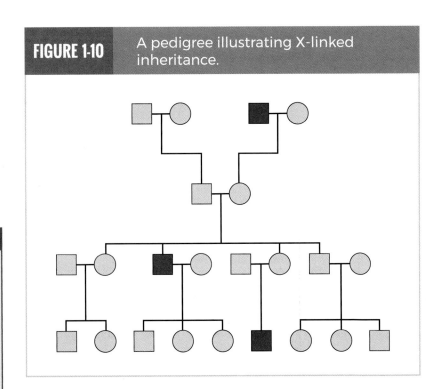

KEY TERM

Hemizygous: describes an individual who has only one member of a chromosome pair or chromosome segment rather than the usual two; refers in particular to X-linked genes in males who, under usual circumstances, have only one X chromosome.

hemizygous for the mutant allele on that chromosome. Therefore, they are more likely to develop the mutant phenotype, regardless of whether the mutation is dominant or recessive. A female with two X chromosomes may be either heterozygous or homozygous for the mutant allele, which may be

BOX 1-3	Characteristics of X-Linked Inheritance

» There is no male-to-male transmission of the phenotype.
» Unaffected males do not transmit the phenotype.
» All daughters of an affected male are heterozygous carriers.
» Males are usually more severely affected than females.
» Whether a heterozygous female is counted as affected—and whether the phenotype is called "recessive" or "dominant"—often depends on the sensitivity of the assay or examination.
» Some mothers of affected males will not themselves be heterozygotes (i.e., they will be homozygous normal) but will have a germinal mutation. The proportion of heterozygous (carrier) mothers is negatively associated with the severity of the condition.
» Heterozygous women transmit the mutant gene to 50% of their sons, who are affected, and to 50% of their daughters, who are heterozygotes.
» If an affected male mates with a heterozygous female, 50% of the male offspring will be affected, giving the false impression of male-to-male transmission. Among the female offspring of such matings, 50% will be affected as severely as the average hemizygous male; in small pedigrees, this pattern may simulate autosomal dominant inheritance.

Data from Pyeritz, R. E. Medical genetics. In L. Tierney et al. *Current medical diagnosis & treatment,* 42nd ed. 2003.

dominant or recessive. Therefore, the terms "X-linked dominant" and "X-linked recessive" are applicable to expression of the mutant phenotype only in women (**Box 1-3**).

The characteristics of X-linked inheritance depend on phenotypic severity. For some disorders, affected males do not survive to reproduce. In such cases, approximately two-thirds of affected males have a carrier mother; in the remaining third, the disorder arises by new germinal mutation in an X chromosome of the mother. When the disorder is nearly always manifested in heterozygous females (X-linked dominant inheritance), females tend to be affected approximately twice as often as males; on average, an affected female transmits the phenotype to 50% of her sons and 50% of her daughters.

The Y chromosome has a relatively small number of genes. One gene, the sex-region determining Y factor (*SRY*), encodes the testis-determining factor that is crucial for normal male development. Normally there is infrequent exchange of sequences on the Y chromosome with the X chromosome.

Mitochondrial Inheritance

As described earlier, transmission of genes encoded by DNA contained in the nuclear chromosomes follows the principles of Mendelian inheritance. In addition, each mitochondrion contains several copies of a small circular chromosome that encodes tRNA, **ribosomal RNA (rRNA)**, and proteins that are involved in oxidative phosphorylation and ATP generation. The mitochondrial genome does not recombine and is inherited through the maternal line because sperm does not contribute significant cytoplasmic components to the

KEY TERM

Ribosomal RNA (rRNA): a type of RNA molecule that is a component of the ribosomal subunits.

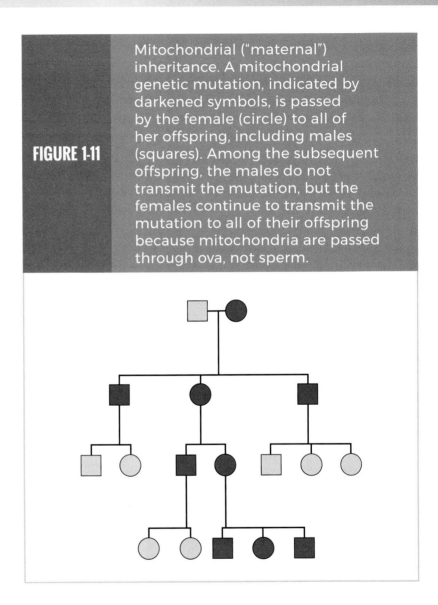

FIGURE 1-11 Mitochondrial ("maternal") inheritance. A mitochondrial genetic mutation, indicated by darkened symbols, is passed by the female (circle) to all of her offspring, including males (squares). Among the subsequent offspring, the males do not transmit the mutation, but the females continue to transmit the mutation to all of their offspring because mitochondria are passed through ova, not sperm.

zygote. Mutations in the genes encoded by the mitochondrial chromosome cause a variety of diseases that affect (in particular) organs highly dependent on oxidative metabolism, such as the retina, brain, kidneys, and heart. An affected woman can pass the defective mitochondrial chromosome to all of her offspring, whereas an affected man has little risk of passing his mutation to a child (**Figure 1-11**).

Human Genome Project

Genomics is the study of all the genes in a person as well as the interactions of these genes with one another and with the individual's environment. All people are 99.9% identical in genetic makeup, but differences in the remaining 0.1% offer important clues about health and disease. The goals of the Human Genome Project were to determine the complete sequence of the 3 billion DNA subunits (bases), identify all human genes, and make that information accessible for further biological study. The project was completed in 2003 and identified approximately 25,000 genes in human DNA (**Box 1-4**).

The completion of the Human Genome Project has inspired much excitement regarding the many potential applications using this information: (1) improved disease diagnosis, (2) ability to detect genetic predispositions to disease, (3) development of drugs based on molecular information, (4) use of gene therapy and control systems as drugs, and (5) creation of "custom drugs" based on individual genetic profiles. In addition, the creation of more detailed genome maps has helped researchers seeking genes associated with dozens of

---

BOX 1-4   Genomic Sequencing Highlights

» The human genome contains 3.2 billion chemical nucleotide bases (A, C, T, and G).
» The average gene consists of 3,000 bases, but sizes vary greatly. The largest known human gene is dystrophin, which has 2.4 million base pairs.
» Functions are unknown for more than 50% of discovered genes.
» The human genome sequence is almost exactly (99.9%) the same in all people.
» Approximately 2% of the genome encodes instructions for the synthesis of proteins.
» Repeat sequences that do not code for proteins make up at least 50% of the human genome.
» Repeat sequences are thought to have no direct functions, but they shed light on chromosome structure and dynamics. Over time, these repeats reshape the genome by rearranging it, thereby creating entirely new genes or modifying and reshuffling existing genes.
» The human genome has a much greater portion (50%) of repeat sequences than the mustard weed (11%), the worm (7%), and the fly (3%).
» More than 40% of the predicted human proteins share similarity with fruit fly or worm proteins.
» Genes appear to be concentrated in random areas along the genome, with vast expanses of noncoding DNA occurring between these areas.
» Chromosome 1 (the largest human chromosome) has the most genes (3,168), and the Y chromosome has the fewest (344).
» Particular gene sequences have been associated with numerous diseases and disorders, including breast cancer, muscle disease, deafness, and blindness.
» Scientists have identified millions of locations where single-base DNA differences occur in humans. This information promises to revolutionize the processes of finding DNA sequences associated with such common diseases as cardiovascular disease, diabetes, arthritis, and cancers.

Reproduced from U.S. Department of Energy Genome Programs, Insights from the Human DNA Sequence. Available at http://www.ornl.gov/sci/techresources/Human_Genome/publicat /primer2001/4. shtml. Accessed August 13, 2010.

genetic conditions, including myotonic dystrophy, fragile X syndrome, neurofibromatosis types 1 and 2, inherited colon cancer, Alzheimer's disease, and familial breast cancer. Even though the concept of using this genetic information to treat and/or cure many diseases is very exciting, many challenges must be overcome before viable and safe treatments are available for human diseases.

Chapter Summary

» Genetics is the study of biologically inherited traits determined by genes that are transmitted from parents to offspring during the course of reproduction.

» Chromosomes are how the genes are transmitted from generation to generation.

» The human genome is estimated to contain 20,000–25,000 genes. A germinal mutation occurs during formation of an egg or a sperm, but if change occurs after conception, it is termed a somatic mutation.

» Advanced maternal and paternal age are associated with different types of mutations.

» Phenotypes due to alterations at a single gene are characterized as Mendelian, and monogenic human diseases are frequently referred to as Mendelian disorders.

» Genomics is the study of all the genes in a person as well as the interactions of these genes with one another and with an individual's environment.

Chapter Review Questions

1. The _____ encodes a few of the proteins for oxidative metabolism and all of the _____ used in translation of proteins within this organelle.
2. A change in DNA that could adversely affect the host that occurs after conception is termed a _____.
3. The three types of aneuploidy are _____, _____, and _____.
4. Autosomal recessive phenotypes are often associated with deficient activity of enzymes and, therefore, are termed _____.
5. Because of the presence of one X chromosome, males are said to be _____ for the mutant allele on that chromosome.

Bibliography

American College of Obstetricians and Gynecologists. (2017, March). *Committee opinion: Carrier screening in the age of genomic medicine.* Retrieved from https://www.acog.org/Clinical-Guidance-and-Publications/Committee-Opinions/Committee-on-Genetics/Carrier-Screening-in-the-Age-of-Genomic-Medicine

Chial, H. (2008). DNA sequencing technologies key to the Human Genome Project. *Nature Education 1*(1): 219. Retrieved from https://www.nature.com/scitable/nated/article?action=showContentInPopup&contentPK=828

U.S. Department of Energy Office of Science. (n.d.). *Genomics and its impact on science and society.* [PDF file]. Retrieved from https://web.ornl.gov/sci/techresources/Human_Genome/publicat/primer2001/primer11.pdf

Hartl, D. L., & Ruvolo, M. (2019). *Genetics: Analysis of genes and genomes* (9th ed.). Burlington, MA: Jones & Bartlett Learning.

Jameson, J. L., & Kopp, P. (2012). Principles of human genetics. In A. S. Fauci, E. Braunwald, D. L. Kasper, S. L. Hauser, D. L. Longo, J. L. Jameson, & J. Loscalzo (Eds.), *Harrison's principles of internal medicine* (18th ed., pp. 1122–1125). New York, NY: McGraw-Hill Medical.

Jorde, L. B., Carey, J. C., Bamshad, M. J., & White, R. L. (2016). *Medical genetics* (5th ed.). Philadelphia, PA: Elsevier.

National Down Syndrome Society. (n.d.). Retrieved from http://www.ndss.org/index.php

National Library of Medicine, National Institutes of Health, U.S. Department of Health and Human Services. (n.d.). *Genetics home reference.* Retrieved from http://ghr.nlm.nih.gov/

National Office of Public Health Genomics, Centers for Disease Control and Prevention. (n.d.). *Public health genomics.* Retrieved from http://www.cdc.gov/genomics/update/current.htm

Nussbuam, R. L., McInnes, R. R., & Willard, H. F. (2016). *Thompson & Thompson genetics in medicine* (8th ed.). Philadelphia, PA: Elsevier.

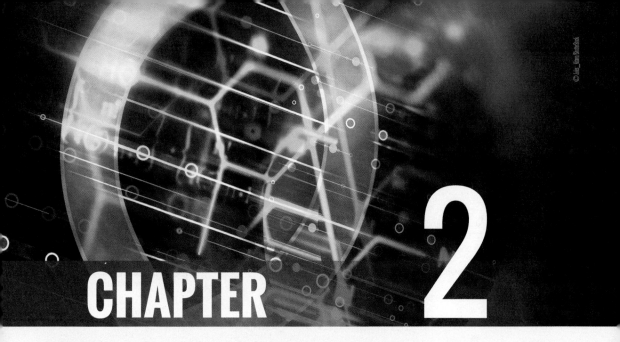

CHAPTER 2

Diagnostic Techniques in Medical Genetics

Hereditary disorders can affect different organ systems and people of all ages, making it important for healthcare providers to be familiar with genetic testing methodology. These tests range from taking a thorough family history that includes several (at least three) familial generations (i.e., pedigree), to DNA sequencing, to hybridization with specific probes. Although it is impractical to construct a detailed pedigree with every patient visit because of time constraints, it is important to know how to map out a pedigree in case there is some concern about a specific disease within a family.

Family History

Clinicians are well trained in and well aware of the importance of taking a good family history and should, at the very least, ask about the medical history of all first-degree relatives (parents, siblings, and offspring) and, if possible, more distant relatives. Pertinent information includes age, sex, ethnicity, general health status, major illnesses, and cause of death. Once this information is obtained, it can further be analyzed using a pedigree diagram to identify the mode of inheritance for a disease process.

Pedigree Analysis

A pedigree is a diagram representing the familial relationships among relatives. It can be used to analyze Mendelian inheritance of certain traits, whether autosomal dominant, autosomal recessive, sex-linked dominant, sex-linked recessive, or familial clustering. Some patients may be offended by the term "pedigree," so using the term "family tree" when interviewing patients may yield better results. A pedigree should have at least three generations of relatives. The pedigree symbols have been standardized so that females are represented by circles and males by squares (**Figure 2-1**). A diamond is used if the sex is

| FIGURE 2-1 | Conventional symbols used in depicting human pedigrees. |

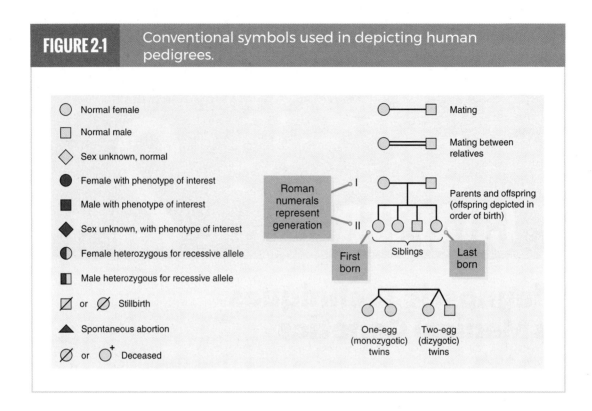

Normal female

Normal male

Sex unknown, normal

Female with phenotype of interest

Male with phenotype of interest

Sex unknown, with phenotype of interest

Female heterozygous for recessive allele

Male heterozygous for recessive allele

or Stillbirth

Spontaneous abortion

or Deceased

Mating

Mating between relatives

Roman numerals represent generation

I

II

Parents and offspring (offspring depicted in order of birth)

First born

Siblings

Last born

One-egg (monozygotic) twins

Two-egg (dizygotic) twins

KEY TERMS

Consanguineous: mating between related individuals.

Sibling (sib): a brother or sister, each having the same parents.

unknown. In the case of a miscarriage, a triangle is used. Colored or shaded symbols show individuals with the phenotype of interest, and half-filled symbols show heterozygous *carriers* of recessive alleles of said phenotype of interest.

Mating between a male and a female is indicated by a horizontal line; a vertical line is then drawn from this horizontal line to join a second horizontal line. The first horizontal line joins the mother and father, and the second horizontal line joins the offspring together. The vertical line joins the offspring to their parents (mates). Mating between related (**consanguineous**) individuals is indicated with a double horizontal line. The offspring, called **sibs or siblings**, are represented from left to right in order of birth; each row corresponds to a generation that is labeled with a Roman numeral.

Figure 2-2 shows an example of a pedigree for a family in which some members have Huntington's disease. Within any generation, the individuals are numbered consecutively from left to right. The pedigree starts with the woman I-1, and the man is I-2. The man has Huntington's disease, as indicated by the shaded symbol (shaded symbols represent the phenotype).

FIGURE 2-2	Pedigree of a human family showing the inheritance of the gene for Huntington's disease. Females and males are represented by circles and squares. Shaded symbols indicate people affected by the disease.

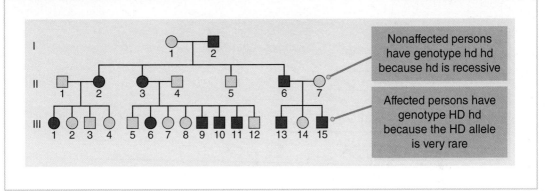

Nonaffected persons have genotype hd hd because hd is recessive

Affected persons have genotype HD hd because the HD allele is very rare

Because this disease is due to a dominant mutation, all affected individuals will have the heterozygous genotype *HD hd*, and all nonaffected people will have the homozygous genotype *hd hd*. The disease has complete **penetrance**, which means the trait is expressed in 100% of people with that genotype.

For example, in the case of a rare dominant allele with complete penetrance, the following characteristics are observed:

1. Females and males are affected equally.
2. Affected offspring typically have one affected parent, with the same likelihood ratio of the affected parent being the mother or the father.
3. Approximately 50% of siblings with the same parents are affected.

An example of a pedigree for a homozygous recessive allele is albinism (**Figure 2-3**). In comparison, inheriting a rare recessive allele with complete penetrance would yield the following observed characteristics:

1. Females and males are affected equally.
2. Affected individuals would not have affected offspring.
3. Affected individuals typically have *no* affected parents.
4. Parents of those affected may be related.
5. Approximately 25% of siblings with the same parents are affected.

In the case of inheritance of a rare recessive trait, the mates of homozygous affected persons are usually homozygous for the normal allele, so all the offspring will be heterozygous and not affected. Because it is more likely that a person will inherit only one copy of a rare mutant allele rather than two copies, heterozygous carriers of mutant alleles are more common than

KEY TERM

Penetrance: the proportion of organisms having a particular genotype that actually expresses the corresponding phenotype. If the phenotype is always expressed, penetrance is complete; otherwise, it is incomplete.

FIGURE 2-3 Pedigree of albinism. With recessive inheritance, affected persons (filled symbols) often have unaffected parents. The double horizontal line indicates a mating between relatives—in this case, first cousins.

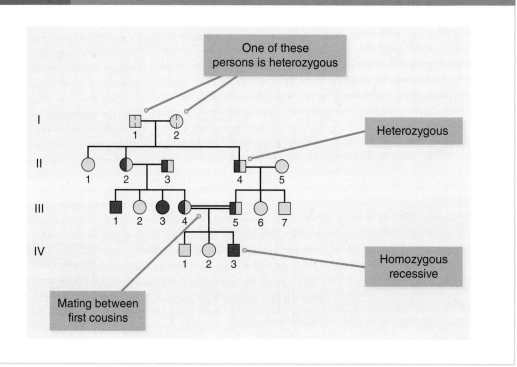

homozygous affected individuals. Therefore, most homozygous recessive genotypes result from mating between heterozygous carriers, in which each offspring has a 25% chance of being affected. This can occur especially if parents of affected individuals are related (Hartl & Jones, 2005).

A rare recessive allele (i.e., albinism) is more likely to be expressed when mating between related heterozygous individuals occurs (Figure 2-3). The offspring resulting from this mating have a 25% chance of inheriting the homozygous recessive allele and will express the albino trait.

A pedigree analysis can be of particular importance for diseases such as sickle cell and sickle cell trait, cystic fibrosis, and Marfan syndrome. For example, when mapping out a family pedigree, if it is discovered that two mates both have sickle cell trait (both are carriers without exhibiting the disease), there is an increased probability of their offspring inheriting both recessive alleles and suffering from sickle cell disease. A geneticist or specialized genetics nurse can offer genetic counseling so that patients can learn about the implications of genomic information for clinical care and future offspring.

Several organizations provide genomic materials and meetings for patients looking for information on genetic disorders, including The Jackson Laboratory (www.jax.org).

Cytogenetic Studies

Cytogenetics is the study of chromosomes using light microscopy. Chromosomal analysis is done by growing human cells in tissue culture, chemically inhibiting mitosis, and staining, observing, photographing, sorting, and counting the chromosomes. Samples can be obtained from peripheral blood, amniotic fluid, trophoblastic cells from the chorionic villus, bone marrow, and cultured fibroblasts (usually obtained from a skin biopsy). In a **karyotype**, the chromosomes (during metaphase) are rearranged systematically in pairs from longest to shortest and numbered from 1 (the longest) through 22 to represent the autosomes (**Figure 2-4**). The sex chromosomes are usually

KEY TERM

Karyotype: the chromosome complement of a cell or organism; often represented by an arrangement of metaphase chromosomes according to their lengths and the positions of their centromeres.

FIGURE 2-4 Human chromosome painting, in which each pair of chromosomes is labeled by hybridization with a different fluorescent probe. (A) Metaphase spread showing the chromosomes in a random arrangement as they were squashed onto the slide.

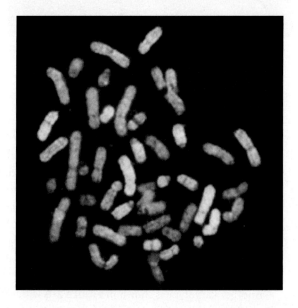

FIGURE 2-4   (B) A karyotype, in which the chromosomes have been grouped in pairs and arranged in conventional order. Chromosomes 1–20 are arranged in order of decreasing size, but for historical reasons, chromosome 21 precedes chromosome 22, even though chromosome 21 is smaller.

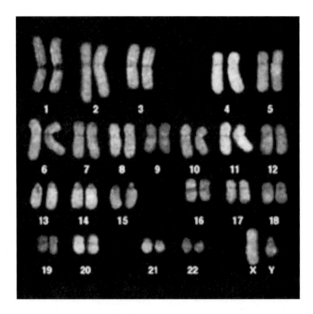

Courtesy of Johannes Wienberg, Ludwig-Maximilians-University, and Thomas Ried, National Institutes of Health.

KEY TERM

Chromosome painting: use of differentially labeled, chromosome-specific DNA strands for hybridization with chromosomes to label each chromosome with a different color.

set off at the bottom right. The karyotype of a normal human female has a pair of X chromosomes instead of an X and a Y. **Chromosome painting**, as shown in Figure 2-4, helps to identify pairs of homologous chromosomes. The different colors are "painted" on each chromosome by hybridization with DNA strands labeled with different fluorescent dyes. The only downside to karyotyping is that if there is an abnormal or missing gene, it cannot be seen using this method. If a whole or part of a chromosome is abnormal or missing, this would be the appropriate genetic test.

Another karyotype is shown in **Figure 2-5** with chromosome banding. These chromosomes have been treated with Giemsa stain, which causes chromosomes to exhibit transverse bands (G-bands) that are specific for each pair

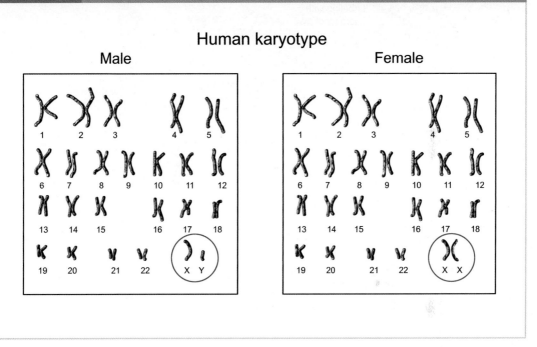

FIGURE 2-5 A karyotype of a normal human male and female. Blood cells arrested in metaphase were stained with Giemsa and photographed with a microscope. (A) The chromosomes as seen in the cell by microscopy. (B) The chromosomes have been cut out of the photograph and paired with their homologs.

© Kateryna Kon/Shutterstock.

of homologs. These G-bands allow smaller segments of each chromosome arm to be identified as well. Chromosomal abnormalities, as well as autosomes and sex chromosomes, can be identified using this technique.

Fluorescence in Situ Hybridization

Chromosome staining and painting provides a way to visualize banding patterns and pairs of homologous chromosomes. However, this interpretation can be rather difficult given that a "standard" karyotype reveals approximately 400 to 500 bands per set of haploid chromosomes. Thus, individual gene

| **FIGURE 2-6** | Diagram showing fluorescence in situ hybridization. |

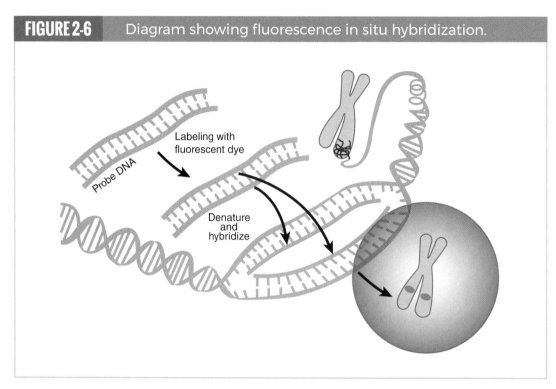

Courtesy of National Human Genome Research Institute. Retrieved from https://www.genome.gov /10000206/fish-fact-sheet.

KEY TERM

Probe: a labeled DNA or RNA molecule used in DNA-RNA or DNA-DNA hybridization assays.

mutations cannot be seen during chromosome staining. The development of fluorescence in situ hybridization (FISH) has made it easier to visualize and map chromosomal and gene abnormalities.

"Fluorescent" means emitting light that comes from a reaction within the emitter, and "in situ" refers to this technique being performed within the chromosomes, cells, or tissue in place (in situ) on a microscope slide ("Fluorescent in situ hybridization," n.d.). A short sequence of nucleic acid—a sequence that matches a portion of the gene in question—is labeled with a fluorescent dye and is referred to as a **probe**. The probe is then allowed to hybridize to suitably prepared cells or histological sections; hybrids are formed with complementary sequences of nucleic acids in a chromosome (**Figure 2-6**). Through nucleic acid hybridization, the degree of sequence identity can be determined, in addition to detecting specific sequences located on specific chromosomes ("Fluorescent in situ hybridization," n.d.). This technique is frequently used to look for localization of genes on specific chromosomes.

INDICATIONS FOR CYTOGENETIC ANALYSIS

- Malformations associated with a particular syndrome or aberration
- Serious mental or physical developmental problems
- Maldefined genitalia (internal or external)
- Primary amenorrhea or delayed pubertal development
- Males with learning or behavioral disorders who are taller than expected
- Malignant or premalignant disease
- Parents of a patient with a chromosome translocation
- Parents of a patient with a suspected syndrome
- Couples with a history of multiple spontaneous abortions of unknown cause
- Infertility not caused by obstetric or urogenital problems
- Prenatal diagnosis

Data from Pyeritz, R. E. Medical genetics. In L. Tierney et al. *Current medical diagnosis & treatment*, 42nd ed. 2003.

DNA Analysis

Molecular genetics involves understanding the expression of genes by studying DNA sequences of chromosomes. Once a particular gene is shown to be defective in a given disease, sequencing the nucleotides and comparing them with those of a normal allele can elucidate the nature of the mutation. Molecular testing is available for more than 1,000 hereditary conditions and has had a significant impact on the diagnosis of Mendelian disorders.

Similar to the use of specific probes in a FISH analysis of chromosomal abnormalities, probes are used to identify specific genes that may be mutated in a certain hereditary disease. The probe may be a piece of the actual gene, a sequence close to the gene, or just a few nucleotides at the actual mutation. The closer the probe is to the actual mutation, the more accurate and the more useful the information. When even a minute amount of DNA from a patient (e.g., from a few leukocytes, buccal mucosal cells, or hair bulbs) is combined with the primers in a reaction mixture that replicates DNA—called **polymerase chain reaction (PCR)**—the region of DNA between the primers will be amplified exponentially after about a dozen cycles. For example, the presence of early HIV infection can be detected after PCR amplification of a portion of the viral genome.

KEY TERM

Polymerase chain reaction (PCR): repeated cycles of DNA denaturation, renaturation with primer oligonucleotide sequences, and replication, resulting in exponential growth in the number of copies of the DNA sequence located between the primers.

KEY TERMS

Phenylketonuria (PKU): a hereditary human condition resulting from inability to convert phenylalanine into tyrosine. It causes severe intellectual disability unless treated in infancy and childhood by a low-phenylalanine diet.

Phenylalanine hydroxylase (PAH): the enzyme that converts phenylalanine to tyrosine and that is defective in phenylketonuria.

Cystic fibrosis: a congenital metabolic disorder, inherited as an autosomal recessive trait, in which secretions of exocrine glands are abnormal. Excessively viscid mucus causes obstruction of passageways (including pancreatic and bile ducts, intestines, and bronchi), and the sodium and chloride content of sweat is increased throughout the patient's life.

EXAMPLE INDICATIONS FOR DNA ANALYSIS

- Presymptomatic detection of Huntington's disease or adult polycystic kidney disease
- Screening for cystic fibrosis and thalassemias
- Screening for X-linked conditions such as Duchenne muscular dystrophy and hemophilia A and B
- Screening for familial polyposis coli

Data from Pyeritz, R. E. Medical genetics. In L. Tierney et al. *Current medical diagnosis and treatment*, 42nd ed. 2003.

Biochemical Analysis

The primary goal of biochemical testing is to determine whether certain proteins are present or absent. Biochemical testing also identifies the proteins' characteristics and effectiveness in vitro. This kind of analysis is used to look for enzymatic defects because these important catalysts are made of protein. For example, **phenylketonuria (PKU)** is an inherited disorder caused by the absence of or a defect in the enzyme **phenylalanine hydroxylase (PAH)**. In the absence of PAH, the amino acid phenylalanine accumulates and can lead to severe intellectual disability. If this deficiency is diagnosed early in life, however, children can be placed on low-phenylalanine diets, and intellectual disability can be avoided. Based on this knowledge, all babies in the United States are screened for PKU.

Another disease process associated with a defective protein is **cystic fibrosis (CF)**. In this disease, a mutation in the **CFTR gene** disrupts chloride and water transport across membranes. The end result is production of thick and sticky mucus that obstructs the airways in the lungs and the ducts in the pancreas. In addition to breathing difficulty, people with CF have problems with nutrient digestion because the buildup of mucus prevents pancreatic digestive enzymes from reaching the intestine.

Both PKU and CF are examples of **inborn errors of metabolism**, which refers to an inherited defect in one or more enzymes. Currently, the state of Georgia screens newborns for 24 metabolic disorders plus sickle cell anemia. Not all states test for all the same disorders in their screening of infants, however, and in some cases, parents can refuse to have the tests done. For a more detailed listing and description of inborn errors of metabolism, refer to the

United States National Newborn Screening Status Report at https://genes
-r-us.uthscsa.edu/sites/genes-r-us/files/nbsdisorders.pdf

Ethical Issues with Genetic Testing

Genetic testing is very valuable in confirming certain diagnoses that otherwise cannot be obtained. This can lead to earlier screenings for cancer or other genetic defects. For example, someone with hereditary non-polyposis colorectal cancer will have screenings for colon cancer much earlier than the average person, ultimately finding and treating colon cancer early in these individuals. However, it is important to always obtain informed consent before genetic testing and to review with patients the risks and benefits of such testing. For example, genetic testing can be very expensive and not always conclusive. However, when genetic testing is conclusive, it cannot be modified. Once a patient has a positive diagnosis, he or she cannot do anything to change it. Diet, exercise, and lifestyle modifications can do nothing to change one's genome. Sometimes this can lead to anger, depression, and blame. It is also important to warn the patient before genetic testing that nobody is "genetically perfect"—that minor genetic mutations do not always lead to disease or pathology. Also, there are no laws preventing insurance rate spikes that may follow genetic testing; insurance companies cannot deny people coverage, but they can raise premiums.

Another ethical issue with genetic testing is the risk of HIPPA violation. The right to know one's genetic risk and the right to *not* know one's genetic risk are both valid and are the patient's decision. However, if a patient's grandfather has Huntington's disease and the patient tests positive because of the inheritance pattern, it is known that the patient could have inherited Huntington's disease only through his or her mother. This violates HIPPA if the mother wishes not to know her genetic risk because now she knows her genetic status without being tested.

KEY TERMS

CFTR gene: a gene that codes for a protein involved in chloride and water transport across membranes. In patients with cystic fibrosis, a mutation in this gene disrupts chloride and water transport across membranes. The end result is production of thick and sticky mucus that obstructs the airways in the lungs and the ducts in the pancreas.

Inborn error of metabolism: a genetically determined biochemical disorder, usually in the form of an enzyme defect that produces a metabolic block.

Chapter Summary

» A good family history should, at the very least, involve asking a patient about the medical history of all first-degree relatives (parents, siblings, and offspring) and, if possible, more distant relatives.

» A pedigree can be used to analyze Mendelian inheritance of certain traits.

» Cytogenetics is the study of chromosomes using light microscopy.

» Once a particular gene is shown to be defective in a given disease, the nature of the mutation can be elucidated by sequencing the nucleotides and comparing this sequence with that of a normal allele.

» The primary goal of biochemical testing is to determine whether certain proteins are present or absent as well as to identify their characteristics and effectiveness in vitro.

Chapter Review Questions

1. Mating between related individuals, also known as _____, is indicated with a double horizontal line in a pedigree diagram.
2. Siblings of individuals who carry the recessive gene for albinism have a _____ percent chance of inheriting and being affected by this trait.
3. In a _____, the chromosomes are rearranged systematically in pairs, from longest to shortest, and numbered from 1 (the longest) through 22.
4. _____ with a fluorescent probe is one method used to assess the degree of sequence identity as well as detect and locate specific sequences on a specific chromosome.
5. In the absence of _____, the amino acid phenylalanine accumulates and can lead to severe intellectual disability.

Bibliography

The American Heritage Dictionary of the English Language (4th ed.). (2006). Boston, MA: Houghton Mifflin.

Bennett, R. L., French, K. S., Resta, R. G., & Doyle, D. L. (2008). Standardized human pedigree nomenclature: Update and assessment of the recommendations of the National Society of Genetic Counselors. *Journal of Genetic Counseling, 17*, 424–433.

Fluorescent in situ hybridization. (n.d.). *MedicineNet*. Retrieved from https://www.medicinenet.com/script/main/art.asp?articlekey=3486

Hartl, D. L., & Jones, E. W. (2005). *Genetics: Analysis of genes and genomes* (6th ed.). Sudbury, MA: Jones and Bartlett Publishers.

Hartl, D. L., & Jones, E. W. (2006). *Essential genetics: A genomic perspective* (4th ed.). Sudbury, MA: Jones and Bartlett Publishers.

Ignatavicius, D. D., & Workman, M. L. (2010). *Medical-surgical nursing: Patient-centered collaborative care* (6th ed., pp. 62–79). St. Louis, MO: Saunders Elsevier.

National Newborn Screening & Global Resource Center. (n.d.). Retrieved from http://genes-r-us.uthscsa.edu/

Pyeritz, R. E. (2003). Medical genetics. In L. J. Tierney, Jr., S. J McPhee, & M. A. Papadakis (Eds.), *Current medical diagnosis and treatment* (42nd ed., pp. 1643–1666). New York, NY: McGraw-Hill.

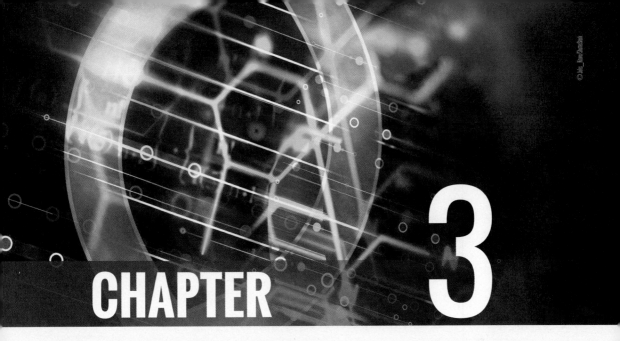

CHAPTER 3

Prenatal Genetics

Overview

Three to five percent of live births are associated with a birth defect, intellectual disability, or genetic condition. **Aneuploidy** (any extra or missing chromosome) occurs in approximately 1 in 350 live births and includes trisomy 21 (Down syndrome), trisomy 18, trisomy 13, and sex chromosome aneuploidies such as Klinefelter syndrome and Turner syndrome. However, 50–60% of miscarriages and stillbirths are due to chromosome imbalances. Aneuploidies are rarely inherited, but often result from a nondisjunctional event that occurs during meiosis. Therefore, a family history of aneuploidy does not typically raise a couple's risk, and infants with aneuploidy are usually born to parents with no family history of aneuploidy. An exception is if the couple experienced a previous pregnancy with aneuploidy, or if a parent is a carrier of a **Robertsonian translocation** involving chromosome 13 or 21. The likelihood of maternal nondisjunction increases as a woman ages. Age 35 or older at the time of delivery is designated as **advanced maternal age**. Although in the past, screening for aneuploidy was offered only to women in this category, the American College of Obstetricians and Gynecologists (ACOG) now recommends that screening and testing options be available to all women regardless of age. Patients should be aware there is not a dramatic increase in risk that occurs at age 35, but that this risk slowly increases each year. The reason age 35 was originally chosen as the cutoff is explained in **Box 3-1**.

The prenatal genetic landscape has become increasingly complex. With the advent of newer screening methods, better ultrasounds, and panel testing for carrier screening, it can be hard for any provider to stay up to date on all the nuances. That said, the typical pregnant patient is offered screening for aneuploidy and open neural tube defects (ONTDs), as well as some degree of carrier screening.

BOX 3-1 Why Is 35 or Older Considered Advanced Maternal Age?

Age 35 was chosen as the cutoff because the chance that a woman will have a fetus with Down syndrome at this age is approximately 1 in 200, and this used to be the risk for miscarriage from amniocentesis. Therefore, it was thought that an invasive diagnostic test should be offered to women who were as least as likely to have an affected pregnancy as to have an adverse outcome from the procedure itself.

Prenatal Screening

Prenatal genetic screening refers to any "test" that is not diagnostic. Screens provide a modified risk number for one or more aneuploidies by taking into account the mother's age and other factors. Screening methods cannot provide a prenatal diagnosis of aneuploidy. Prenatal genetic screening falls into three major categories: ultrasound, maternal serum screening, and noninvasive prenatal screening (NIPS).

Ultrasound

An ultrasound can be the most exciting appointment for a pregnant patient. Many, though, do not realize that ultrasound is a genetic screen. There are many types of ultrasounds that a patient may encounter during her pregnancy. The standard ultrasound, sometimes called the anatomy scan, includes an evaluation of fetal number and presentation, amniotic fluid volume, fetal biometry, cardiac activity, placental position, and anatomic survey. If this is the only ultrasound that a patient receives, the best time to do it is between 18 and 22 weeks of gestation. As a genetic screen, it is assessing the presence or absence of birth defects and soft markers. Soft markers are not birth defects, but subtle changes that alter a woman's risk for specific types of aneuploidy. Echogenic intracardiac foci, echogenic bowel, and shortened long bones (humerus or femur) are examples of soft markers. Approximately 95% of fetuses with trisomy 18 or trisomy 13 will have some feature identified on an anatomy scan, whether a birth defect or a soft marker. In contrast, only approximately 50–60% of fetuses with Down syndrome will have an identifiable feature on ultrasound. Therefore, it is important for patients to understand that a normal ultrasound does not guarantee the birth of a healthy child.

As a genetic screen, the first trimester ultrasound measures the nuchal translucency (NT). This needs to be done when the fetus is measuring between 11 weeks and 1 day and 13 weeks and 6 days. The technician performing the ultrasound and the doctor reading the ultrasound should be certified to accurately assess the genetic risk. Approximately 30% of fetuses with Down syndrome will have a normal NT measurement. Additional reasons that the NT can be thick include a structural anomaly, such as a cardiac defect, a sign of pending fetal demise, and normal variation. A fetal echocardiogram is recommended in the second trimester when a thickened NT is identified in the first trimester.

Bedside ultrasounds are done during routine office visits to quickly assess the fetus's heartbeat and well-being. They are often done early in pregnancy to help determine the due date. Patients should be made aware that this ultrasound does not assess genetic risk.

The biophysical profile (BPP) and growth ultrasounds are used later in pregnancy to assess fetal well-being and aid doctors in caring for the pregnancy. Not all patients need to have a BPP or growth ultrasound. These do not assess a genetic risk.

Maternal Serum Screening

Maternal serum screening involves the analysis of various analytes, such as human chorionic gonadotrophin (hCG) and alpha-fetoprotein (AFP), found in a pregnant woman's blood. These are used to statistically provide a risk number that is specific to the current pregnancy. These screens compare the amount of analytes found in the mother's blood with what the average pregnancy produces at that specific gestational age. Analyte levels closer to average will lower the woman's age-related risk for aneuploidy. Specific patterns of these analytes are associated with increased risk for aneuploidy and ONTDs. **Table 3-1** shows these patterns.

TABLE 3-1	Typical Analyte Pattern for Down Syndrome, Trisomy 18/ Trisomy 13, and Open Neural Tube Defects						
	First Trimester			**Second Trimester**			
	hCG	PAPP-A	AFP	hCG	Inhibin	uE3	AFP
Down Syndrome	↑	↓	↓	↑	↑	↓	↓
Trisomy 18	↓	↓	↓	↓	↓	↓	↓
Trisomy 13	↓	↓	↓	NA	NA	NA	NA
ONTD	NA	NA	NA	-----	-----	-----	↑

AFP: alpha-fetoprotein; hCG: human chorionic gonadotrophin; ONTD: open neural tube defect; PAPP-A: pregnancy-associated plasma protein A; uE3 = estriol.

First Trimester Screen

The first trimester screen (FTS) measures pregnancy-associated plasma protein A (PAPP-A), human chorionic gonadotrophin (hCG), and alpha-fetoprotein (AFP) from the mother's blood to provide a risk for Down syndrome and a combined risk for trisomy 18/trisomy 13. Various factors can affect the levels of these analytes in the mother's blood. Therefore, the lab will need to know the mother's race, the mother's age, the gestational age, and if the mother is an insulin-dependent diabetic. Additionally, if an egg donor was used, the lab will need to know the age of the egg donor at the time of donation. Typically, the blood for the first trimester screen can be drawn between 10 weeks 0 days and 13 weeks 6 days. **Table 3-2** shows the detection and false positive rates.

Combined First Trimester Screen (with Ultrasound)

The combined first trimester screen takes the biochemical portion of the first trimester screen described earlier and combines it with the first trimester ultrasound (nuchal translucency) to provide a risk for Down syndrome and a combined risk for trisomy 18/trisomy 13. Table 3-2 shows the detection and false positive rates.

Quad Screen

The quadruple screen, often called the quad screen, measures hCG, estriol (uE3), inhibin, and AFP from the mother's blood to provide a risk for Down syndrome, trisomy 18, and ONTDs such as spina bifida and anencephaly.

TABLE 3-2	Summary of the Detection Rates and False Positive Rates for the Maternal Serum Screens			
Screen	**Detection Rate**			**False Positive Rate**
	T21	**T18/T13**	**ONTDs**	
First Trimester Screen (biochemical only)	60–70%	60–70%	NA	5%
First Trimester Screen with Ultrasound	91%	95%	NA	5%
Quad Screen	80%	80% (T18 only)	85%	5%
Sequential Screen	88–94%	95%	85%	5%
Integrated Screen	96%	95%	85%	5%

Note that neural tube defects do not increase with maternal age, but occur in approximately 1–2/1,000 pregnancies. As with the first trimester screen, the lab will need to know the mother's race, the mother's age, the gestational age, and if the mother is an insulin-dependent diabetic. Typically, the blood for the quad screen can be drawn between 15 weeks 0 days and 22 weeks 6 days; however, 16 to 18 weeks is considered ideal because it optimizes screening for ONTDs. Table 3-2 shows the detection and false positive rates.

Sequential/Integrated Screening

Sequential and integrated screening combines first trimester screening and second trimester screening to provide risks for Down syndrome, trisomy 18/trisomy 13, and ONTDs. The added benefit of these types of screens is that they have the highest detection rates of the maternal serum screens; the downside is that they require two blood draws—one in the first trimester and one in the second trimester—to receive results. Therefore, if a patient does not return for the second part, no results will be given. Sequential screening will typically release results only after the two blood draws; however, if the first results are higher than a certain cutoff, those results will be released, and the patient will not need to have the second part done. This way, the patient has the option for earlier diagnostic testing. Integrated screening provides the risk results only after the two blood draws. Table 3-2 shows the detection and false positive rates.

Noninvasive Prenatal Screening

Noninvasive prenatal screening, also referred to as cell-free DNA (cfDNA), evaluates fragments of DNA in the mother's blood that come from the placenta to provide a risk for Down syndrome, trisomy 18, trisomy 13, and sex chromosome aneuploidy. It can also reveal the fetal sex. Some companies offer risk evaluations for certain microdeletions syndromes, such as *22q11.2* deletion syndrome, and additional trisomies. NIPS can be drawn any time after 9–10 weeks' gestation. There is no upper limit for when NIPS can be drawn. Although NIPS offers higher detection rates (99%) and lower false positive rates (0.5%) than the maternal serum screens, it is important to remind your patients that it is not diagnostic and does not replace invasive diagnostic testing. Therefore, patients should not make pregnancy decisions based on these results alone. For example, in a 40-year-old woman, the positive predictive value (PPV), or the chance that a positive screen is a true positive, is approximately 93% for Down syndrome, 64% for trisomy 18, 44% for trisomy 13, and 39% for the sex chromosomes aneuploidies. However, these PPVs are based on the prevalence of the condition and thus can be much lower for women at younger ages. The important risk information to provide the patient is not the sensitivity or specificity, but the likelihood that the fetus actually has the condition if the screen result is positive (the PPV).

Some laboratories provide this information, but clinicians can also calculate it by using online programs.[1]

Twins and Prenatal Screening

Twin pregnancies present unique issues in prenatal screening. With the exception of ultrasound, prenatal screening cannot give risks for individual fetuses, but instead will provide just one risk number for the entire pregnancy. If the risk comes back high, one cannot know from the screen alone if one or both twins are affected, or if it is just a false positive for the entire pregnancy. Additionally, it is possible that if one twin is euploid and the other twin is aneuploid, the euploid twin's normal analytes mask the aneuploid twin's abnormal analytes, leading to a false negative result. Therefore, the detection rates are lower for twin pregnancies when compared with singleton pregnancies. The benefit of using a maternal serum screen that takes into account the NT measurement for twin pregnancies is that each twin will have its own NT measurement. Additionally, maternal serum screens have been extensively studied in twin pregnancies. Although NIPS has higher detection rates and lower false positive rates than maternal serum screens, even for twin pregnancies, there are limited data on NIPS in twin pregnancies because it is a newer screening option. For higher multiples (triplets, quadruplets, and so on), screening options, outside of ultrasound, are currently unavailable. For more information on NIPS, please see **Box 3-4**.

Prenatal Diagnostic Testing

Prenatal diagnostic testing refers to the techniques in which placental or fetal cells are obtained for genetic testing. Unlike prenatal screens, false positive or false negative results do not occur. These tests are diagnostic; however, because they are invasive, there is a risk of adverse outcome, such as miscarriage. The two most common prenatal diagnostic tests are chorionic villus sampling (CVS) and amniocentesis (See **Table 3-3**). For more information on Prenatal Diagnostic Testing, please see **Boxes 3-2** and **3-3**.

Chorionic Villus Sampling

Chorionic villus sampling is a prenatal diagnostic test in which chorionic villi cells from the placenta are removed for genetic testing. Depending on the placement of the placenta and the physician performing the procedure, the cells will be removed transabdominally via a needle or transcervically via a flexible catheter, all under ultrasound guidance. This procedure can be performed between 10 weeks and 13 weeks 6 days. The risk of miscarriage is truly dependent on the physician performing the procedure; however,

---

[1] See https://www.perinatalquality.org/vendors/nsgc/nipt/.

TABLE 3-3	Comparing and Contrasting CVS and Amnio

Procedure	Facts	Advantages	Disadvantages
CVS	Performed between 10 weeks and 13 weeks 6 days	Done earlier in pregnancy	Risk for confined placental mosaicism Slightly higher risk of miscarriage
Amnio	Performed after 15–16 weeks	Slightly lower risk of miscarriage Can test for ONTDs	Done later in pregnancy

ONTDs: open neural tube defects.

BOX 3-2	Note on Prenatal Testing Laboratories

Note that many laboratories offer these various prenatal screens. The purpose of the descriptions in this chapter is to summarize the various products currently on the market; it is recommended that you check with the laboratory you are using for specifics.

BOX 3-3	Note on Prenatal Testing

If a mother has had a first trimester screen, noninvasive prenatal screening, or the diagnostic chorionic villus sampling, maternal serum alpha-fetoprotein can be drawn to provide a risk for ONTDs only. The quad screen should not be ordered if any of these tests have been done previously.

BOX 3-4	A Word of Caution Regarding NIPS

Many patients have a misunderstanding of the limitations of NIPS and do not realize that the possibility of a false positive as well as a false negative exists. It is important to remind your patients of these limitations. For example, a patient with a low risk of NIPS who presents with ultrasound findings suggestive of trisomy 13 during the anatomy scan should still be offered amniocentesis despite the low-risk NIPS result.

in skillful hands, the risk of miscarriage ranges from 1 in 200 to 1 in 450. Patients may ask about the association between CVS and limb-reduction defects. If the CVS is performed after 10 weeks, the risk for limb-reduction defects does not appear to be greater than the risk in the general population. CVS also has a 1–2% risk for **confined placental mosaicism**, in which more than one cell line is present in the placenta but not found in the fetus. Therefore, if mosaicism is detected during a CVS, following up with amniocentesis is recommended to determine if the mosaicism is confined to the placenta, or if it is found in the fetus as well. ONTDs cannot be tested for via CVS. Therefore, maternal serum alpha-fetoprotein is recommended for patients who had CVS.

Amniocentesis

Amniocentesis, often shortened to *amnio*, is a prenatal diagnostic test in which amniocytes are removed through the amniotic fluid for genetic testing. The procedure is done transabdominally under ultrasound guidance using a needle to remove ~20–30 cc of amniotic fluid, which contains the amniocytes needed for genetic testing. Amniocentesis can be done once the amnion has fused to the uterine wall, typically after 15–16 weeks. There is no upper limit to when the amnio can be performed. Like CVS, the risk of miscarriage is truly dependent on the physician performing the procedure; however, in skillful hands, the risk of miscarriage ranges from 1 in 300 to 1 in 900.

What Can Be Done with the Sample?

Fluorescence In Situ Hybridization

Fluorescence in situ hybridization (FISH) can be ordered to give a patient quick results on a limited number of chromosomes. It is considered preliminary because it only provides information on five chromosomes (13, 18, 21, X, and Y). Because FISH is done on interphase cells, results can be available in one to two days. This can be very helpful in reducing patient anxiety; however, the patient needs to be reminded that these are just preliminary results, and the final results are needed for confirmation and to provide information on the other chromosomes. FISH is not a standalone test; chromosome analysis and/or microarray must be performed as well.

Chromosomes

Chromosome analysis, also called a karyotype, is considered the gold standard for diagnosing aneuploidy. It provides information on all the chromosomes and can report large chromosome deletions or duplications. Cells need to be cultured (metaphase), so it can take 10–14 days for results to be returned.

Microarray

Microarray uses comparative genomic hybridization to report on gains or losses throughout the genome. It can typically detect smaller gains or losses than can be seen through chromosome analysis. DNA needed for the microarray can be extracted from uncultured cells; however, cultures are often needed to obtain enough DNA for testing. Therefore, the turnaround time is typically between two and four weeks. Microarray has been found to detect a pathogenic gain or loss in approximately 1.7% of patients with a normal karyotype and a normal ultrasound. It is important to note that many of these pathogenic gains or losses have widely variable phenotypes that often cannot be predicted. Thus, couples may be faced with making a decision about the pregnancy when they do not know the severity of the condition. Although the microarray can detect smaller gains and losses than chromosome analysis, it is unable to detect balanced rearrangements, such as balanced translocations and balanced inversions, and, depending on the type of microarray, it may or may not be able to detect triploidy. Additionally, there is a chance that a variant of uncertain significance (VOUS) will be found. Therefore, parental blood is always recommended when ordering a prenatal microarray.

Although there is literature that suggests microarray be offered to any woman who is undergoing an invasive procedure, some insurance companies will pay for microarray only when congenital anomalies are found on ultrasound. Therefore, it is recommended, as with all prenatal screening and testing options, that a patient check with her insurance company to be aware of potential out-of-pocket costs.

Known Mutation Analysis

Prenatal diagnostic testing can be done for any genetic condition in the family in which known pathogenic mutations have been previously identified. Examples include when one parent has an autosomal dominant condition, such as Huntington's disease, or when both parents are carriers for an autosomal recessive condition, such as cystic fibrosis. One always needs to check with the laboratory before obtaining and sending the sample because various requirements differ among laboratories and between tests. Typically, labs will not accept the case if there is a VOUS. Additionally, labs typically will not do full gene sequencing for disorders during pregnancy.

Ethical issues surround prenatal diagnostic testing. An example is when a patient wants to test a fetus for an adult-onset condition such as

Huntington's disease or hereditary breast and ovarian cancer syndrome. Because it is not recommended that minors be tested for adult-onset conditions, laboratories may feel uncomfortable accepting a sample if the patient will not terminate an affected fetus. Additionally, laboratories often perform identity testing as part of their prenatal test to ensure that a sample switch does not occur. Identity testing is not paternity testing, but nonpaternity could be revealed during this process.

Carrier Screening

We are all thought to be carriers of approximately five to eight different autosomal recessive conditions. Most of us do not know any of the conditions for which we are carriers. Carriers are typically healthy and usually do not have any features of the condition. Additionally, there is often no family history of genetic diseases that are inherited in an autosomal recessive manner. We know that some conditions are more prevalent in certain ethnicities, and recommendations for carrier testing have been established by professional organizations.

ACOG guidelines recommend that all women, regardless of ethnicity, be offered screening for cystic fibrosis (CF), spinal muscular atrophy (SMA), and hemoglobinopathies, such as sickle cell anemia and thalassemias, via hemoglobin electrophoresis and a complete blood count. Additionally, if there is a family history of fragile X (a genetic syndrome that causes intellectual disability, behavioral problems, and various physical characteristics) or intellectual disability, fragile X screening should be offered. It is recommended that carrier screening occur preconceptionally. This allows more time for carrier testing of the partner and, if both are carriers, provides the couple with more reproductive options. However, pregnant women should also be offered carrier screening. ACOG also notes that, in addition to the mentioned conditions, providing ethnic-specific, panethnic, and expanded carrier screening is an acceptable strategy for carrier screening. **Table 3-4** shows a breakdown of recommended ethnic-specific conditions.

Because of new technology, larger panels called panethnic carrier screening and expanded carrier screening have become available, some testing for up to 100 or more conditions. It is recommended that laboratories include only conditions that are frequent in the general population, that are severe, and that are not primarily adult-onset conditions. The benefit of these panels to the patient is that they are often equally or less expensive than carrier screening for just CF and SMA. Additionally, the patient may be comforted knowing that she has been screened for several conditions and not just a select few. The downside to this type of screening is that more individuals will be found to be carriers for at least one condition

TABLE 3-4	Ethnicity-Based Carrier Screening Recommendations

Ethnicity	Condition
African American	Sickle cell disease (ACOG, ACMG) Hemoglobinopathies (ACOG, ACMG)
Ashkenazi Jewish	Tay-Sachs disease (ACOG, ACMG) Canavan disease (ACOG, ACMG) Familial dysautonomia (ACOG, ACMG) Cystic fibrosis (ACOG, ACMG) Bloom syndrome (ACMG, ACOG–considered) Familial hyperinsulinism (ACOG–considered) Fanconi anemia (ACMG, ACOG–considered) Gaucher disease (ACMG, ACOG–considered) Glycogen storage disease type I (ACOG–considered) Joubert syndrome (ACOG–considered) Maple syrup urine disease (ACOG–considered) Mucolipidosis type IV (ACMG, ACOG–considered) Niemann-Pick disease (ACMG, ACOG–considered) Usher syndrome (AGOG–considered)
Asian	Hemoglobinopathies (ACOG, ACMG)
Cajun	Tay-Sachs (ACOG, ACMG)
Caucasian (non-Hispanic)	Cystic fibrosis (ACOG, ACMG)
French-Canadian	Tay-Sachs (ACOG)
Mediterranean	Hemoglobinopathies

ACMG: American College of Medical Genetics; ACOG: American College of Obstetricians and Gynecologists.

on the panel. This can result in patient anxiety while the partner is tested. It also increases the number of abnormal results than need to be reported to patients.

Residual Risk

It is important to review with your patient that negative carrier screening does not completely eliminate the possibility of the individual still being a carrier. The **residual risk** is the risk that an individual is still a carrier for a condition despite a negative (normal) screen for that condition. These risks will differ based on the condition being screened and the patient's ethnicity. For example, when a Caucasian individual has a normal CF common mutation panel, her residual risk for being a carrier is ~1 in 290, which is decreased from her starting population risk of 1 in 29.

KEY TERM

Residual risk: the risk that an individual carries an abnormal gene after a negative (normal) screening test result.

Carrier Screening of Reproductive Partner

If a patient is found to be a carrier for an autosomal recessive condition, the reproductive partner of that patient should be offered carrier screening for the specific condition(s) to accurately determine the risk to offspring. If there are time constraints, such as desiring carrier screening while already pregnant, concurrent screening of both partners can be suggested.

Consanguinity

Couples with **consanguinity** should be offered genetic counseling to review the increased risk of autosomal recessive conditions for their children. The benefits and limitations of carrier screening should also be discussed.

In-Vitro Fertilization with Preimplantation Genetic Diagnosis and Preimplantation Genetic Screening

For patients undergoing in-vitro fertilization (IVF), preimplantation genetic diagnosis (PGD) and preimplantation genetic screening (PGS) are options.

PGD is an option when there is a genetic condition in the family and the mutation(s) is known. IVF is performed, and cells are removed from the embryos at day 3 or day 5 and sent for genetic analysis for the familial mutation(s). Only unaffected embryos are selected for implantation. Because of the chance of mosaicism, PGD is not perfect, and errors have been reported. The chance that an affected embryo is transferred ranges from 1 to 10% depending on the inheritance of the genetic condition. Therefore, prenatal testing is always recommended for patients who use PGD.

In PGS, embryos are screened for aneuploidy before implantation. Similar to PGD, this is done at day 3 or day 5. Only euploid embryos are selected for implantation. Because of the risk of mosaicism, prenatal screening and/or testing is recommended for patients who use PGS.

Family History

Family history information should also be collected on all couples currently pregnant or who are considering pregnancy. Referral for genetic counseling should be offered to any individual or couple who answers yes to any of the questions in **Box 3-5**.

BOX 3-5   Family History Questions

All patients (and partners) should be asked if there is a family history of:

» Birth defects
» Multiple pregnancy losses
» Intellectual disability
» Hearing or vision loss at birth
» Known genetic conditions
» Consanguinity

Chapter Summary

» There are various means of prenatal screening for aneuploidy, including ultrasound, maternal serum screens, and NIPS.

» Prenatal screens are not diagnostic and have false positives and false negatives.

» Prenatal diagnostic testing involves an invasive procedure (CVS or amnio) and has a risk of miscarriage.

» Carrier screening should be offered to all couples who are pregnant or considering pregnancy; however, it is ideal to offer carrier screening before pregnancy.

» All couples should be asked some basic family history questions to determine if a referral to a genetic counselor is needed.

Chapter Review Questions

1. Which of the following screens for ONTDs?
   A. First trimester screen
   B. Quad screen
   C. CVS
   D. NIPS

2. True or False: Amniocentesis has a risk of confined placental mosaicism.

3. Which of the following aneuploidies is not analyzed via FISH?
   A. Trisomy 18
   B. Trisomy 13
   C. Klinefelter syndrome (XXY)
   D. Trisomy 16

4. True or False: If a patient screens negative for cystic fibrosis, there is no chance that she will have a child affected with cystic fibrosis.

5. Which of the following screens has the best detection rate for Down syndrome?
    A. First trimester screen
    B. Quad screen
    C. Sequential screen
    D. Integrated screen

6. True or False: Noninvasive prenatal test results are considered diagnostic.

Bibliography

American College of Medical Genetics. (2013a). ACMG policy statement: ACMG position statement on prenatal/preconception expanded carrier screening. *Genetics in Medicine, 15*(6), 482–483.

American College of Medical Genetics. (2013b). ACMG policy statement: ACMG statement on noninvasive prenatal screening for fetal aneuploidy. *Genetics in Medicine, 15*(5), 395–398.

American College of Obstetricians and Gynecologists. (2016a, May). ACOG Practice Bulletin Number 162: Prenatal diagnostic testing for genetic disorders. *Obstetrics and Gynecology, 127,* e108–e122.

American College of Obstetricians and Gynecologists. (2016b, May). ACOG Practice Bulletin Number 163: Screening for fetal aneuploidy. *Obstetrics and Gynecology, 127,* e123–e137.

American College of Obstetricians and Gynecologists. (2016c, December). ACOG Practice Bulletin Number 175: Ultrasound in Pregnancy. *Obstetrics and Gynecology, 128,* e241–e256.

American College of Obstetricians and Gynecologists. (2017a, March). ACOG Committee Opinion Number 690: Carrier screening in the age of genomic medicine. *Obstetrics and Gynecology, 129,* e35–e40.

American College of Obstetricians and Gynecologists. (2017b, March). ACOG Committee Opinion Number 691: Carrier screening for genetic conditions. *Obstetrics and Gynecology, 129,* e41–e55.

Lazarin, G. A., Hague I. S., Nazareth, S., Iori, K., Patterson, A. S., Jacobson, J. L., Marshall, J. R., . . . Srinivasan, B. S. (2013). An empirical estimate of carrier frequencies for 400+ causal Mendelian variants: Results from an ethnically diverse clinical sample of 23,453 individuals. *Genetics in Medicine, 15*(3), 178–186.

National Society of Genetic Counselors. (2016). NSGC position statement: Prenatal cell-free DNA screening. Retrieved from https://www.nsgc.org/p/bl/et/blogaid=805

Resnik, R., Creasy, R., Iams, J., Lockwood, C., Moore, T., & Green, M. (2013). *Creasy & Resnik's maternal-fetal medicine principles and practice* (7th ed.). Philadelphia, PA: Saunders Elsevier.

Tanner, A. K., Valencia, C. A., Rhodenizer, D., Espirages, M., Da Silva, C., Borsuk, L., Caldwell, S., . . . Hegde, M. (2014). Development and performance of a comprehensive targeted sequencing assay for pan-ethnic screening of carrier status. *Journal of Molecular Diagnostics, 16*(3), 350–360.

Wang, J. C., Sahoo, T., Schonberg, S., Kopita, K. A., Ross, L., Patek, K., & Strom, C. M. (2015). Discordant noninvasive prenatal testing and cytogenetic results: A study of 109 consecutive cases. *Genetics in Medicine, 17*, 234–236.

Wapner, R. J., Martin, C. L., Levy, B., Ballif, B. C., Eng, C. M., Zachary, J. M., Savage, M., . . . Scholl, T. (2012). Chromosomal microarray versus karyotyping for prenatal diagnosis. *New England Journal of Medicine, 367*, 2175–2184.

Yao, R., & Goetzinger, K. R. (2016). Genetic carrier screening in the twenty-first century. *Clinics in Laboratory Medicine, 36*(2), 277–288.

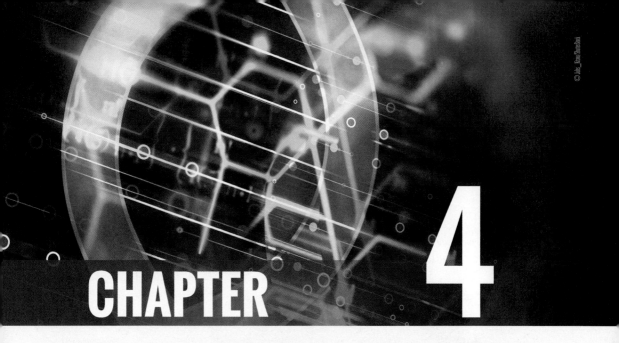

CHAPTER 4

Development and Teratogenesis

During fertilization, sperm come into contact with the plasma membrane of the oocyte. This interaction triggers meiotic division, which results in the formation of the ovum or egg. Once the sperm enters the ovum, the nuclei combine to form a **zygote** that contains 46 chromosomes. The next step is the first mitotic division—one of many billions of such divisions that will occur during human growth and development. Throughout this process, a clear distinction is made between weeks of pregnancy and weeks of development. Pregnancy starts with the first day of the last menstrual period, whereas development starts at fertilization (usually two weeks after the last menstrual period).

Embryonic Development

Human development consists of three stages, labeled as pre-embryonic, embryonic, and fetal. The pre-embryonic stage includes all the changes that occur from fertilization to the time just after an embryo becomes implanted in the uterine wall. During this phase, the zygote undergoes rapid cellular division and is converted into a solid ball of cells called a **morula (Figure 4-1)**. Three to four days after fertilization, repeated cell cleavages yield a total of 16–32 cells. By this time, the morula has reached the uterus; during the next three to four days, it floats in the intrauterine fluid as more cell divisions occur.

Fluid soon begins to accumulate in the morula and creates a hollow sphere of cells called a **blastocyst**. This stage consists of a clump of cells, the **inner cell mass (ICM)**, which will eventually become the **embryo**, and a ring of flattened cells, the **trophoblast**. The trophoblast will further develop into the embryonic portion of the **placenta** that supplies nutrients to and removes wastes from the embryo.

FIGURE 4-1	Formation of the morula and blastocyst during pre-embryonic development.

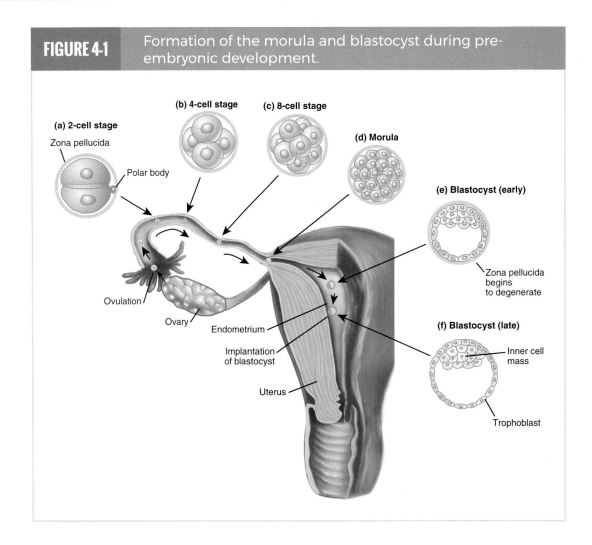

Implantation

The blastocyst attaches to the uterine wall six or seven days after fertilization. For the next few weeks, cells of the trophoblast secrete enzymes that digest the adjacent endometrial cells so that the embryo can obtain nourishment. However, if the endometrium is not ready for any reason, the blastocyst cannot implant. This implantation can be prevented by the presence of an endometrial infection, an intrauterine device, or use of a **morning-after pill**. Blastocysts may also fail to implant if their cells contain certain genetic mutations. Unimplanted blastocysts are absorbed by the endometrium through a process called phagocytosis or expelled during menstruation.

If implantation does occur, by day 14, the uterine endometrium grows over the blastocyst, enclosing it and walling it off from the rest of the uterine cavity. Endometrial cells respond to the attached blastocyst by producing **paracrines**, such as prostaglandins, that promote local changes in the endometrial tissue. These changes include increased development of uterine blood vessels, which helps to ensure delivery of oxygen and other nutrients to the area. Soon after this stage, the maternal (endometrium) and embryonic (trophoblast) tissues combine to form the placenta.

Early in the development of the placenta, a layer of cells separates from the ICM to form the **amnion**, and a small cavity forms between the ICM and the amnion. This amniotic cavity fills with amniotic fluid that, in addition to providing nutrients, acts like a "shock absorber" to protect the fetus from injury during development. After the amnion is formed, the cells of the ICM differentiate to create three distinct germ layers: the **ectoderm**, the **mesoderm**, and the **endoderm**. These are known as the primary germ layers, and their formation marks the beginning of embryonic development and will give rise to the organs by a process called **organogenesis**. **Table 4-1** shows the organs that form from each layer.

TABLE 4-1	Organs and Tissues Associated with Embryonic Germ Layers	
Endoderm	**Mesoderm**	**Ectoderm**
Lining of digestive system	Dermis	Epidermis
Lining of respiratory system	All muscles of the body	Hair, nails, sweat glands
Urethra and urinary bladder	Cartilage	Brain and spinal cord
Gallbladder	Bone	Cranial and spinal nerves
Liver and pancreas	Blood	Retina, lens, and cornea of eye
Thyroid gland	All other connective tissue	Inner ear
Parathyroid gland	Blood vessels	Epithelium of nose, mouth, and anus
Thymus	Reproductive organs	
Kidneys	Enamel of teeth	

Modified from Chiras, D. D. (2005). *Human biology* (5th ed.). Sudbury, MA: Jones and Bartlett Publishers.

The formation of the central nervous system (spinal cord, brain) is one of the first steps of organogenesis. Early in embryonic development, the ectoderm located along the back of the embryo folds inward. This creates a long trench—the neural groove that runs the length of the back surface of the embryo. During the next few weeks, this neural groove deepens and eventually closes off, thereby creating the neural tube. The walls of the neural tube thicken to form the spinal cord. In the head region, the neural tube expands to form the brain. The spinal and cranial nerves develop from small aggregations of ectodermal cells (the neural crest) that are found on either side of the neural tube. These cells eventually develop into axons that grow throughout the body and attach to organs, muscle, bone, and skin. The ectoderm is also the precursor for the epidermis.

The mesoderm is the middle germ layer, which gives rise to body tissues such as muscle, cartilage, bone, and dermis. The endoderm contributes to the formation of a large pouch under the embryo called the **yolk sac**. The uppermost part of the yolk sac develops into the lining of the intestinal tract. It also gives rise to blood cells and primitive germ cells. During organogenesis, the germ cells migrate from the wall of the yolk sac to the developing testes or ovaries. These cells eventually become spermatogonia or oogonia.

Fetal development involves ongoing organ development and growth as well as changes in body proportions. It begins in the eighth week of pregnancy and ends at **parturition** (birth). The fetus grows rapidly during this period, increasing in length from approximately 2.5 to 35–50 cm and increasing in weight from 1 to 3,000–4,000 g. The fetus also becomes more humanlike in physical appearance with each month of gestation. The organ development that started during the embryonic stage is completed during the fetal stage.

Congenital Abnormalities

It has been estimated that 31% of all successful fertilizations end in miscarriage or spontaneous abortion. Approximately 66% of these miscarriages occur before a woman is even aware that she is pregnant. This high frequency is thought to reflect how nature deals with defective embryos. This system of dealing with abnormalities is not perfect, however, given that many children are born each year with birth defects. Between 10 and 12% of all newborns have some kind of birth defect, ranging from a minor biochemical problem to some sort of gross physical deformity. Such defects may be caused by a variety of biological, chemical, and physical agents. Some contributors to these congenital abnormalities include mutant genes, chromosomal defects, and multifactorial components. Unfortunately, the largest cause of these defects is of unknown etiology.

Teratology is the study of abnormal development (**Box 4-1**). Teratogens include anything capable of disrupting embryonic or fetal development

BOX 4-1	Principles of Teratology

1. Susceptibility to teratogens is variable.
2. Susceptibility to teratogens is specific for each developmental stage.
3. The mechanism of teratogenesis is specific for each teratogen.
4. Teratogenesis is dose dependent.
5. Teratogens produce death, growth retardation, malformation, or functional impairment.

Data from Rubin E. (2001). *Essential pathology* (3rd ed.). Baltimore, MD: Lippincott Williams & Wilkins.

TABLE 4-2	Types of Teratogens	
Pharmacological	Thalidomide
	Diethylstilbestrol
	Retinoic acid
Infectious agents	*Toxoplasma gondii*
	Rubella
	Cytomegalovirus
	Herpes
	Congenital syphilis
	Zika virus
Industrial agents	Lead
	Mercury
	Pesticides/herbicides
Recreational	Alcohol
	Tobacco
	Cocaine

KEY TERMS

Mesoderm: the middle of the three primary germ layers of the embryo (the others being ectoderm and endoderm). The mesoderm is the origin of connective tissues, myoblasts, blood, the cardiovascular and lymphatic systems, most of the urogenital system, and the lining of the pericardial, pleural, and peritoneal cavities.

Endoderm: the innermost of the three primary germ layers of the embryo (ectoderm, mesoderm, endoderm). The epithelial lining of the primitive gut tract and the epithelial component of the glands and other structures (e.g., lower respiratory system) that develop as outgrowths from the gut tube are derived from the endoderm.

Organogenesis: formation of organs during development.

and producing malformations (i.e., birth defects). A host of chemical, physical, and biological agents may cause developmental anomalies (see **Tables 4-2** and **4-3**). Most complex developmental abnormalities affecting several organ systems result from injuries inflicted from the time of implantation of the blastocyst through early organogenesis. During the stage of primordial organ system formation, the embryo is extremely vulnerable to negative effects of teratogens.

The critical period for teratogenic effects is between 3 and 16 weeks of gestation. Three major factors that affect the likelihood and extent of

TABLE 4-3	Common Drugs That Are Teratogenic or Fetotoxic	
ACE inhibitors	Diethylstilbestrol	Progestins
Alcohol	Disulfiram	Radioiodine
Amantadine	Ergotamine	Reserpine
Androgens	Estrogens	Ribavirin
Anticonvulsants	Griseofulvin	Sulfonamides
Aspirin and other salicylates (third trimester)	Hypoglycemics, oral (older drugs)	SSRIs
Benzodiazepines	Isotretinoin	Tetracycline (third trimester)
Carbarsone	Lithium	Thalidomide
Chloramphenicol (third trimester)	Methotrexate	Tobacco smoking
Cyclophosphamide	NSAIDs (third trimester)	Trimethoprim (third trimester)
Diazoxide	Opioids (prolonged use)	Warfarin (Coumadin) and other anticoagulants

ACE: angiotensin-converting enzyme; NSAIDs: nonsteroidal anti-inflammatory drugs; SSRIs: selective serotonin reuptake inhibitors.
Reproduced from Crombleholme, W. R. (2009). Obstetrics and obstetric disorders. In S. J. McPhee, M. A. Papadakis, & L. M. Tierney, Jr. (Eds.), *Current medical diagnosis and treatment* (48th ed., Chapter 19). Copyright © The McGraw-Hill Companies, Inc. All rights reserved.

teratogenesis are dosage, time of exposure, and genotype of the embryo. Because organ systems develop at different times, the timing of exposure determines which systems are affected by a given agent (**Figure 4-2**). During its critical development period, an organ is vulnerable to toxins, viruses, and genetic abnormalities. Any alteration of normal development may cause birth defects. The central nervous system begins to develop during the third week of pregnancy, whereas the teeth, palate, and genitalia do not begin to form until about the sixth or seventh week of pregnancy. Therefore, exposure to some teratogen during the seventh week of pregnancy may affect the genitalia, palate, or teeth but have little effect on the central nervous system because it has entered a less sensitive phase of development.

Thalidomide

Thalidomide is used today to treat illnesses such as multiple myeloma, erythema nodosum leprosum, HIV wasting, and aphthous ulcers. It was originally developed in the 1950s for the treatment of pregnancy-associated

FIGURE 4-2	Human development is divided into three stages: pre-embryonic, embryonic, and fetal. Organogenesis occurs during the embryonic stage. Each bar indicates when an organ system develops. The dark-shaded area indicates the periods most sensitive to teratogenic agents.

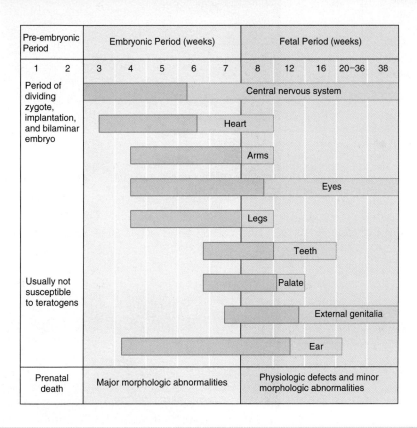

Pre-embryonic Period	Embryonic Period (weeks)					Fetal Period (weeks)				
1 2	3	4	5	6	7	8	12	16	20–36	38
Period of dividing zygote, implantation, and bilaminar embryo	Central nervous system								
	Heart								
	Arms								
	Eyes								
	Legs								
	Teeth								
Usually not susceptible to teratogens	Palate								
	External genitalia								
	Ear								
Prenatal death	Major morphologic abnormalities					Physiologic defects and minor morphologic abnormalities				

morning sickness but was withdrawn from the market because of the tragic consequences of its teratogenicity, which included stunted limb growth in affected fetuses. This drug was given to pregnant women to prevent morning sickness between weeks 4 and 10 of pregnancy, which is the critical period for limb formation. Among babies who survived, birth defects included deafness, blindness, disfigurement, cleft palate, and many other internal disabilities. However, the disabilities most closely associated with thalidomide involved defective development of arms, legs, or both so that the hands and feet were attached close to the body, resembling the flippers of a seal (**phocomelia**; see **Figure 4-3**).

KEY TERM

Parturition: the process of birth.

FIGURE 4-3   Baby with malformed limbs due to in utero thalidomide exposure.

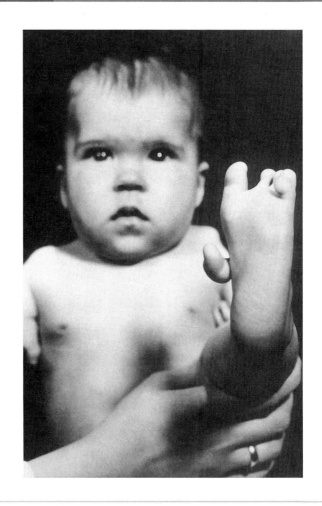

© National Cancer Institute/Science Source.

The numbers vary from source to source because no proper census was ever taken, but it has been claimed that there were between 10,000 and 20,000 babies born disabled as a consequence of thalidomide. There are approximately 5,000 survivors alive today around the world (Thalidomide Victims Association of Canada, 2010).

The number of babies who were miscarried or stillborn as a consequence of thalidomide has never been counted.

TORCH Complex

A complex of similar signs and symptoms produced by fetal or neonatal infection with a variety of microorganisms is referred to as TORCH. This collection of infectious organisms includes *Toxoplasma* (T), rubella (R), cytomegalovirus (C), and herpes simplex virus (H); the letter "O" in the acronym represents "others." Children infected in utero with any of these agents have very similar symptoms.

Asymptomatic toxoplasmosis is common, with 25% of women in their reproductive years exhibiting antibodies to this organism. However, intrauterine *Toxoplasma* infection occurs in only 0.1% of all pregnancies.

Early in the 1960s, an epidemic of rubella occurred over a period of approximately two years; 20,000 children developed congenital rubella syndrome, and there were 30,000 stillbirths from this infection. "Rubella syndrome, or congenital rubella, is characterized by rash at birth, low birth weight, small head size, heart abnormalities (i.e., patent ductus arteriosis), visual problems (i.e., cataracts), and bulging fontanelle" ("Rubella Syndrome," 2010). Fortunately, the introduction of the rubella vaccine in the United States has virtually eliminated congenital rubella.

"Cytomegalovirus (CMV) is a virus found around the world. It is related to the viruses that cause chickenpox and infectious mononucleosis. Once CMV is in a person's body, it stays there for life" ("Cytomegalovirus infections," 2010). Approximately 66% of childbearing-age women test positive for CMV immunoglobulin G, and as many as 2% of newborns in the United States are congenitally infected with this virus. Newborns who survive are at increased risk for hearing loss and mental retardation. "However, only 3% of newborns infected with CMV during pregnancy experience problems from the virus. Most are born healthy or with only mild CMV symptoms" ("Cytomegalovirus," 2010).

Clinical and pathological findings in the symptomatic newborn with TORCH complex vary. Only a few present with multisystem disease and the entire spectrum of abnormalities. Lesions of the brain represent the most serious pathological changes in TORCH-infected children. Acute encephalitis is associated with foci of necrosis. **Microcephaly**, **hydrocephalus**, and abnormally shaped gyri and sulci are frequently observed. As mentioned earlier, ocular defects are prominent in children infected with rubella, with more than two-thirds of these patients presenting with cataracts. In addition, congenital rubella often leads to cardiac anomalies, such as patent ductus arteriosus and various septal defects.

Zika virus can be included in the category of "O" for other viruses that cause fetal infection. Zika virus is an arthropod-borne flavivirus transmitted by mosquitoes. In 2016, outbreaks occurred in the Americas,

---

KEY TERMS

Microcephaly: abnormal smallness of the head; a term applied to a skull with a capacity of less than 1,350 mL. Microcephaly is usually associated with mental retardation.

Hydrocephalus: a condition marked by an excessive accumulation of cerebrospinal fluid, resulting in dilation of the cerebral ventricles and raised intracranial pressure; it may also result in enlargement of the cranium and atrophy of the brain.

the Caribbean, and the Pacific. The first U.S. case of Zika-related microcephaly was reported January 2016 in Hawaii, in a baby born to a woman who had resided in Brazil during her pregnancy. The first U.S. case of sexually transmitted Zika virus infection was reported in Texas in February 2016. The Zika virus has been reported in the blood, urine, semen, saliva, female genital tract secretions, cerebral spinal fluid, amniotic fluid, and breast milk of infected individuals. Greatest risk of serious fetal sequelae occurs in the first trimester. Complications of Zika virus infection include fetal losses among women infected during pregnancy, congenital microcephaly, development problems among babies born to women infected during pregnancy, Guillain-Barre syndrome, myelitis, and meningoencephalitis. There is no specific treatment for Zika virus infection. Suggested prevention is wearing long sleeves and long pants, using insect repellent, staying indoors as feasible, and following safe sex practices. Currently there is no vaccine available.

Fetal Alcohol Syndrome

Ethyl alcohol (also known simply as alcohol) is one of the most potent teratogens known. Its use during pregnancy varies by population. A safe threshold dose for alcohol use during pregnancy has never been established (Crombleholme, 2007). Fetal alcohol syndrome comprises a complex of abnormalities caused by maternal consumption of alcohol and includes growth retardation, central nervous system dysfunction, and characteristic facial dysmorphology. Because not all children adversely affected by maternal alcohol abuse exhibit the entire spectrum of abnormalities, the term **fetal alcohol effect** is also used to describe this condition.

Children with fetal alcohol effect have milder degrees of mental deficiency and emotional disorders; this outcome is more common than the full fetal alcohol syndrome scenario. The minimum amount of alcohol that results in fetal injury is not well established, but children afflicted with fetal alcohol syndrome are usually the offspring of mothers with chronic alcoholism. Characteristic features associated with this syndrome are outlined in **Box 4-2**.

It has been reported that 20% of children with fetal alcohol syndrome have IQs lower than 70, and 40% of the children have IQs between 70 and 85. (Normal IQ values are in the vicinity of 100.) The affected child may have congenital heart and joint defects and demonstrate failure to thrive and persistent irritability during the early years of life. These problems are followed by developmental delay, growth deficiency, and poor coordination. Other comorbid conditions include mental retardation, attention-deficit/hyperactivity disorder, learning disorders, sensory impairment, cerebral palsy, and epilepsy.

> ## BOX 4-2 — Characteristic Features Associated with Fetal Alcohol Syndrome
>
> Behavior disturbances
> Brain defects
> Cardiac defects
> Spinal defects
> Craniofacial anomalies
>   Absent or hypoplastic philtrum
>   Broad upper lip
>   Flattened nasal bridge
>   Hypoplastic upper lip vermilion
>   Micrognathia
>   Microphthalmia
>   Short nose
>   Short palpebral tissues
>
> Data from Cunningham, F. G., Leveno, K. L., Bloom, S. L., Hauth, J. C., Gilstrap, L. C., III, Wenstrom, K. D. (2006). Teratology, Drugs, and Other Medications; Cunningham, F. G., Leveno, K. L., Bloom, S. L., Hauth, J. C., Gilstrap, L. C., III, Wenstrom, K. D. (2009). *Williams obstetrics*, 22nd ed.

Tobacco

Cigarette smoke contains a number of potential teratogens, including nicotine, cotinine, cyanide, thiocyanate, carbon monoxide, cadmium, lead, and various hydrocarbons. In addition to being fetotoxic, many of these substances have vasoactive effects that reduce oxygen levels. A well-documented reproductive outcome related to smoking is a direct dose-response reduction in fetal growth. Newborns of mothers who smoke weigh, on average, 200 g less than newborns of nonsmoking mothers, and heavy smoking results in more severe weight reduction. Smoking doubles the risk of low birth weight and increases the risk of a small-for-gestational age newborn by 2.5-fold. Women who stop smoking early in pregnancy generally have neonates with normal birth weights. Smoking also may cause a slightly increased incidence of subfertility, spontaneous abortion, placenta previa and abruption, and preterm delivery.

Cocaine

Cocaine is currently one of the most widely abused drugs in the United States. This central nervous system stimulant exerts its effects through sympathomimetic action via dopamine. Cocaine is a highly effective topical anesthetic and local vasoconstrictor, and most of the adverse outcomes noted in offspring associated with pregnant women's use of cocaine result from the drug's vasoconstrictive and hypertensive effects. Maternal complications include myocardial infarction, arrhythmias, aortic rupture, stroke, seizure, bowel ischemia, and sudden death. Placental abruption is the most frequently cited cocaine-related pregnancy complication in cocaine abusers: Its incidence is fourfold greater in users than in nonusers.

The risk of vascular disruption within the embryo, fetus, or placenta is highest after the first trimester of pregnancy and likely accounts for the increased incidence of stillbirth. A number of cocaine-related congenital anomalies resulting from vascular disruption have been described, including skull defects, cutis aplasia, **porencephaly**, subependymal and periventricular cysts, ileal atresia, cardiac anomalies, and visceral infarcts. Because few reports address dosage or total fetal exposure during pregnancy, it is difficult to estimate the precise fetal risk associated with antenatal cocaine use.

Vitamin A

Beta-carotene is a precursor of vitamin A that is found in fruits and vegetables; it has not been shown to cause birth defects. Many foods contain the fat-soluble vitamin A, but animal liver contains the highest amounts. Excessive dietary intake of vitamin A has been associated with teratogenicity in humans. Therefore, caution must be used to avoid unnecessary supplementation of women of childbearing age.

Some vitamin A isomers are used for dermatological disorders because they stimulate epithelial cell differentiation. Isotretinoin, which is 13-*cis*-retinoic acid, is effective for treatment of cystic acne. It is also considered one of the most potent teratogens in widespread use. First-trimester exposure to this isomer is associated with a high rate of fetal loss, and the 26-fold increased malformation rate in survivors is similar to that observed among children exposed to thalidomide in utero. Abnormalities have been described only with first-trimester use of isotretinoin, however. Because isotretinoin is rapidly cleared from the body (its mean serum half-life is 12 hours), anomalies are not increased in women who discontinue therapy with this drug before conception.

Although any organ system can be affected by isotretinoin exposure, malformations typically involve the cranium and face, heart, central nervous system, and thymus. These defects frequently appear in conjunction with agenesis of the external ear canal. Other defects include cleft palate and maldevelopment of the facial bones and cranium. The most frequently noted cardiac anomalies are outflow tract defects, and hydrocephalus is the most common central nervous system defect.

Diethylstilbestrol

From 1940 to 1971, between 2 million and 10 million pregnant women took diethylstilbestrol (DES) to "support" high-risk pregnancies. This drug later was shown to have no beneficial effects, and its use for this purpose was abandoned. In 1971, however, it was reported that eight women who had prenatal exposure to DES had developed vaginal clear-cell adenocarcinoma. Subsequent studies showed that the absolute cancer risk in prenatally exposed women is substantially increased, to about 1 per 1,000. Malignancy is not dose related, and there is no relationship between the location of the tumor and the timing of exposure.

In the years since the first reports of a DES–cancer link surfaced, researchers have shown that DES produces both structural and functional abnormalities. Because DES interrupts the transition of cells within the developing vagina/cervix in as many as half of exposed female fetuses, DES-exposed women have a twofold increase in vaginal and cervical intraepithelial neoplasia. One-fourth of exposed females have structural abnormalities of the cervix or vagina; the embryological mechanism underlying these defects is unknown. The most commonly reported abnormalities include a hypoplastic, T-shaped uterine cavity; cervical collars; hoods, septa, and coxcombs; and "withered" fallopian tubes. Affected women are at increased risk for poor pregnancy outcomes related to uterine malformations, decreased endometrial thickness, and reduced uterine perfusion. Exposed male fetuses have normal sexual function and fertility but are at increased risk for epididymal cysts, microphallus, cryptorchidism, testicular hypoplasia, and hypospadias.

Chapter Summary

» Human development proceeds through three stages: pre-embryonic, embryonic, and fetal.

» The ectoderm, mesoderm, and endoderm are the primary germ layers; their formation marks the beginning of embryonic development. As the embryo develops, these layers give rise to the organs by a process called organogenesis.

» An estimated 31% of all successful fertilizations end in miscarriage or spontaneous abortion; 66% of these miscarriages occur before a woman is even aware that she is pregnant.

» Teratology is the study of abnormal development; teratogens include anything capable of disrupting embryonic or fetal development and producing malformations.

» The critical period for teratogenic effects is between 3 and 16 weeks of gestation.

» Three factors known to affect the likelihood and extent of teratogenesis are dosage, time of exposure, and genotype of the embryo.

» Fetal alcohol syndrome is perhaps the most common cause of acquired mental retardation.

» Isotretinoin is effective for treatment of cystic acne, but is also considered to be one of the most potent teratogens in widespread use.

Chapter Review Questions

1. The _____ attaches to the uterine wall six or seven days after fertilization.
2. After the amnion is formed, the cells of the inner cell mass differentiate to create three distinct germ layers: the _____, the _____, and the _____.
3. The critical period for teratogenic effects is between _____ of gestation.
4. Which drug was given to pregnant women to prevent morning sickness between weeks 4 and 10 and caused severe birth defects?
5. _____ doubles the risk of low birth weight and increases the risk of a small-for-gestational age newborn by 2.5-fold.

Bibliography

Azaïs-Braesco, V., & Pacal, G. (2000). Vitamin A in pregnancy: Requirements and safety limits. *American Journal of Clinical Nutrition, 71*(Suppl.): 1325S–1333S.

Chabner, B. A., Amrein, P. C., Druker, B. J., Michaelson, M. D., Mitsiades, C. S., Goss, P. E., Ryan, D. P., ... Wilson, W. H. (2005). Antineoplastic agents. In L. L. Brunton, J. S. Lazo, & K. L. Parker (Eds.), *Goodman & Gilman's the pharmacological basis of therapeutics* (11th ed., pp. 1315–1404). New York, NY: McGraw-Hill.

Chiras, D. D. (2005). *Human biology* (5th ed.). Sudbury, MA: Jones and Bartlett Publishers.

Crombleholme, W. R. (2007). Obstetrics. In S. J. McPhee, M. A. Papadakis, & L. M. Tierney, Jr. (Eds.), *Current medical diagnosis and treatment* (46th ed., pp. 782–806). New York, NY: McGraw-Hill.

Cunningham, F. G., Leveno, K. L., Bloom, S. L., Hauth, J. C., Gilstrap, L. C., III, & Wenstrom, K. D. (2006). Teratology, drugs, and other medications. *Williams obstetrics* (22nd ed., pp. 341–372). New York, NY: McGraw-Hill.

Cytomegalovirus. (2010). *Familydoctor.org*. Retrieved from https://familydoctor.org/condition/cytomegalovirus/

Cytomegalovirus infections. (2010). *MedlinePlus*. Retrieved from http://www.nlm.nih.gov/medlineplus/cytomegalovirusinfections.html

Franks, M. E., Macpherson, G. R., & Figg, W. D. (2004). Thalidomide. *Lancet, 363,* 1802–1811.

Germann, W. J., & Stanfield, C. L. (2005). *Principles of human physiology* (2nd ed.). San Francisco, CA: Benjamin Cummings.

IQ Comparison Site. (n.d.). *IQ basics*. Retrieved from http://www.iqcomparisonsite.com/IQBasics.aspx

Rubella. (n.d.). *MedlinePlus*. Retrieved from http://www.nlm.nih.gov/medlineplus/rubella.html

Rubella syndrome: disease and conditions. (2010). *AllRefer.com*. Retrieved from http://health.allrefer.com/health/congenital-rubella-rubella-syndrome.html

Rubin, E. (2001). *Essential pathology* (3rd ed.). Baltimore, MD: Lippincott Williams & Wilkins.

Sadler, T. W. (2015). *Langman's medical embryology* (13th ed.). Philadelphia, PA: Wolters Kluwer Health.

Smithells, R. W., & Newman, C. G. (1992). Recognition of thalidomide defects. *Journal of Medical Genetics, 29,* 716–723.

Thalidomide Victims Association of Canada. (2010). *The Canadian tragedy: The tragedy of thalidomide in Canada.* Retrieved from https://thalidomide.ca/en/the -canadian-tragedy/

‹ Describe the history, role, and function of genetic counselors within the healthcare system.

‹ Evaluate the impact of advances in genetics and genomics on the practice of medicine.

‹ Understand the complexities associated with genetic testing and provision of genetic counseling.

‹ Compare and contrast the application of genetics and genomics in various medical specialties.

‹ Determine when a referral to a genetic counselor is appropriate.

KEY TERMS

Clinicians

Counselors

Educators

Information gathering

Information giving

Investigators

Psychosocial and support

Risk assessment

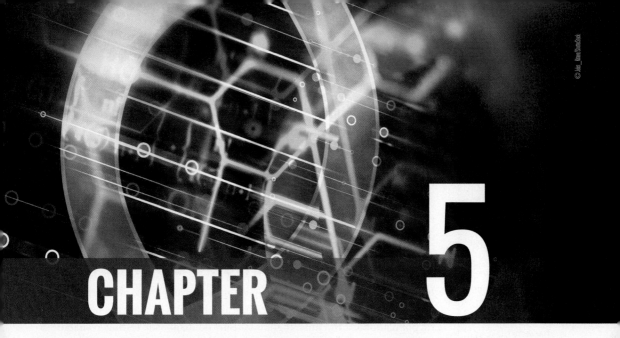

CHAPTER 5

Genetic Counseling

Definition and History of Genetic Counseling

According to Runge, Patterson, & McKusick (2006), "Genetic counseling is the process of helping people understand and adapt to the medical, psychological and familial implications of genetic contributions to disease. This process integrates:

» Interpretation of family and medical histories to assess the chance of disease occurrence or recurrence.
» Education about inheritance, testing, management, prevention, resources and research.
» Counseling to promote informed choices and adaptation to the risk or condition" (p. 46).

The profession of genetic counseling was born in 1971 with the first graduating class of master's-level genetics counselors from Sarah Lawrence College. The term *genetic counseling*, however, was coined by Sheldon Reed in 1947, and *genetics* as the "science of heredity" at the turn of the century. Early genetics "advising," unfortunately, was focused on a eugenics model with the goal of "improving the human race" through forced sterilization of individuals considered "undesirable." In the 1950s, geneticists were using our relatively simplified understanding of inheritance patterns to explain risks of recurrence to families and chromosome analysis to diagnose conditions such as Down syndrome. It was the advent of amniocentesis for prenatal diagnosis of aneuploidy and newborn screening in the 1960s that created the need for a nonphysician clinician to provide information, support, and options for families impacted by genetic conditions.

The National Society of Genetic Counselors was formed in 1979. At the time, there were fewer than 100 counselors and just a handful of training programs. Accreditation of training programs and certification were originally established under the American College of Medical Genetics. In 1994, the American Board of Genetic Counseling (ABGC) took over these activities, and in 2012, the Accreditation Council for Genetic Counseling (ACGC) split off from ABGC as an independent body. Now there are over 4,000 board-certified genetic counselors in the United States and 41 ACGC-accredited training programs. Training programs also now exist in more than 15 countries around the world. Fueled by the exponential rate of human and medical genetic and genomic discoveries, the demand for genetic counselors is now at an all-time high.

Essentials of Genetic Counseling

In the early days of the profession, genetic counselors primarily worked in university settings as assistants to medical geneticists treating the pediatric population. At the time, there was really no diagnostic testing available beyond karyotypes, and genetic diagnoses were made solely on the basis of medical/developmental issues and dysmorphic features. The role of genetic counselors focused on creating and interpreting pedigrees, providing education and support, and assisting families in adjusting to the diagnosis or situation. Genetic counselors also provided information regarding risks for chromosome aneuploidies for pregnant women of "advanced maternal age." At this time, amniocentesis was the only available testing option, often performed without the benefit of ultrasound guidance.

The profession has changed dramatically over the last three decades in parallel with the continuous advances in genetic and genomic technology, as described in the next section. Genetic counseling, however, retains the essence of the fundamental roles that existed at the beginning: clinician, investigator, educator, and counselor.

Genetic counselors are **clinicians**, trained in the fundamentals of human disease and healthcare; they use the most current genetic knowledge and testing to facilitate diagnoses and provide information regarding medical/developmental implications and management. Genetic counselors are **investigators**, deciphering medical and family histories to identify possible genetic etiologies and accessing the most current literature and research to ensure that their patients receive the most up-to-date information and options. Genetic counselors are **educators**, transforming complex genetic information and translating it to a form that is understandable and meaningful to patients and audiences of all levels of literacy. Genetic counselors are **counselors**, trained in psychological techniques and empathetic communication to help individuals and families adjust to and cope with the genetic condition or risk in question. The philosophy of genetic counseling is to empower the patient with the knowledge, tools, and support to facilitate decision making and the adjustment process, as opposed to telling the patient what to do or advising a single course of action.

Components of Clinical Genetic Counseling Sessions

As with most clinical appointments, all genetic counseling sessions begin with **information gathering**. The primary data-gathering tool of the genetic counselor is the family history, formatted as a pedigree. At minimum, creation of the pedigree involves three generations, includes all individuals—both healthy and those with health issues—age and sex, ages of diagnosis, treatment of relevant medical/developmental issues, and ages and causes of death. Pregnancies and previous pregnancy losses (miscarriages/stillbirths/terminations of pregnancy), including weeks of gestation, are recorded. Ancestry and ethnicity of both sides of the family are ascertained and consanguinity ruled out. This is because some genetic conditions/gene alterations are more prevalent in certain populations, and consanguinity increases the probability for the occurrence of an autosomal recessive condition. **Figure 5-1**

> **KEY TERM**
>
> **Counselors:** genetic counselors who are trained in psychological techniques and empathetic communication to help individuals and families adjust to and cope with the genetic condition or risk in question.

FIGURE 5-1   Detailed pedigree.

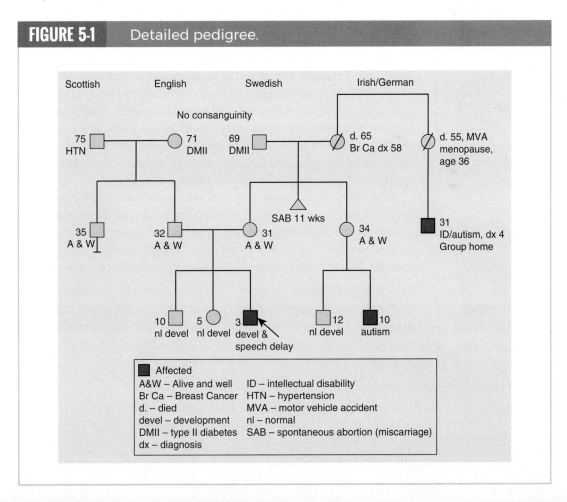

shows a detailed pedigree of the type that might be collected for a general genetics referral.

The second major component of a genetic counseling session is **risk assessment**. The pedigree and medical history/characteristics of the proband are used to identify possible genetic diagnoses and hereditary patterns, for both rare genetic conditions and common diseases. This assessment assists the counselor in determining if genetic testing is appropriate and which genetic tests should be considered.

The bulk of the genetic counseling session is **information giving**. Basic information about chromosomes, genes, and gene mutations is presented in language tailored to the individual's understanding, often with the use of diagrams and illustrations to enhance comprehension. Patients are provided with information regarding the genetic condition, including, as appropriate, inheritance patterns and risks of occurrence or reoccurrence. Communication of risk is a particularly challenging aspect of genetic counseling that is complicated by issues of both numeracy and genomic literacy. It is important to provide risks in multiple formats and reframe so that the magnitude of the risk is better understood (**Box 5-1**).

Options for genetic testing are explained, including possible test results, limitations of available testing, and insurance issues. It is not uncommon for people to be concerned about undergoing genetic testing for fear of insurance discrimination, although both state and federal laws exist protecting against this possibility (**Box 5-2**). It should be noted that many insurance companies do cover the cost of genetic counseling and testing for appropriate indications. Indeed, several insurance companies require genetic counseling by a qualified professional in order to cover genetic testing costs.

If the patient elects to undergo genetic testing, it is the role of the counselor to determine the available testing options and counsel the patient on the advantages and disadvantages of each. In addition, the counselor often coordinates the testing and works with the patient and the laboratory on insurance coverage. When results are complete, a follow-up counseling session occurs.

BOX 5-1 Communicating Genetic Risk

Case: A 35-year-old woman who is 12 weeks pregnant undergoes first-trimester screening. Her result is "screen positive," indicating a 1/200 risk for her baby to have Down syndrome.

Examples of risk communication:

» This is a screening test; it does not mean your baby has Down syndrome.
» The chance is 1/200, which is one-half of 1%. This means that there is a 99.5% likelihood that your baby does *not* have Down syndrome.
» If there were a room full of 200 women your exact age with the same screening result, 1 of them would have a baby with Down syndrome, but the remaining 199 would *not*.

BOX 5-2 Genetic Discrimination Laws

» All 50 states have laws that prohibit making health insurance and employment decisions on the basis of genetic testing (www.ncsl.org/research/health/genetic-nondiscrimination-in-health -insurance-laws.aspx).

» The federal Genetic Information Nondiscrimination Act (GINA) was passed in 2008. It provides protection against health insurance denial or rate hikes on the basis of genetic information, including family history. GINA also applies to employment (http://ginahelp.org/).

» The Affordable Care Act (ACA) prohibits health insurance discrimination based on any "preexist-ing" condition, including those with a genetic cause.

Life insurance and long-term disability insurance are not covered by these laws. Patients should be made aware of this before undergoing genetic testing.

Depending on the indication and results, this may be either in person or by phone. The result session involves explanation of the genetic findings, including discussion of the condition, disease risks or manifestations, inheritance pattern, and medical management recommendations. If test results are negative or uncertain, options for further testing or evaluation and opportunities for participation in clinical research are discussed. A unique and powerful aspect of genetic counseling is that these issues are relevant not only to the individuals undergoing testing, but to their extended family members as well. Thus, patients are provided with implications of the test results for family members, including how they may access genetic counseling and testing.

The final and perhaps most important component of genetic counseling is the **psychosocial and support** aspect. Individuals experience a myriad of feelings when a genetic diagnosis is made. For parents, this may run from relief at finally putting an end to the diagnostic odyssey with a diagnosis, to fear for what the future may hold for their child, to guilt if the condition was inherited. In the prenatal setting, the parents may be grieving the loss of the "normal healthy" child they had been expecting, while facing the agonizing decision over whether to end or continue the pregnancy. A father who learns his daughter developed breast cancer at a young age because of a *BRCA1* gene mutation he passed on to her may find himself weighed down with guilt and alienated from his children. A brother who learns that he received the flip of the coin without the familial mutation for Huntington's disease struggles between feelings of relief for himself and his family, and survivor guilt in relation to his sister who did inherit the mutation. Genetic counselors are trained in the technique of providing anticipatory guidance, helping families to come to terms with, and gain some sense of control over, the genetic situation by understanding what to expect from a physical, developmental, and emotional perspective. An example is anticipating heightened feelings of grief or loss on the anniversary of the death of a

KEY TERMS

Information giving: the process in which patients are provided with information regarding the genetic condition, including, as appropriate, inheritance patterns and risks of occurrence or reoccurrence.

Psychosocial support: the support provided by genetic counselors which may include incorporating empathy and compassion into their sessions and making sure individuals and families have access to appropriate health and educational interventions.

child or other loved one. Parents of children with disabilities may experience chronic grief; over time, their child does not experience "normal" life milestones such as learning to ride a bike, learning to drive, and going to the prom. The absence of each of these milestones may be accompanied by renewed feelings of loss. Although genetic counselors are not trained as psychologists per se, they are trained to assess and recognize psychosocial challenges that may warrant referral to a mental health professional.

The support provided by genetic counselors can take many forms, from incorporating empathy and compassion into their sessions to making sure individuals and families have access to appropriate health and educational interventions. One of the advantages of receiving a genetic diagnosis is the ability to connect with others going through a similar experience. The Internet has allowed even those with very rare conditions to find a common community (see the list of resources in this chapter).

Because of the content and complexity involved with genetic counseling, most appointments last between 30 and 90 minutes, and sometimes longer. The length, of course, will depend on the genetic condition involved and the educational and support needs of the individual/family. A description of the difference between provision of genetic counseling care and standard medical appointments suggested by Hsia in 1979 still remains applicable today. He suggested that whereas in most nongenetics clinician–patient encounters, the central topic is treatment or cure, in genetic counseling (where cure and treatment is rarely available), information giving and education may be considered the treatment itself.

Impact of Advances in Genetics/Genomics on Genetic Counseling

Although the essence of genetic counseling as provision of education remains the same, the technological advances over the last two decades have dramatically altered the content of these sessions and options available to patients and families.

The $3 billion Human Genome Project (HGP), started in 1995, was undoubtedly the spark that launched the genomic revolution. This revolution shows no signs of ending, with genetic technologies and discoveries continuing to be developed at ever-increasing levels of complexity and speed.

The ahead-of-schedule completion of the HGP led us to understand that humans have only approximately 20,000 genes, rather than the estimated 100,000 believed to exist as recently as 1988. To date, the function of about 8,000 of these genes is known. Sanger sequencing allowed for the development of genetic laboratories that could economically provide gene sequencing and analysis on a clinical basis. The number of genes for which clinical testing is available has risen from 100 in 1993 to close to 6,000 in 2017. New genes are being discovered on literally a daily basis and are added quickly to laboratory test menus.

Karyotype analysis has been replaced by microarray in the pediatric setting, a technique that uses comparative genomic hybridization to pinpoint submicroscopic deletions and duplications of the chromosomes, which are termed "copy number variants," or CNVs. Microarray has led to a substantial improvement in our ability to provide a diagnosis for individuals with a variety of health, developmental, and cognitive challenges. Microarray is not, however, without its challenges. In 5–6% of cases, CNVs are identified that have not been previously described in association with a particular phenotype. Although we may be able to determine which genes are extra or missing in a particular CNV, in many cases, we cannot determine if these are related to the phenotype, or indeed have any impact at all. Microarray is becoming more common for prenatal diagnosis, with a diagnostic yield of 1–7%. In prenatal settings, finding a CNV of unknown significance creates particular counseling challenges.

Next-generation sequencing techniques emerging in the mid-2000s accelerated our ability to sequence genes with increasing rapidity and accuracy. In the past, testing was offered one gene at a time, based on the clinician's assessment of the most likely diagnosis. Now, however, multiple genes can be sequenced for the same cost as a single gene in the past. These "panel tests" may include several hundred genes that have been associated with a particular phenotype, such as hearing loss, epilepsy, autism, and cancer.

In the last five years, sequencing of the entire exome (regions of the genome that code for specific proteins) and whole genome sequencing (WGS) have greatly influenced the ability to find a genetic diagnosis in individuals for whom standard genetic testing failed for years to find an answer. Between 25% and 35% of children with a combination of birth defects, developmental delay, and dysmorphic features receive a diagnosis through this technology. Whole exome sequencing (WES) is now being explored in prenatal situations in which an ultrasound finding is observed, and studies are under way that evaluate the efficacy and utility of using WES in place of routine newborn screening.

One of the most significant challenges associated with these advances in genomic and genetic technology is the significant frequency with which genetic findings of uncertain significance are encountered. Although we are able to sequence a person's DNA in its entirety, we are far from understanding the implications of most of the variation in the human genome. When we sequence the DNA, there is always the possibility of finding what is known as a "variant of uncertain significance," or VOUS. When testing for *BRCA1/2* first became available, the rate of finding a VOUS was as high as 20%. Twenty years later, this rate is closer to 5% as our understanding and classification of variation in DNA sequence of the gene have improved. However, now that

BOX 5-3	Classification of Variants Identified on Gene Sequencing

» **Pathogenic**—strong evidence that the variant is disease causing
» **Likely Pathogenic**—moderate to strong evidence that the variant is disease causing
» **Uncertain Significance**—insufficient or contradictory evidence regarding disease association
» **Likely Benign**—moderate to strong evidence that the variant is not associated with disease
» **Benign**—strong evidence that the variant is not associated with disease

large panels are being more frequently used, the overall likelihood of a VOUS is multiplied by the number of genes involved. **Box 5-3** illustrates the range of results that can be obtained through sequencing of a gene. Alterations in medical management or testing of relatives should be offered *only* if pathogenic or likely pathogenic results are obtained.

Although the discovery of pathogenic and likely pathogenic variants can be highly informative, the other categories do not allow us to explain or predict the genetic implications of the condition. One of the most significant concerns of nongenetic health professionals interpreting these results is the mistaken assumption that any DNA variation found is disease causing. Indeed, women have received recommendations to undergo prophylactic mastectomy based on a VOUS in a gene associated with hereditary breast cancer, only to have that variation reclassified as benign a year later. More concerning, however, are the more recent findings indicating that several genes previously thought to be associated with disease are not actually causative (genes of uncertain significance, or GOUSs). Pretest genetic counseling must include the possibility of finding one or more VOUSs, along with the potential implications of both a pathogenic mutation and no mutation identified. Each of these results has significantly different implications. Families also need to be made aware that changes in our understanding of the genome could result in changes in the interpretation of their results in the future.

WES and WGS are even more complicated because testing might reveal deleterious mutations in genes not associated with the phenotype—so-called incidental findings. These may be in genes associated with adult-onset conditions or carrier status for recessive conditions. The American College of Medical Genetics has issued recommendations for mandatory reporting of mutations in 56 specific genes associated with high penetrance and medical management implications. Most laboratories will report clearly deleterious mutations in any gene not related to the phenotype that is well described and has medical management implications, along with select pharmacogenomics variants. Pretest counseling for WES/WGS must therefore include a thorough discussion of this possibility and ascertainment of the desire of the individuals/parents to receive this information. The posttest counseling session involves providing for *each reportable variant,* information regarding the certainty of the finding, the disease/condition associations and risks, inheritance pattern, medical management recommendations, and implications for family members.

Healthcare providers also need to be aware that not all genetic testing companies are created equal. There is little to no regulation of these laboratories with respect to which genes they test and how the results are curated, interpreted, and reported. Indeed, one laboratory may report a variant as pathogenic, whereas another classifies it as a VOUS. Although the Clinical Laboratory Improvement Amendments (CLIA) ensure analytical validity, they do not require evidence of clinical validity or utility. Technology and profit are the driving forces, with genes being added to testing menus and panels often before any reliable information is available regarding disease-associated risks or evidence-based management recommendations. Interpretation of genetic test results therefore requires the healthcare professional to use available database and literature resources to determine the relevance and implications of each finding for his or her patient.

Genetic Counseling Practice Areas

The technological advances in genetic and genomic testing have led to involvement of genetic counselors in multiple areas of clinical practice. Genetic counselors are being increasingly viewed as essential members of the healthcare team in the treatment and management of patients in many subspecialty clinics, such as oncology, neurology, cardiovascular, and ophthalmology clinics, in addition to the more traditional pediatric genetic and maternal-fetal medicine settings. When genetic counseling came into being, conditions with a genetic component were considered to impact only a very small minority of the population. Now, we know that genetics plays a role in virtually every human disease.

An exhaustive description of the impact of genetic conditions in these various clinical settings is, of course, beyond the scope of this text. **Table 5-1** provides examples of the genetic contribution and conditions associated with several clinical specialties. In larger academic settings, multidisciplinary specialty clinics exist to care for patients with specific genetic conditions, such as muscular dystrophy, lysosomal storage diseases, Turner syndrome, tuberous sclerosis, and cystic fibrosis. An important role of these specialty clinics is to involve patients in the increasing number of clinical trials available to treat genetic disease. These range from enzyme replacement therapy for diseases such as Fabry disease, to exon-skipping therapies for individuals with specific mutations in genes associated with Duchenne muscular dystrophy and cystic fibrosis. It is indeed an exciting time for those of us in genetics, knowing that there will be increasing opportunities to provide not just education

TABLE 5-1   Impact of Genetics in Various Clinical Settings

Clinical Setting	Genetic Contribution	Applications/Examples/Implications
Oncology	‹ 5–10% of cancer is hereditary ‹ All cancer results from genetic alteration	‹ Panel testing of both high- and moderate-penetrance genes ‹ Tumor gene profiling is being used to guide chemotherapy decisions
Ear, Nose, & Throat	‹ Over 50% of early onset hearing loss has a genetic etiology	‹ 1/30 individuals carry a mutation in the *connexin* genes associated with AR hearing loss ‹ Most children identified with hearing loss at birth have no family history
Cardiology	‹ 1/150 individuals have an inherited cardiovascular disease ‹ 5–15% of SIDS cases are due to inherited channelopathies	‹ Panel testing for hypertrophic cardiomyopathy will identify a mutation in over 75% of cases ‹ Most inherited cardiovascular disease is AD
Epilepsy	‹ 40% of pediatric epilepsy has a genetic etiology	‹ Over 150 genes are included on epilepsy panels ‹ Identification of genetic etiology can direct pharmaceutical intervention
Neurology	‹ 5–10% of ALS, Alzheimer's disease, PD, and FTD are caused by single-gene mutations	‹ Panel testing of over 35 genes associated with these conditions is available ‹ The APOE4 allele is associated with late-onset alzheimer's disease, but risk and age of diagnosis vary widely
Ophthalmology	‹ Over 200 genes have been associated with retinal dystrophies	‹ Retinitis pigmentosa can be inherited as AR, AD, and XL ‹ 5 SNPs explain 50% of the heritability of age-related macular degeneration

AD: autosomal dominant; ALS: amyotrophic lateral sclerosis; AR: autosomal recessive, FTD: frontotemporal dementia; PD: Parkinson's disease; SIDS: sudden infant death syndrome; SNPs: single nucleotide polymorphisms

but treatment, and possibly cures, for individuals and families impacted by genetic conditions.

In addition to clinical practice, the skills of genetic counselors are being used more and more in nonclinical settings. With the increasing array of genetic tests and testing companies over the last several years, genetic counselors have become an integral part of the majority of genetic testing laboratories. Laboratory counselors act as the liaison between the lab and the ordering provider. In this setting, they also assist with variant interpretation, report writing, and marketing.

An important responsibility of genetic counselors is the education of nongenetic clinicians and the lay public. Genomic literacy remains significantly low in this country, which can lead to inappropriate testing, misunderstanding of test results, mistrust of genetic advances, and waste of healthcare dollars. As an example, any consumer can go online and order direct-to-consumer tests that claim to tell them their athletic prowess, optimum diet and supplements to take, and even how quickly they are aging based on telomere length.

Genetic counselors have long worked in public health settings, primarily in the arena of newborn screening. Many states also now employ genetic counselors as part of their health prevention programs in such areas as cancer and cardiovascular genetics. Population screening for individuals at increased risk for hereditary cancers, and families impacted by sudden cardiac death of the young, have the potential to improve health outcomes for significant portions of the population. Health insurance companies, pharmaceutical companies, and the Food and Drug Administration are increasingly seeking professionals with genetic expertise to evaluate test coverage, conduct clinical trials on treatments for genetic conditions, and advise on issues related to genetic testing and pharmacogenetics.

Referral and Access to Genetic Counselors

There is no doubt that primary care clinicians will have an increasing role in provision of genetic healthcare as we move deeper into the era of personalized medicine. However, as with all medical care, it is the responsibility of the clinician to understand his or her limits and know when to refer to a specialist. **Table 5-2** provides examples of when clinicians should consider referring a patient to a qualified genetic healthcare provider.

The genetic counseling community recognizes that access to genetic counselors is limited by numbers and geography. Although the profession continues to grow rapidly, it is unlikely that there will be enough genetic counselors to meet the expanding need. One effort to address this issue is through the use of telegenetics. Genetic counseling is very amenable to provision by either telephone alone or with video conferencing. Several companies that provide telegenetic services have sprung up in recent years (see the resources list in this chapter), and clinics and hospitals are using these technologies to reach patients who live in remote or rural areas. Video education is also being used to provide basic educational content, allowing the counselor to serve more patients by focusing on their individual needs. Genetic counselors will likely

TABLE 5-2	Indications for Genetic Counseling Referral
Family History	**Test/Screening Results**
Multiple affected individuals in multiple generations with the same or related conditions	Mutation identified on carrier screening (e.g., cystic fibrosis)
Unusually early onset of disease (e.g., dementia)	Abnormal prenatal screening or testing results
Bilateral disease (e.g., renal cysts)	Uncertainty regarding appropriateness of genetic testing, or which test/lab to consider
Multiorgan/system involvement	Identification of a pathogenic or likely pathogenic mutation on genetic testing
Developmental delay/intellectual disability/autism	Identification of variants of uncertain significance on genetic testing
Known birth defects or genetic conditions	Negative genetic test results when there is a high level of suspicion for genetic disease
Sudden unexplained deaths	Tumor gene profiling indicating a mutation in a gene associated with hereditary cancer
Nonsyndromic hearing loss, epilepsy, early vision loss	Abnormal newborn screening results, including carrier status

become central to the use of genetic testing within healthcare systems by providing education and training to other clinicians, reviewing and approving genetic tests ordered by nongenetic healthcare providers, and being the go-to resource for complicated genetic test results or situations.

Conclusion

Genetic and genomic technological and medical advances have become an ever-greater component of the provision of quality healthcare. Along with these advances, however, have come a dizzying array of genetic testing options. In addition, the complexity of interpreting genetic test results and the substantial probability of uncertain or ambiguous findings necessitate adequate patient education in the form of pretest and posttest counseling. Genetic counseling involves far more than just providing recurrence risks for dominant or recessive conditions; it requires a thorough understanding of genetic etiology for disease, genetic testing options and result interpretation, disease manifestation and management, and the ability to communicate complex information in clear, simplified language while providing psychosocial support.

Genetic counselors are an integral part of the healthcare team who can assist nongenetic healthcare providers in the responsible and appropriate application of genomic medicine to improve the health of their patients.

Genetic Counseling Resources

» National Society of Genetic Counselors—www.nsgc.org
  • Find a counselor: www.nsgc.org/page/find-a-gc-search
» Gene Tests—International directories of genetic testing laboratories and genetic clinics: www.genetests.org
» Gene Reviews—Expert authored, peer-reviewed disease descriptions: www.ncbi.nlm.nih.gov/books/NBK1116/
» Genetic Alliance—Organization focused on advocacy, education, and support for genetic and rare diseases: www.geneticalliance.org
» Genetics Home Reference—Your Guide to Understanding Genetic Conditions, appropriate for patients: https://ghr.nlm.nih.gov/
» OMIM—Online Mendelian Inheritance in Man.® An Online Catalog of Human Genes and Genetic Disorders: www.omim.org
» Telegenetic Counseling
  • Informed DNA: http://informeddna.com
» Genetic Counseling Services: www.geneticcounselingservices.com

Chapter Summary

» Advances in genetic and genomic technology have led to the availability of genetic testing for several thousand conditions, both rare and common.

» Testing technologies, including microarray, gene panels, and whole exome/genome testing provide genetic diagnoses in an increasing number of situations, but are associated with substantial likelihoods of uncertain/ambiguous results and incidental findings.

» Genetic counseling involves information gathering in the form of health and family history; risk assessment to determine the likelihood of genetic disease, common disease risk and recurrence risk; ascertainment of appropriateness of genetic testing, which tests to consider and which laboratory to use; interpretation of genetic test results in the context of medical and family history; information giving regarding disease manifestations, risks, management recommendations and implications of test results for family members; and provision of psychosocial counseling and support.

» Genetic medicine is being integrated into virtually every medical subspecialty, with genetic counselors as a part of the healthcare team.

» Interprofessional education and collaboration between genetic counselors and other healthcare providers will be essential to ensure appropriate application of genomic medicine advances.

Chapter Review Questions

1. The roles of genetic counselors include clinician, _____, _____, and _____.
2. Components of the genetic counseling session include _____, risk assessment, _____, and _____.
3. Individuals who undergo genetic testing are at risk for health insurance discrimination.   True   False
4. A counseling challenge for next-generation sequencing panel results is _____.
5. Genetic testing and counseling are being integrated into many medical subspecialties.   True   False

Bibliography

Bernhardt, B. A., Biesecker B. B., & Mastromarino, C. L. (2000, September 18). Goals, benefits, and outcomes of genetic counseling: Client and genetic counselor assessment. *American Journal of Medical Genetics, 94*(3), 189–197.

Biesecker B. B. (2001). Goals of genetic counseling. *Clinical Genetics, 60*(5), 323–330.

Burke K., & Clarke A. (2016). The challenge of consent in clinical genome-wide testing. *Archives of Disease in Childhood, 101*, 1048–1052.

Green, R. C., Berg, S. B., Grody, W. W., Kalia, S. S., Korf, B. R., Martin, C. L., . . . Biesecker, L. G. (2013). ACMG recommendations for reporting of incidental findings in clinical exome and genome sequencing. *Genetics in Medicine,15*(7), 565–574.

Hsia, Y. E. (1979). The genetic counselor as information giver. In A. M. Capron, M. R. F. Lappé, T. M. Powledge, S. B. Twiss, & D. Bergsma (Eds.), *Genetic counseling: Facts, values and norms* (Vol. 15, No. 2, pp. 169–186). Birth Defects: Original Article Series. New York, NY: Alan R. Liss.

LeRoy, B. S., McCarthy Veach, P., & Bartels, D. M. (2010). *Genetic counseling practice.* Hoboken, NJ: Wiley.

Meiser, B., Irle, J., Lobb, E., & Barlow-Stewart, K. (2008). Assessment of the content and process of genetic counseling: A critical review of empirical studies. *Journal of Genetic Counseling, 17*(5), 434–451.

Pangalos, C., Hagnefelt, B., Lilakos, K., & Konialis, C. (2016). First applications of a targeted exome sequencing approach in fetuses with ultrasound abnormalities reveals an important fraction of cases with associated gene defects. *PeerJ.* doi:10.7717/peerj.1955

Richards, S., Aziz, N., & Bale, S. (2015). Standards and guidelines for the interpretation of sequence variants: A joint consensus recommendation of the American College of Medical Genetics and Genomics and the Association for Molecular Pathology. *Genetics in Medicine, 17*(5), 405–424.

Roche, M. I., & Berg J. S. (2015). Incidental findings with genomic testing: Implications for genetic counseling practice. *Current Genetic Medicine Reports, 3*, 166–176.

Runge, M. S., Patterson, C., & McKusick, V. A. (2006). *Principles of molecular medicine* (2nd ed., p. 46). Totowa, NJ: Human Press.

Schaffer, L. G., Dabell, M. P., Fisher A. J., Coppinger, J., Bandholz, A. M., Ellison, J. W., . . . Rosenfeld, J. A. (2012). Experience with microarray-based comparative genomic hybridization for prenatal diagnosis in over 5,000 pregnancies. *Prenatal Diagnosis, 32*(10), 976–985.

Skirton, H., Cordier, C., Ingvoldstad, C., Taris, N., & Benjamin, C. (2015). The role of the genetic counsellor: A systematic review of research evidence. *European Journal of Human Genetics, 23*(4), 452–458.

Uhlmann, W. R., Schuette, J. L., & Yashar, B. (2009). *A guide to genetic counseling.* Hoboken, NJ: Wiley.

< Describe the etiology and various forms of Alzheimer's disease.
< Detail symptoms associated with Alzheimer's disease.
< Describe the etiology and symptoms of Huntington's disease.
< Review current treatment recommendations for both degenerative diseases.

KEY TERMS

Allele
Chorea

Dyskinesia
Huntingtin

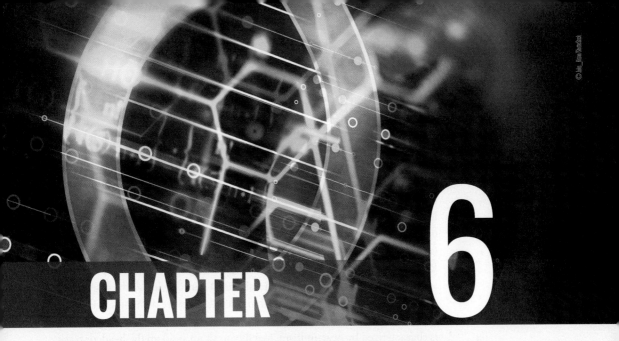

CHAPTER 6

Neurodegenerative Diseases

Alzheimer's Disease

Dementia is a brain disorder that seriously affects a person's ability to perform daily activities. The most common form of dementia in older people is Alzheimer's disease (AD), which involves progressive mental deterioration manifested by memory loss, inability to calculate, loss of visual–spatial orientation, confusion, and disorientation. The disease usually begins after age 60, and the risk increases with age; AD typically results in death within 5–10 years.

People affected by AD have a loss of cholinergic neurons in certain brain areas and exhibit the formation of beta-amyloid plaques and neurofibrillary tangles in these neurons. Science has been unable to determine the exact roles of the plaques and tangles relative to the disease—only that patients with AD develop far more of them. The brain is also atrophic. Both of these effects are believed to block the normal communication between nerve cells.

AD accounts for approximately 65% of dementia cases in the United States, with the rest primarily attributable to vascular dementia. It is officially listed as the sixth leading cause of death in the United States in 2016. Risk factors for AD include greater age, family history, lower education level, and female gender. Some measures that may slow down the progression of the disease include nonsteroidal anti-inflammatory drugs, HMG-CoA reductase inhibitors (statins), moderate ethanol intake, and strong social support. Unfortunately, there is no cure for this devastating disease; it gets worse over time and is inevitably fatal. It has been predicted that AD will become a public health crisis of the 21st century as baby boomers grow older. The total number of people with this disease in the United States will explode, from an estimated 5.4 million in 2016 to as many as 11–16 million by 2050. It is further estimated that by 2050, someone in the United States will develop the disease every 33 seconds (www.alz.org).

Diagnostic Clues

Progressive impairment of intellectual function, including short-term memory loss and one or more deficits in at least one other area (such as aphasia, apraxia, agnosia, or a disturbance in executive functioning) is a common clinical feature of AD. It is important to note that AD typically presents with early problems in memory and visuospatial abilities (e.g., becoming lost in familiar surroundings, inability to copy a geometric design on paper), but that changes have been occurring in the brain at the microscopic level well before memory loss is noted (www.alz.org). Social graces may be retained despite advanced cognitive decline. Personality changes and behavioral difficulties (e.g., wandering, inappropriate sexual behavior, agitation, and aggressiveness) may develop as the disease progresses. Hallucinations may occur in moderate to severe dementia. It is important to note that delirium is not usually associated with AD. End-stage disease is characterized by near-mutism; inability to sit up, hold up the head, or track objects with the eyes; difficulty with eating and swallowing; weight loss; bowel or bladder incontinence; and recurrent respiratory or urinary tract infections.

Genetic Progress

Because of the prevalence of AD, AD research is at an all-time high. It has been estimated that 90% of all research findings relative to AD have occurred within the last 15 years. Research has shown that those persons who have a parent, brother or sister, or child with AD are more likely to develop AD. These observations support the involvement of genetics and/or environment as factors influencing the development of AD. In fact, several different genes appear to predispose persons to development of AD when they are mutated.

Two forms of Alzheimer's genes have been identified. In *familial Alzheimer's disease*, many family members in multiple generations are affected. This type of AD is also referred to as "early onset" because symptoms start before age 65 and are caused by mutations on chromosomes 1, 14, or 21. All these genes influence production of beta-amyloid, a sticky protein fragment that clumps together in the brain. Fortunately, mutations in these genes are rare and account for less than 5% of all AD cases. Because all children have a 50% chance of developing early-onset AD if one of their parents had it, the inheritance pattern is autosomal dominant.

The second form of AD is late-onset or sporadic AD; this variation, which accounts for the majority of cases, usually develops after age 65. Even though a specific gene has not been identified as a specific cause of this form of the disease, one gene appears to influence the risk of developing the disease. The *apolipoprotein E (APOE)* gene found on chromosome 19 is involved in making a protein that helps carry cholesterol in the bloodstream; this protein may also be involved in determining the structure and function of the fatty membrane surrounding a brain cell.

Although the *APOE* gene has several different forms (**alleles**), three occur most frequently: *APOE e2*, *APOE e3*, and *APOE e4*. People inherit one *APOE* allele from each parent. The presence of one or two copies of *e4* increases AD risk in an individual. Although having this allele is a risk factor, it does not mean that AD will always develop. Some people with two copies of *e4* do not develop clinical signs of AD, whereas others with no *e4*s do. Between 35 and 50% of people with AD have at least one copy of *APOE e4*. These results suggest that other currently unidentified genes are also involved in the propensity to develop AD, as well as environmental factors.

Diagnostic Testing

Even though individuals who carry the *APOE e4* allele are at increased risk of developing late-onset AD, *APOE* testing is not recommended because there is no way to tell whether a person with this allele will definitely develop the disease. The only definitive way to diagnose AD is to microscopically examine brain tissue (from a postmortem autopsy) to determine if there are plaques and tangles present. Clinical evaluation should include a family history, medical history, laboratory tests, mini-mental status exam, and neuro-imaging. If no other cause for the dementia is identified, a person is said to have "probable" or "possible" AD.

Treatment

In recognition of the loss of cholinergic neurons associated with this disease (i.e., loss of the neurotransmitter acetylcholine), acetylcholinesterase inhibitors (donepezil, galantamine, rivastigmine) have been used to treat patients with mild to moderate AD. These drugs increase the amount of acetylcholine available in the brain by blocking its destruction by acetylcholinesterase in synaptic spaces. These medications have been shown to produce modest improvements in cognitive function.

Patients with moderate to severe disease have shown benefit from the use of memantine, which is an *N*-methyl-D-aspartase (NMDA) receptor antagonist. It is believed that too much of the neurotransmitter glutamate in the brain can lead to nerve degeneration and contribute to AD. Memantine blocks the glutamate receptor (NMDA), thereby decreasing the excess stimulatory effect of glutamate. Its use has produced moderate improvement in cognitive function when compared with baseline. In addition, memantine can be combined with use of an acetylcholinesterase inhibitor in one treatment (e.g., memantine + donepezil).

Huntington's Disease

Huntington's disease (HD; also known as Huntington's chorea) is a fatal, progressive neuro-degenerative disease that impacts the nerve cells in the brain and is not reversible. This autosomal dominant disorder is characterized by involuntary movements of all parts of the body, deterioration of cognitive

KEY TERMS

Chorea: from the Greek word for "dance"; the incessant, quick, jerky, involuntary movements that are characteristic of Huntington's disease.

Huntingtin: the product of the Huntington's disease gene on chromosome 4.

function, and, often, severe emotional disturbance. As in other autosomal dominant disorders, if one parent has HD, each offspring has a 50% chance of developing the disease. Similar to the relationship between AD and plaque, HD involves microscopic deposits of amyloid-related protein in the basal ganglia. The name **chorea** refers to "ceaseless rapid complex body movements that look well-coordinated and purposeful but are, in fact, involuntary" ("Chorea," 2017). The period of time from the onset of symptoms to death averages 15 years.

Genetics

This disorder primarily affects Caucasian people of northwestern European ancestry. The HD gene on chromosome 4 codes for a novel protein termed **Huntingtin**; the mutation in HD consists of an expanded and unstable trinucleotide (CAG) repeat. In most autosomal dominant diseases, heterozygotes tend to be less severely affected than homozygotes. However, HD is an exception and appears to be the only human disorder of complete dominance (**Figure 6-1**). Most cases are inherited, but some new cases occur as spontaneous mutations.

The genetic injury remains latent for three to five decades, after which it manifests itself in the form of progressive neuronal dysfunction. The sex of the affected parent exerts a strong influence on the expression of HD. Specifically, inheritance of the HD allele from an affected father results in clinical disease three years earlier than inheritance of the allele from an affected mother. Furthermore, children with juvenile-onset HD have almost always inherited the mutated gene from the father. It is thought that a process that differentially labels maternal and paternal chromosomes (genomic imprinting) plays a role in this early expression.

FIGURE 6-1   Pedigree of a human family showing the inheritance of the dominant gene for Huntington's disease. Females and males are represented by circles and squares. Shaded symbols indicate people affected with the disease.

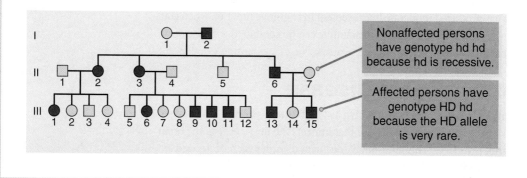

Nonaffected persons have genotype hd hd because hd is recessive.

Affected persons have genotype HD hd because the HD allele is very rare.

Diagnostic Clues

Initial symptoms may consist of either abnormal movements or intellectual changes, but eventually both of these will occur. Onset of symptoms usually occurs between 30 and 50 years of age. The earliest mental changes are often behavioral (i.e., irritability, moodiness, antisocial behavior, or psychiatric disturbance), followed by subsequent dementia. The **dyskinesia** initially may be no more than restlessness, but eventually choreiform movements and dystonic posturing occur. "Progressive rigidity and akinesia (rather than chorea) sometimes occur in association with dementia, particularly in cases of childhood onset" (Aminoff, 2007). **Table 6-1** summarizes the early and late signs and symptoms associated with HD.

> **KEY TERM**
>
> **Dyskinesia:** difficulty in performing voluntary movements.

Diagnostic Testing

Clinical evaluation should include a thorough family history and medical history. In established cases of HD, computerized tomography scanning usually demonstrates cerebral atrophy and atrophy of the caudate nucleus. Magnetic resonance imaging and positron emission tomography have shown reduced glucose utilization in an anatomically normal caudate nucleus. Offspring of known HD-affected parents should be offered genetic counseling. Genetic testing provides for presymptomatic detection and definitive diagnosis of the disease.

Treatment

Unfortunately, there is no cure for HD, and disease progression cannot be halted. Treatment is offered purely for symptomatic relief and is aimed at

TABLE 6-1	Physical Signs and Symptoms Associated with Huntington's Disease

Early	Late
Personality changes	Sudden jerky, involuntary movements throughout body
Decreased cognitive abilities	
Mild balance problems	Wide, prancing gait
Clumsiness	Severe balance and coordination problems
Involuntary facial movements	Unable to shift gaze without moving head Hesitant, halting, or slurred speech Difficulty swallowing or unable to swallow Dementia

Data from Huntington's Disease Symptoms. MayoClinic.com website. Available at http://www.mayo clinic.com/health/huntingtons-disease/DS00401/DSECTION=symptoms. Accessed January 24, 2017.

known biochemical changes that suggest underactivity of neurons that contain gamma-aminobutyric acid (GABA) and acetylcholine or a relative overactivity of dopaminergic neurons. Drugs that block dopamine receptors, such as phenothiazines or haloperidol, may control dyskinesia and any behavioral disturbances. However, a common side effect is sedation, and in some cases, these medications may cause additional stiffness and rigidity. Attempts to compensate for the relative GABA deficiency by enhancing central GABA activity or to compensate for the relative cholinergic underactivity by giving choline chloride have not proved therapeutic.

Because speech can be impaired and affect the ability to express complex thoughts, speech therapy may be beneficial for patients with symptomatic HD. Physical therapy can keep muscles stronger and more flexible, which helps the patient maintain balance and may lessen the risk of falling. Occupational therapy can help make the home safer and provide strategies for coping with memory and concentration problems. Furthermore, later in the course of the disease, occupational therapy can assist with eating, dressing, and hygiene challenges.

Chapter Summary

» The most common form of dementia in older people is Alzheimer's disease, which involves progressive mental deterioration manifested by memory loss, an inability to calculate, loss of visual–spatial orientation, confusion, and disorientation.

» Alzheimer's disease typically presents with early problems in memory and visuospatial abilities.

» The majority of Alzheimer's disease cases are late onset or sporadic, usually developing after age 65.

» Acetylcholinesterase inhibitors have been used to treat patients with mild to moderate Alzheimer's disease.

» Huntington's disease is an autosomal dominant disorder characterized by involuntary movements of all parts of the body, deterioration of cognitive function, and, often, severe emotional disturbance.

» There is no cure for Huntington's disease, and disease progression cannot be halted.

Chapter Review Questions

1. Alzheimer's disease accounts for approximately 65% of dementia cases in the United States, with the rest primarily attributable to _____.

2. Early problems associated with Alzheimer's disease typically include _____ and _____.

3. The majority of Alzheimer's disease is _____, as it usually develops after age 65.

4. The Huntington's disease gene on chromosome 4 codes for a novel protein called _____.

5. The earliest mental changes associated with Huntington's disease are often behavioral, followed by subsequent _____.

Bibliography

Aminoff, M. J. (2007). Nervous system. In S. J. McPhee, M. A. Papadakis, & L. M. Tierney, Jr. (Eds.), *Current medical diagnosis and treatment* (46th ed., pp. 998–1062). New York, NY: McGraw-Hill.

Bird, T. D. (2008). Alzheimer disease overview. *GeneReviews*. Retrieved from https://www.ncbi.nlm.nih.gov/books/NBK1161/

Chorea. (2017). *MedicineNet*. Retrieved from http://www.medterms.com/script/main/art.asp?articlekey=10029

Couturié, B. (Director & Producer), & Sandkuhler, A. (Producer). (2009).*The Alzheimer's Project* [Television documentary]. United States: HBO Documentaries. Retrieved from http://www.hbo.com/alzheimers/index.html

Germann, W. J., & Stanfield, C. L. (2005). *Principles of human physiology* (2nd ed.). New York, NY: Pearson/Benjamin Cummings.

Hartl, D. L., & Jones, E. W. (2005). *Genetics: Analysis of genes and genomes* (6th ed.). Sudbury, MA: Jones and Bartlett Publishers.

Hartl, D. L., & Jones, E. W. (2006). *Essential genetics: A genomic perspective* (4th ed.). Sudbury, MA: Jones and Bartlett Publishers.

Hughes, M. D. (2006). Multiple sclerosis, Alzheimer's disease, and dementia. *Audio-Digest Family Practice, 54*(16).

Huntington's disease. (n.d.). *MayoClinic.org*. Retrieved from http://www.mayoclinic.com/health/huntingtons-disease/DS00401

Huntington's Disease Society of America. (n.d.). http://www.hdsa.org/

Johnston, C. B., Covinsky, K. E., & Landefeld, C. S. (2005). Geriatric medicine. In L. M. Tierney, S. J. McPhee, & M. A. Papadakis (Eds.), *Current medical diagnosis and treatment* (44th ed., pp. 1238–1240). New York, NY: McGraw-Hill.

McConnell, T. H. (2007). *The nature of disease: Pathology for the health professions* (p. 639). Baltimore, MD: Lippincott Williams & Wilkins.

Memantine. (n.d.). *MedicineNet.com*. Retrieved from http://www.medicinenet.com/memantine/article.htm

Rubin E. (2001). *Essential pathology* (3rd ed.). Baltimore, MD: Lippincott Williams & Wilkins.

U.S. National Institutes of Health, National Institute on Aging, Alzheimer's Disease Education and Resource Center. (n.d.). *Alzheimer's disease and related dementias*. Retrieved from http://www.nia.nih.gov/alzheimers

‹ Describe the genes involved in hereditary breast and ovarian cancer.
‹ Identify risks associated with mutations in breast cancer genes.
‹ Detail the impacts of the founder effect and penetrance.
‹ Discuss management options for patients at risk for or affected by hereditary breast and/or ovarian cancer.

KEY TERMS

BRCA1
BRCA2
Cowden syndrome
Founder effect
Germline mutation

Kindred
Li-Fraumeni syndrome (LFS)
Peutz-Jeghers syndrome (PJS)

PTEN hamartoma tumor syndrome (PHTS)
Tumor suppressor gene
Tumorigenesis

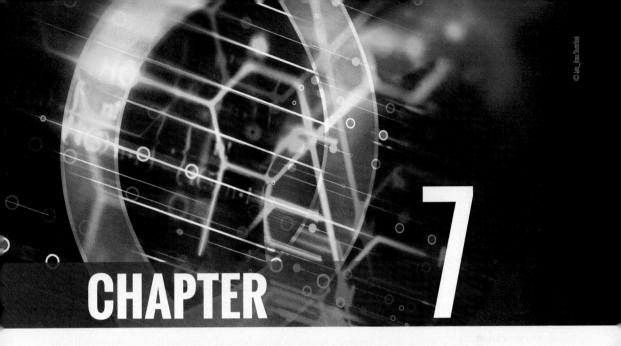

CHAPTER 7

Hereditary Breast and Ovarian Cancer Syndrome

According to the American Cancer Society, cancer is the second most common cause of death in the United States and accounts for nearly 1 of every 4 deaths. Although genetics certainly plays a role in many different cancers, it is known that most cancer is not inherited. Rather, it is the *predisposition* to cancer that is inherited. Of the women with breast cancer, about 10–20% have one or more first-degree relatives who have been affected by breast cancer, and about 5–10% of all breast cancers are attributable to a hereditary form.

The lifetime risk for a woman developing breast cancer is about 12% (1 in 8), while the lifetime risk of developing ovarian cancer is a little more than 1% (1 in 75). The lifetime risk for males to develop breast cancer is less than 1%. Epidemiological studies have established the role of family history as an important risk factor for both breast and ovarian cancer. Besides gender and age, a positive family history of breast cancer continues to be one of the strongest known predictive risk factors for the development of breast cancer.

Major phenotypic features of hereditary breast and ovarian cancer syndrome include early age (often before age 50) of breast cancer onset, triple-negative (estrogen receptor negative, progesterone receptor negative, and human epidermal growth factor receptor 2 negative) breast cancer at or before age 60, family history of both breast and ovarian cancer, increased chance of multiple primary cancers (i.e., bilateral tumors), or development of both breast cancer and ovarian cancer in the same individual. Other diagnostic clues include an autosomal dominant pattern of inheritance, which means a vertical transmission of cancer through either the maternal or paternal side of the family. An increased incidence of tumors in other specific organs, such as the ovary, prostate, or pancreas, in family members is also consistent with this syndrome. Other factors that increase the likelihood of hereditary breast and ovarian syndrome are a family history of male breast cancer and Ashkenazi Jewish ancestry.

KEY TERMS

Kindred: an aggregate of genetically related persons.

BRCA1: a tumor suppressor gene on chromosome 17 that prevents cells with damaged DNA from dividing. Carriers of germline mutations in *BRCA1* are predisposed to develop both breast and ovarian cancer.

BRCA2: a tumor suppressor gene on chromosome 13. Carriers of germline mutations in *BRCA2* have an increased risk, similar to that of carriers of *BRCA1* mutations, of developing breast cancer and a moderately increased risk of ovarian cancer. *BRCA2* families also exhibit an increased incidence of male breast, pancreatic, prostate, stomach, skin, and uterine cancer.

Tumor suppressor gene: a gene whose function is to suppress cellular proliferation. Loss of a tumor suppressor gene through chromosomal aberration leads to heightened susceptibility to neoplasia.

Breast Cancer Genes

The study of large **kindreds** with multiple individuals affected with breast cancer led to the identification of two major cancer susceptibility genes. In 1990, the first gene associated with breast cancer was identified on chromosome 17. This gene was named "breast cancer 1," or **BRCA1**. Mutations in this gene are transmitted through an autosomal dominant pattern in a family. The *BRCA1* gene was found to encode for a protein that contained 1,863 amino acids. Even after this significant finding, it was soon apparent that not all families with hereditary breast cancer possessed the *BRCA1* gene. In 1994, another gene (**BRCA2**) was identified on chromosome 13 that encoded a protein consisting of 3,418 amino acids. Mutations in this gene are also transmitted in an autosomal dominant familial pattern and are associated with male breast cancer, ovarian cancer, prostate cancer, and pancreatic cancer. Other genes that have been found to be associated with hereditary susceptibility to breast cancer include *TP53*, *PTEN*, and *STK11*. In addition, *MLH1*, *MSH2*, *MSH6*, and *PMS2* are all mismatch repair genes that have been found to be associated with increased risk of ovarian cancer.

Both *BRCA1* and *BRCA2* are **tumor suppressor genes**, which normally control cell growth and cell death. In addition, both genes are involved in other important cell functions, including DNA repair, genomic stability, transcriptional regulation, and cell cycle control. Each individual has two *BRCA1* genes (one on each chromosome 17) and two *BRCA2* genes (one on each chromosome 13). When a person has one altered or mutated copy of either *BRCA1* or *BRCA2*, his or her risk for various types of cancer increases (**Table 7-1**).

Before cancer will develop in a person, both copies of a tumor suppressor gene (i.e., *BRCA*) must be mutated. For example, in the case of hereditary breast and ovarian cancer syndrome, the first mutation is inherited from either the mother or the father and is present in all body cells. This is called a **germline mutation**. Whether a person with a germline mutation develops cancer and where the cancer appears will depend on where the second mutation occurs. If the second mutation is in the ovary, then ovarian cancer may develop. If it manifests in the breast, then breast cancer may develop.

Even though mutations in tumor suppressor genes are known to increase the risk of developing cancer, tumor development requires mutations in multiple growth control genes to become manifest. Loss of both copies of *BRCA1* or *BRCA2* is just the first step in the overall process of **tumorigenesis**. The causes of these additional mutations are unknown. It has been suggested that chemical, physical, or biological environmental exposures or chance errors in cell replication may be involved.

In addition, even though an individual may have inherited a germline *BRCA1* or *BRCA2* mutation, that person may never develop cancer because

TABLE 7-1	Risks Associated with Either a *BRCA1* or *BRCA2* Mutation
***BRCA1* Mutation**	***BRCA2* Mutation**
Lifetime risk for breast cancer (females): 55–70%	Lifetime risk for breast cancer (females): 45–70%
Lifetime risk of breast cancer (males): 1%	Lifetime risk for breast cancer (males): 8%
Lifetime risk for ovarian cancer: approximately 40%	Lifetime risk for ovarian cancer: approximately 50%
Lifetime risk for contralateral (opposite) breast cancer: up to 63%	Lifetime risk of pancreatic cancer: 5%
Increased risk for other cancer types (i.e., prostate)	Increased risk for other cancer types (i.e., prostate, stomach, melanoma, and uterine serous carcinoma)

Data from Peshkins, B. N., & Isaacs, C. (2017). BRCA1 and BRCA2-associated hereditary breast and ovarian cancer. In T. W. Post (Ed.), *UpToDate*. Retrieved from http://www.uptodate.com/

he or she may never get the second mutation that knocks out the function of the gene and starts the process of tumor formation. This phenomenon can make it appear that the cancer has "skipped" a generation within a family, when, in reality, the mutation is present. Regardless of whether they develop cancer, individuals with a mutation have a 50:50 chance of passing the mutation on to the next generation.

Approximately 2,000 distinct mutations and sequence variations in *BRCA1* and *BRCA2* have been described. Complete analysis of *BRCA1* and *BRCA2* is commercially available, and this type of testing is most desirable because it can exclude both known and novel *BRCA1* and *BRCA2* gene mutations. Another testing option available is targeted mutational analysis, which can be used for patients who have a relative who has tested positive for a deleterious *BRCA1* or *BRCA2* gene mutation. Current routine analysis of *BRCA* genes assesses large genomic rearrangements, which account for 6% of all deleterious *BRCA1* and *BRCA2* gene mutations. It was not until after 2006 that these large genomic rearrangements were analyzed on a regular basis. Another *BRCA* testing option is next-generation sequencing panels. The testing for *BRCA* gene mutations was added to these next-generation sequencing panels after the *BRCA* patent was invalidated by the Supreme Court in 2013. According to UpToDate, multigene testing in the clinical setting has shown that about 5–10% of women have a *BRCA1* or *BRCA2* gene mutation, and about

KEY TERMS

Germline mutation: a change in a gene in the body's reproductive cell (egg or sperm) that becomes incorporated into the DNA of every cell in the body of the offspring.

Tumorigenesis: production of a new growth or growths.

4–7% have a harmful mutation in another gene that predisposes them to breast and/or ovarian cancer. Unfortunately, 10–15% of all individuals undergoing full sequencing of *BRCA1* and *BRCA2* will not show a known deleterious gene mutation but may show a gene mutation of unknown significance.

Founder Effect

Among those affected with *BRCA1* or *BRCA2* mutations, most families express mutations specific to that family. Mutations in such families that recur for generation after generation have been studied in families of Ashkenazi Jewish heritage as well as in families originating from the Netherlands, Hungary, Iceland, Sweden, Italy, France, South Africa, Pakistan, and Asia, and in French Canadians, Hispanics, and African Americans. This pattern represents the **founder effect**. Three mutations account for the majority of the *BRCA* mutations in individuals of Ashkenazi Jewish ancestry (**Table 7-2**). These three mutations are thought to occur at an increased rate because of a combination of founder effect and genetic drift. In other words, these mutations are assumed to have originated in a common ancestor shared by many Ashkenazi Jews. Founder effect mutations for *BRCA1* and *BRCA2* are also seen in Icelandic, French Canadian, U.S. Hispanic, and Black American populations. Based on this information, some laboratories offer "ethnic-specific" mutation genetic testing panels. Such tests look for specific mutations based on the ethnicity of a patient rather than searching through the entire gene sequence.

In the general population, it has been estimated that 1 in 400–800 individuals has a *BRCA1* or *BRCA2* mutation. In contrast, because of the founder

TABLE 7-2	Mutations Associated with Breast and Ovarian Cancer in the Ashkenazi Jewish Population	
Mutation	**Gene**	**Carrier Frequency in Ashkenazi Jewish Population**
185delAG	*BRCA1*	1.0%
5382insC	*BRCA1*	0.13%
6174delT	*BRCA2*	1.52%

Data from *BRCA1* and *BRCA2*. AmbryGenetics. Aliso Viejo, CA, 2017. Retrieved from http://www.ambrygen.com/tests/brca1-and-brca2

effect, 1 in 40 Ashkenazi individuals has one of the recurring mutations. Obviously, this knowledge has important implications in terms of assessing family history for breast and ovarian cancer in Ashkenazi versus non-Ashkenazi individuals.

Penetrance

Penetrance is defined as the probability of developing disease in a carrier of a deleterious mutation; it is usually defined in terms of a given age (e.g., to age 70). In general, individuals with rare genetic mutations have a higher penetrance, whereas individuals with a common genetic mutation have a lower penetrance. To estimate risk, penetrance of certain mutations must be understood. Modifiers are also affected by penetrance.

Thus, the relative risk of developing a major disorder is calculated by comparison of the incidence of a condition associated with a specific gene mutation among carriers of that mutation in relationship to the incidence among noncarriers of the mutation. The risk of cancer among individuals who carry a mutation in *BRCA1* or *BRCA2* may be modified by a second gene or by an environmental factor. Examples of these environmental factors include exposure to carcinogens (i.e., tobacco) and hormonal factors. For modifying factors, the relative risk is the penetrance of the disease among individuals with the modifying factor compared with the penetrance of the disease among those without the modifying factor. According to the National Cancer Institute, estimates of penetrance by age 70 years for *BRCA1* were 55–65% and *BRCA2* were 45–47% for breast cancer, while the estimates of penetrance by age 70 for *BRCA1* were 39% and *BRCA2* were 11–17% for ovarian cancer.

Other Syndromes Associated with Breast and Ovarian Cancer

Li-Fraumeni syndrome (LFS) is a rare syndrome associated with a germline mutation of the tumor suppressor tumor protein gene *TP53* on chromosome 17. It is characterized by premenopausal breast cancer in combination with childhood sarcoma, brain tumors, leukemia, and adrenocortical carcinoma. Tumors in families who carry the Li-Fraumeni syndrome mutation tend to occur in childhood and early adulthood and often present as multiple primary tumors in the same individual. The average age of onset of breast cancer is under 35 years in families with this mutation. A *TP53* mutation is thought to account for less than 1% of all breast cancer cases, but the lifetime risk of developing breast cancer in patients harboring this mutation by 60 years old is almost 50%.

KEY TERMS

Li-Fraumeni syndrome (LFS): caused by a mutation in the *TP53* gene (a tumor suppressor gene), this syndrome is associated with an increased risk for breast cancer, osteosarcoma, and soft tissue sarcomas, as well as leukemias and adrenal carcinoma.

Cowden syndrome: caused by mutations in the *PTEN* gene (a tumor suppressor gene), this syndrome is associated with noncancerous growths known as hamartomas and malignancies such as breast, thyroid, colorectal, kidney, and endometrial cancer.

***PTEN* hamartoma tumor syndrome (PHTS)** includes **Cowden syndrome** and Bannayan-Riley-Ruvalcaba syndrome, with Cowden syndrome being the predominant disorder. This syndrome is associated with germline mutations in the phosphatase and tensin homolog (*PTEN*) tumor suppressor gene on chromosome 10. Cowden syndrome is characterized by multiple hamartomas, trichilemmomas, oral fibromas, punctate palmoplantar keratoses, as well as an excess of breast cancer, colorectal malignancies, endometrial cancer, malignant thyroid disease, and kidney cancer. Lifetime estimates for breast cancer among women with this syndrome range between 25% and 50%. Onset of breast cancer is often at a young age, with a mean diagnosis between 38 and 46 years of age. Also, women with this syndrome have an increased incidence of multifocal and bilateral breast cancer. In addition, it is very common for women with Cowden syndrome to manifest benign breast disorders as well.

Peutz-Jeghers syndrome (PJS) is characterized by melanocytic macules on the lips, perioral, and buccal regions, along with multiple gastrointestinal polyps, specifically hamartomatous polyps. This rare syndrome is associated with a germline mutation in the tumor suppressor gene serine/threonine kinase 11 (*STK11*) on chromosome 19. The gastrointestinal tract is commonly affected, with a cumulative incidence of gastrointestinal cancer by age 70. According to UpToDate, the absolute risk of breast cancer is almost 55%. In this syndrome, breast cancer is also diagnosed at a younger age, with a mean age of diagnosis at 37 years. One study showed a 21% prevalence of ovarian cancer in PJS, and this was also diagnosed at an early age.

Hereditary diffuse gastric cancer syndrome (HDGC) is characterized by highly invasive gastric cancer. It is associated with a germline mutation in the cadherin-1 (*CDH1*) gene. This syndrome can present with lobular breast cancer in women. The cumulative lifetime risk of breast cancer in these patients can be as high as 60%.

Lynch syndrome, also called hereditary nonpolyposis colon cancer, is associated with primary cancers of the colon, endometrium, ovaries, and stomach. It is associated with mutations in mismatch repair genes (*MSH2*, *MLH1*, *MSH6*, and *PMS2*) and a mutation in the epithelial cell adhesion molecule (*EPCAM*) gene. *MSH2* and *MLH1* gene mutations have a lifetime risk of ovarian cancer of 4–12%.

Management Options

Patients who do not have a personal history of breast cancer and have also been identified as having the *BRCA* gene mutation are principally managed by breast and ovarian cancer risk-reducing recommendations. For instance, the primary risk-reducing recommendation for these patients is a bilateral salpingo-oophorectomy between the ages of 35 and 40, or once childbearing is complete. This has been shown to significantly decrease the risk of ovarian cancer in this population. Other recommendations include intensive breast cancer screening for these patients, as well as consideration of hormonal and surgical forms of risk reduction, such as bilateral mastectomy. For patients who do not wish to pursue surgical recommendations or would rather delay these recommendations, strict breast cancer and ovarian cancer surveillance should be offered. For men, screening for breast and prostate cancers is recommended.

It is important to note that women with *BRCA* gene mutations who have a personal history of breast cancer also have an increased risk of a new primary breast cancer in the ipsilateral breast and an increased risk of a new contralateral breast cancer. Because of this concern, an ipsilateral mastectomy, a contralateral prophylactic mastectomy, and a prophylactic bilateral salpingo-oophorectomy in premenopausal patients can be recommended to reduce this risk. Moreover, patients who complete adjuvant therapy with tamoxifen or an aromatase inhibitor also decrease their risk of contralateral breast cancer. In contrast, prophylactic bilateral mastectomies are not recommended in patients who are diagnosed with ovarian cancer and have *BRCA* gene mutations because of their high mortality rate at five years postdiagnosis. Instead, prophylactic bilateral mastectomies are recommended at least five years after their ovarian cancer diagnosis.

Breast Cancer Screening

For women with *BRCA* mutations who have not undergone breast risk-reducing surgery, experts recommend self-breast exams performed periodically beginning at age 18 and clinical breast exams every 6–12 months beginning at age 25. Most important, in this population of patients, MRI for breast cancer screening is recommended annually beginning at age 25. The experts also recommend to begin mammography at age 30 or earlier if the age of onset of breast cancer in the family is under 25 years. The MRI of the breast can be scheduled 6 months after the mammogram so that the patient will have some form of breast imaging every 6 months. It is important for mammograms and breast MRIs to be done at a consistent location if possible, or at least to have prior studies to be used for comparison in interpreting new studies.

Because *BRCA1* and *BRCA2* proteins are known to play a role in repairing DNA damage (including radiation damage), it has been suggested that BRCA mutation carriers may be more susceptible to radiation-induced breast cancer compared with women without mutations. However, growing evidence suggests that the effect depends on age during exposure and total dose of radiation exposure. More research is needed to confirm these findings, and the current recommendations still include both mammography and MRI, rather than MRI alone, for breast surveillance.

and symptoms associated with Proteus syndrome, but who do not meet the diagnostic criteria. PTEN hamartoma tumor syndrome is caused by changes (mutations) in the PTEN gene and is inherited in an autosomal dominant manner. Treatment is based on the signs and symptoms present in each person.

Peutz-Jeghers syndrome (PJS): caused by a mutation in the *STK11* gene (a tumor suppressor gene), this syndrome is associated with growths of hamartomas in the stomach and intestine, dark freckling in the axilla, perioral area, and buccal mucosa, and an increased risk for developing pancreatic, gastrointestinal, ovarian, and breast cancers.

Ovarian Cancer Screening

Current recommendations for women with a higher, inherited risk of ovarian cancer include concurrent transvaginal ultrasound and serum CA-125 levels every 6 months beginning at age 30, or 5 years before the earliest family member was diagnosed with ovarian cancer. This guideline is based on the observation that elevated serum CA-125 levels are associated with ovarian tumors. Unfortunately, neither of these screening techniques has been shown to detect ovarian cancer at an early and potentially more treatable stage. Therefore, prophylactic bilateral salpingo-oophorectomy is recommended between the ages of 35 and 40 years or on completion of childbearing as an effective risk-reduction option.

Male Screening

It is recommended that men perform monthly breast self-examinations beginning at age 35 and undergo clinical breast examinations every 12 months starting at age 35. For men with gynecomastia or parenchymal/glandular breast density, annual mammography can be considered. Men with *BRCA1* mutations should have a prostate screening starting at age 40, and men with *BRCA2* mutations should also consider prostate screening.

Chemoprevention

For patients who choose not to have prophylactic bilateral mastectomies, it is reasonable to offer tamoxifen, especially in patients with a *BRCA2* gene mutation. However, chemoprevention is not as effective as prophylactic mastectomies, so the option of prophylactic mastectomies should continue to be discussed with these patients periodically. Chemoprevention is not recommended for use in men.

Genetic Testing

Although genetic tests are available that can identify mutations in *BRCA1/BRCA2*, it is preferable to first test an individual who is affected by cancer before testing unaffected family members. This step is taken to determine whether a detectable *BRCA1* or *BRCA2* mutation is responsible for the breast and/or ovarian cancer within a family. If an unaffected family member is then tested for a known mutation, two results are possible: (1) positive: the individual is at increased risk to develop breast and ovarian cancer; or (2) negative: the individual is not at increased risk but still has the general population risk. Unfortunately, a negative result may also mean that a mutation is present that was not detected because of limitations of the test, or this individual may have a mutation in a different gene that predisposes the person to breast and/or ovarian cancer. In addition, the testing may have revealed a gene alteration, but its significance may not be clear because the gene alteration could be due to an undefined deleterious mutation, a benign polymorphism, or a variant with an intermediate risk of cancer. Clearly, in addition to benefits, there are limitations associated with genetic testing (**Table 7-3**).

There are specific criteria for identifying candidates for genetic counseling and possible testing for hereditary breast and ovarian cancer syndrome that have been developed by the National Comprehensive Cancer Network (NCCN), the American College of Medical Genetics and Genomics, and the National Society of Genetic Counselors. Some of these key criteria include individuals with breast cancer with a known mutation in the family of a gene that increases cancer susceptibility, breast cancer diagnosed ≤50 years, triple-negative breast cancer diagnosed ≤60 years, two or more primary breast cancers, or male sex. Additional criteria include breast cancer diagnosed at any age, in addition to one of the following: ≥1 close blood relative with breast cancer diagnosed ≤50 years; ≥1 close blood relative with ovarian, fallopian tube, or primary peritoneal cancer diagnosed at any age; or ≥2 close blood relatives with breast, pancreatic, and/or prostate cancer diagnosed at any age, or from a population at increased risk. A patient with a personal history of ovarian cancer or a patient of Ashkenazi Jewish descent with breast, ovarian, or pancreatic cancer diagnosed at any age also meets the criteria for genetic testing. Genetic risk evaluation and possible testing should also be done on individuals with no personal history of cancer but with a

TABLE 7-3	Benefits, Risks, and Limitations of *BRCA* Testing	
Benefits	**Limitations**	
Identifies high-risk individuals	Does not detect all mutations	
Identifies noncarriers in families with a known mutation	Continued risk of sporadic cancer	
Allows early detection and prevention strategies	May result in psychosocial and/or economic harm	
May relieve anxiety		

Data from Armstrong et al. (2000) and *BRCA Mutations: Cancer Risk and Genetic Testing.* National Cancer Institute. U.S. National Institutes of Health. Retrieved from http://www.cancer.gov/cancer topics/factsheet/risk/brca

close relative with either a known mutation within the family of a gene that increases susceptibility to cancer, ≥2 breast cancers in a single individual, ≥2 individuals with breast cancers on the same side of family with at least one diagnosed ≤50 years, ovarian cancer, or male breast cancer, or a first- or second-degree relative with breast cancer diagnosed ≤45 years.

Patients should undergo pretest counseling before genetic testing to provide a genetic risk assessment based on their personal and family history. It is also important to discuss options and implications that may be associated with genetic testing, as well as potential benefits, risks, and limitations of testing. The components of pretest counseling should include a pedigree evaluation, the use of risk assessment models, and a discussion of issues for patients who are considering testing, such as financial considerations and genetic discrimination. There are many breast cancer risk prediction models that can be used for assessing the probability that an individual carries a germline deleterious mutation of the *BRCA1* and *BRCA2* genes. For an example, BRCAPRO is a computerized risk prediction model with software available online that incorporates a total of six different predictive models for inherited or familial breast cancer. However, based on the time limitations associated with each patient encounter, it is unlikely that many primary care practitioners would use this type of software to identify appropriate candidates for genetic testing; instead, it is recommended they use the criteria developed by the NCCN. This type of software is more likely to be used by genetic counselors.

Chapter Summary

» After gender and age, a positive family history is the strongest known predictive risk factor for breast cancer.

» Two breast cancer genes—*BRCA1* and *BRCA2*—have been identified as playing roles in hereditary breast and ovarian cancer syndrome.

» Both *BRCA1* and *BRCA2* are tumor suppressor genes that normally control cell growth and cell death.

» Even though an individual may have inherited a germline *BRCA1* or *BRCA2* mutation, the person may never develop cancer because he or she may never get the second mutation that knocks out the function of the gene and starts the process of tumor formation.

Chapter Review Questions

1. After gender and age, what is the strongest known predictive risk factor for breast cancer? _____

2. Vertical transmission of a trait through either the maternal or paternal side of the family is indicative of which type of inheritance? _____

3. _____ is characterized by melanocytic macules on the lips and perioral and buccal regions, along with multiple gastrointestinal polyps.

4. The American Cancer Society recommends annual _____ screening, in addition to mammography for women at hereditary risk for breast cancer.

Bibliography

AmbryGenetics. (2017). *BRCA1 and BRCA2*. Aliso Viejo, CA: Author. Retrieved from http://www.ambrygen.com/tests/brca1-and-brca2

American Cancer Society. (2016). *Cancer facts & figures 2016*. Atlanta, GA: Author.

American Cancer Society. (2017, January 6). *What are the key statistics about ovarian cancer?* Retrieved from https://www.cancer.org/cancer/ovarian-cancer/about/key-statistics.html

American Society of Clinical Oncology. (2015). The genetics of cancer. Cancer.Net. Retrieved from http://www.cancer.net/navigating-cancer-care/cancer-basics/genetics/genetics-cancer

Armstrong, K., Calzone, K., Stopfer, J., Fitzgerald, G., Coyne, J., & Weber, B. (2000). Factors associated with decisions about clinical *BRCA1/2* testing. *Cancer Epidemiology, Biomarkers & Prevention, 9*(11), 1251–1254.

Banerjee, S. (2007). BRCA1 (breast cancer 1, early onset). *Atlas of genetics and cytogenetics in oncology and haematology*. Retrieved from http://atlasgeneticsoncology.org/Genes/BRCA1ID163ch17q21.html

BRCA2 gene. (2017). *Genetics home reference*. Bethesda, MD: U.S. National Library of Medicine. Retrieved from https://ghr.nlm.nih.gov/gene/BRCA2#sources forpage

Elmore, J. G. (2017). Screening for breast cancer: Strategies and recommendations. In T. W. Post (Ed.), *UpToDate*. Retrieved from http://uptodate.com/

Gradishar, W. J. (2017). Breast cancer in men. In T. W. Post (Ed.), *UpToDate*. Retrieved from http://www.uptodate.com

Katsnelson, A. (2010). Breast cancer protein is finally purified. *Nature.* Retrieved from http://www.nature.com/news/2010/100822/full/news.2010.422.html

Narod, S. A. (2001). Modifiers of risk of hereditary breast and ovarian cancer. *Nature Reviews, 2,* 113–123.

National Cancer Institute. (n.d.). *NCI dictionary of cancer terms.* Retrieved from http://www.cancer.gov/dictionary/

National Cancer Institute. (2015). *BRCA1 and BRCA2: Cancer risk and genetic testing.* Retrieved from https://www.cancer.gov/about-cancer/causes-prevention/genetics /brca-fact-sheet

National Cancer Institute. (2017). Genetics of Breast and Gynecologic Cancers (PDQ®) – Health Professional Version. Retrieved from https://www.cancer.gov /types/breast/hp/breast-ovarian-genetics-pdq#section/_88

National Cancer Institute. Genetics of Breast and Ovarian Cancer. https://www .cancer.net/cancer-types/hereditary-breast-and-ovarian-cancer/hereditary -breast-and-ovarian-cancer

NCCN Clinical Practice Guidelines in Oncology. (n.d.). Genetic/familial high-risk assessment: breast and ovarian [Version 2.2017]. Retrieved from https://www.nccn.org/

Peshkins, B. N., & Isaacs, C. (2017). BRCA1 and BRCA2-associated hereditary breast and ovarian cancer. In T. W. Post (Ed.), *UpToDate.* Retrieved from http://www.uptodate.com

Peshkins, B. N., & Isaacs, C. (2017). Genetic counseling and testing for hereditary breast and ovarian cancer. In T. W. Post (Ed.), *UpToDate.* Retrieved from http://www.uptodate.com

Peshkins, B. N., & Isaacs, C. (2017). Overview of hereditary breast and ovarian cancer syndromes. In T. W. Post (Ed.), *UpToDate.* Retrieved from http://www .uptodate.com

PTEN hamartoma tumor syndrome. (n.d.). Retrieved from https://rarediseases.info .nih.gov/diseases/12800/pten-hamartoma-tumor-syndrome

Risk of developing breast cancer. (2016, May 11). *Breastcancer.org.* Retrieved from http://www.breastcancer.org/symptoms/understand_bc/risk/understanding

Saslow, D., Boetes, C., Burke, W., Harms, S., Leach, M. O., Lehman, C. D., . . . American Cancer Society Breast Cancer Advisory Group. (2007). American Cancer Society guidelines for breast screening with MRI as an adjunct to mammography. *CA: A Cancer Journal for Clinicians, 57,* 75–89.

Stanich, P. P., & Lindor, N. M. (2017). *PTEN* hamartoma tumor syndrome, including Cowden syndrome. In T. W. Post (Ed.), *UpToDate.* Retrieved from http://www .uptodate.com

Westman, J. A. (2006). *Medical genetics for the modern clinician.* New York, NY: Lippincott Williams & Wilkins.

< Describe signs and symptoms associated with colorectal cancer.
< Identify colorectal cancer screening tests.
< Differentiate between sporadic and hereditary colorectal cancer.
< Detail genetic causes of familial adenomatous polyposis and hereditary nonpolyposis colorectal cancer.

KEY TERMS

Adenoma
Adenomatous
Adenomatous polyposis coli (APC)
Amsterdam criteria
Apoptosis
Colectomy
Deletion

Familial adenomatous polyposis (FAP)
First-degree relative
Frameshift mutation
Hereditary nonpolyposis colorectal cancer (HNPCC)
Insertion

Microsatellite instability
Nonsense mutation
Polyp
Proctocolectomy

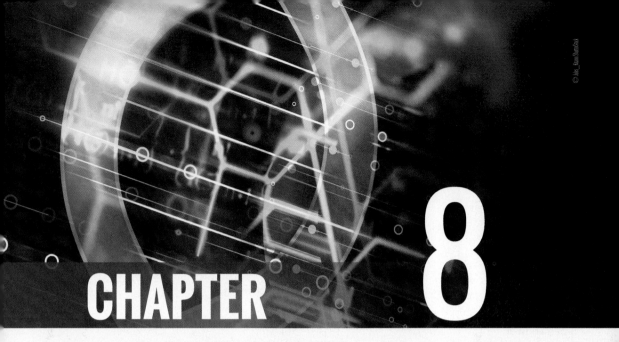

CHAPTER 8

Colorectal Cancer

Colorectal cancer—also called colon cancer or rectal cancer—refers to any cancer in the colon from the beginning (at the cecum) to the end (at the rectum). Colorectal cancer occurs when cells that line the colon or the rectum become abnormal and grow in an out-of-control manner. **Polyps** are usually benign growths that protrude from a mucous membrane in the colon and rectum. If left untreated, these **adenomatous** polyps may eventually evolve into cancer.

Like many cancers, colon cancer may occur sporadically in a population or in a familial pattern. In addition, numerous cancer syndromes involve cancer of the colon. Although the majority of colon cancers are sporadic and occur randomly, it is important to recognize familial or hereditary patterns early in individuals. Based on this knowledge, screening and management guidelines have been developed for both patients and their relatives. The primary goal of these guidelines is to prevent colorectal cancer and other complications associated with these diseases.

Many patients with colorectal cancer do not experience any symptoms until the disease is quite advanced. For this reason, it is important to take a good family history and to assess risk factors for all patients. The risk of colon cancer in a **first-degree relative** of an affected individual can increase an individual's lifetime risk of colon cancer anywhere from 2-fold to 4.3-fold. Signs and symptoms of colorectal cancer are listed in **Box 8-1**. Beginning at age 50, both men and women at average risk for developing colorectal cancer should take the American Cancer Society screening tests identified in **Table 8-1**.

KEY TERMS

Polyp: a usually nonmalignant growth or tumor protruding from the mucous lining of an organ such as the nose, bladder, or intestine, often causing obstruction.

Adenomatous: relating to an adenoma and to some types of glandular hyperplasia.

First-degree relative: any relative who is one meiosis away from a particular individual in a family (i.e., parent, sibling, offspring).

BOX 8-1 Signs and Symptoms Associated with Colorectal Cancer

Blood in the stool
Weight loss with no known reason
Diarrhea that is not the result of diet or illness
A long period of constipation
Crampy abdominal pain
Change in bowel habits
Persistent decrease in the size or caliber of stool
Frequent feeling of distention in the abdomen or bowel region
    (gas pain, bloating, fullness, with or without cramping)
Vomiting and continual lack of energy

Data from American Cancer Society. (2009, May). *Detailed guide: Colon and rectum cancer: How is colorectal cancer diagnosed?* Retrieved from https://www.cancer.org/; Mayo Clinic Staff. (2009, July). *Colon polyps: Symptoms.* Retrieved from http://www.mayoclinic.com/health/colon-polyps/DS00511/DSECTION=symptoms; Johns Hopkins Medicine. (2009). *Familial adenomatous polyposis: Introduction.* Retrieved from https://www.hopkinsmedicine.org/

TABLE 8-1 American Cancer Society Screening Tests

Tests That Find Polyps and Cancer	Tests That Mainly Find Cancer
Flexible sigmoidoscopy every 5 years*	FOBT every year*[†]
Colonoscopy every 10 years	FIT every year*[†]
Double-contrast barium enema every 5 years*	sDNA test, interval uncertain*
CT colonography (virtual colonoscopy) every 5 years*	

*Colonoscopy should be done if test results are positive.
[†]For FOBT or FIT used as a screening test, the take-home multiple sample method should be used. An FOBT or FIT done during a digital rectal exam is not adequate for screening.
CT: computerized tomography; FIT: fecal immunochemical test; FOBT: fecal occult blood test; sDNA: stool DNA test.
Data from American Cancer Society. (2018). *Colorectal Cancer Screening: What Are My Options.* https://www.cancer.org/latest-news/understanding-tests-that-screen-for-colon-cancer.html

Familial Colorectal Cancer

The occurrence of colorectal cancer in more than one family member may be due to chance alone, or it may result from shared exposure to a cancer-causing substance (carcinogen) in the environment or from similar diet or lifestyle factors. It could also mean that the potential for developing colorectal cancer has been passed from one generation to the next, although the exact gene involved has not been identified. Relatives of a person with colorectal cancer may be more likely to develop it themselves. It has been estimated that 15–30% of colorectal cancers are familial. Familial colon cancer may be a result of single-gene mutations, multiple-gene mutations, or the combined effect of gene mutations and environmental risk factors. A family history of one or more members with frank colorectal cancer or premalignant polyps should be considered significant. Additionally, patterns within a family that exist without the identification of a specific mutation are considered familial colorectal cancers.

Hereditary Colorectal Cancer

The hereditary causes of two hereditary colorectal cancer syndromes, **familial adenomatous polyposis (FAP)** and **hereditary nonpolyposis colorectal cancer (HNPCC)**, have been identified. Like other diseases, colon cancer may occur sporadically, in familial patterns, or such that kindreds have the exact same mutations among those persons affected in a family. Mutations in cancer susceptibility genes predispose a person to inherited types of colorectal cancers.

Familial Adenomatous Polyposis

Familial adenomatous polyposis (FAP) is an inherited disorder characterized by the presence of multiple colorectal adenomatous polyps (typically more than 100). In patients affected by this disease, it may be the first case in the family (sporadic). Attenuated FAP is a variant form of FAP in which affected individuals develop fewer polyps (0–500), typically at a later age, than those persons with classical FAP. Although people with attenuated FAP tend to develop colon cancer at a later age than individuals with classical FAP, they still have a near 100% lifetime risk of colon cancer.

People with FAP have a 50% chance of passing the condition to each of their children. The condition can be passed on to offspring even if the patient has had his or her own colon removed. In contrast, children who do not inherit the condition from their parent cannot pass it to their own children. Approximately one-third of people with FAP do not have an affected parent. Individuals who inherit a mutated ***adenomatous polyposis coli (APC)*** gene have a very high likelihood of developing colonic **adenomas**; this risk has been estimated to be more than 90%. Most people with FAP are asymptomatic until they develop cancer. Nonspecific symptoms such as rectal bleeding, diarrhea, and abdominal pain may be suggestive of FAP. Diagnosing presymptomatic patients is essential. The age of onset of adenomas is variable. By age 10 years, only 15% of FAP gene carriers manifest adenomas; by age 20 years, the probability rises to 75%, and by age 30 years, 90% will have presented with FAP.

Genetics of Familial Adenomatous Polyposis

Familial adenomatous polyposis is an autosomal dominant condition caused by mutations in the *APC* tumor suppressor gene on chromosome 5. Most of these mutations lead to premature stop codons that result in truncation of the *APC* gene product, a protein that plays an important role in the regulation of cell adhesion and **apoptosis**. More than 800 different mutations have been reported. The majority of these changes are **insertions**, **deletions**, and **nonsense mutations** that lead to **frameshift mutations** and/or premature stop codons during gene transcription. The location of the mutation affects the number of polyps formed and the type of extracolonic features seen.

Recently, mutations in the *MYH* gene—a gene involved with base excision repair—have been identified in patients with the classic and attenuated forms of FAP who do not have mutations of the *APC* gene. The FAP caused by *MYH* mutation is inherited in an autosomal recessive fashion; hence, a family history of colorectal cancer may not be evident. Of patients with classic FAP, approximately 90% have a mutation in the *APC* gene and 8% in the *MYH* gene. In contrast, among patients with 10–100 adenomatous polyps and suspected attenuated FAP, *APC* mutations are identified in 15%, but *MYH* mutations are identified in 25%.

Genetic Counseling and Testing

Genetic counseling and testing should be offered to patients with a diagnosis of FAP that has been established by endoscopy and to all at-risk relatives of patients with the disease. Testing should also be done to confirm a diagnosis of attenuated disease in patients with 20 or more adenomas. Commercial *APC* gene testing is available. Genetic testing is best performed by sequencing the *APC* gene to identify disease-associated mutations, which are found in approximately 90% of cases of typical FAP. Mutational assessment of *MYH* should be considered in patients with negative test results and in patients with suspected attenuated FAP. Children of patients with FAP should undergo genetic screening beginning at age 10 years.

Screening Recommendations

If genetic testing cannot be done or is not informative, family members at risk should undergo a yearly colonoscopy beginning at 12 years of age. Once the diagnosis has been established, complete **proctocolectomy** or **colectomy** is recommended, usually before age 20 years. Extracolonic manifestations include polyp formation in the upper gastrointestinal tract occurring in 30–100% of patients with FAP. Upper endoscopic evaluation of the stomach, duodenum, and periampullary area should be performed every 1–3 years to look for adenomas or carcinoma. The upper endoscopy is preferred since sulindac and cyclooxygenase-2 selective agents have been shown to decrease the number and size of polyps in the rectum but not in the duodenum.

If attenuated FAP is suspected within a family, it is important that family members be screened with colonoscopy rather than flexible sigmoidoscopy because polyps are not evenly distributed throughout the colon. Given that the number of polyps and age of onset can vary greatly from one family member to another in a family with attenuated FAP, screening should begin at age 15 and be repeated every 1–3 years.

Gardner syndrome was originally used to describe families with colonic polyposis and extracolonic manifestation including desmoid tumors, lipomas, and juvenile nasopharyngeal angiofibromas. A phenotypic variant of FAP, it manifests as bumps or lumps on the bones of the legs, arms, skull, and jaw; cysts of the skin; teeth that do not erupt when they should; and frecklelike spots on the inside lining of the eyes.

Hereditary Nonpolyposis Colorectal Cancer

Hereditary nonpolyposis colorectal cancer is also known as Lynch syndrome. "Nonpolyposis" means that colorectal cancer can occur when only a small number of polyps are present or none at all. In HNPCC, cancer usually affects the right side of the colon. It often occurs at a younger age than sporadic colon cancer. Other cancers may arise in these families as well, including cancer of the uterus, ovaries, stomach, urinary tract, small bowel, and bile ducts.

This autosomal dominant condition accounts for 3–5% of all colorectal cancers. Affected individuals have a 60–80% lifetime risk of developing colorectal carcinoma and a more than 40% lifetime risk of developing endometrial cancer. Unlike individuals with FAP, patients with HNPCC develop only a few adenomas. In contrast to the traditional polyp to cancer progression (which may take several years), the polyps in HNPCC are believed to undergo rapid transformation from normal tissue to adenoma to cancer.

Research criteria used to define Lynch syndrome were originally developed in 1990 and referred to as the **Amsterdam criteria**; these criteria were revised

KEY TERMS

Frameshift mutation: an insertion or deletion involving a number of base pairs that is not a multiple of three and consequently disrupts the triplet reading frame, usually leading to the creation of a premature termination (stop) codon and resulting in a truncated protein product.

Proctocolectomy: a surgical procedure involving the excision of the colon and rectum and the formation of an ileoanal reservoir or pouch.

Colectomy: surgical excision of part or all of the colon.

Amsterdam criteria: research criteria for defining Lynch syndrome established by the International Collaborative Group meeting in Amsterdam.

in 1999 and are now called the Amsterdam criteria II. The latter criteria include the following specifications to warrant a diagnosis of HNPCC:

1. There should be at least three relatives with a Lynch syndrome–associated cancer (colorectal cancer or cancer of the endometrium, small bowel, ureter, or renal pelvis).
2. One should be a first-degree relative of the other two.
3. At least two successive generations should be affected.
4. At least one family member should be diagnosed before age 50 years.
5. Familial adenomatous polyposis should be excluded in the colorectal cancer cases.
6. Tumors should be verified by pathological examination.

Genetics of Hereditary Nonpolyposis Colorectal Cancer

A defect in one of several genes (*MLH1*, *MSH2*, *MSH6*, and *PMS2*) that are important in the detection and repair of DNA base-pair mismatches causes HNPCC. Germline mutations in *MLH1*, *MSH2*, and *MSH6* account for more than 90% of the known mutations in families with HNPCC. Mutations in any of these mismatch repair genes result in a characteristic phenotypic DNA abnormality known as **microsatellite instability**. In more than 95% of cancers in patients with HNPCC, microsatellite instability is readily demonstrated by expansion or contraction of DNA microsatellites (short, repeated DNA sequences). Microsatellite instability also occurs in 15% of sporadic colorectal cancers, usually due to aberrant methylation of the *MLH1* promoter, which results in decreased gene expression.

Genetic Counseling and Testing

A thorough family cancer history is essential to identify families whose members may be affected with HNPCC so that appropriate genetic and colonoscopic screening can be offered. Families with suspected HNPCC should be evaluated first by a genetic counselor and should give informed consent in writing before genetic testing is performed. Patients whose families meet any of the revised Bethesda criteria have an increased likelihood of harboring a germline mutation in one of the mismatch repair genes and should be considered for genetic testing. The Bethesda criteria include the following specifications to warrant a diagnosis of HNPCC:

1. Colorectal cancer before age 50
2. Synchronous or metachronous colorectal or HNPCC-associated tumor regardless of age (endometrial, stomach, ovary, pancreas, ureter and renal pelvis, biliary tract, brain)

3. Colorectal cancer, plus one or more first-degree relatives with colorectal or HNPCC-related cancer, with one of the cancers occurring before age 50
4. Colorectal cancer, plus two or more second-degree relatives with colorectal or HNPCC cancer, regardless of age
5. Tumors with infiltrating lymphocytes, mucinous/signet ring differentiation, or medullary growth pattern in patients younger than 60

These criteria will identify more than 90% of mutation-positive HNPCC families.

Tumor tissues of affected individuals or family members meeting the revised Bethesda criteria should undergo immunohistochemical staining for *MLH1*, *MSH2*, *MSH6*, and *PMS2* (using commercially available assays), testing for microsatellite instability (polymerase chain reaction [PCR] amplification of a panel of DNA markers), or both. Individuals whose tumors have normal immunohistochemical staining or do not have microsatellite instability are unlikely to have germline mutations in mismatch repair genes and do not require further genetic testing. However, if patients have early-age-onset colon cancer or features of hereditary colon cancer syndrome, they should be treated and managed based on their family history; these steps might include intensive cancer surveillance.

Germline testing for gene mutations is positive in greater than 90% of individuals whose tumors show no histochemical staining of one of the mismatch repair genes and in 50% of those patients whose tumors have a high level of microsatellite instability. Germline testing is also warranted in families with a strong history consistent with HNPCC when tumors from affected members are unavailable for assessment. If a mutation is detected in one of the known mismatch genes in a patient with cancer, genetic testing of other at-risk family members is indicated.

Screening Recommendations

If genetic testing documents an HNPCC gene mutation, affected relatives should be screened with colonoscopy every 1–2 years beginning at age 25 (or at an age 5 years younger than the age at diagnosis of the youngest affected family member). If cancer is found, subtotal colectomy followed by annual surveillance of the rectal stump should be performed. Upper endoscopy should be performed every 2–3 years to screen for gastric cancer. Women should undergo screening for endometrial cancer beginning at age 25–35 years with pelvic examination, CA-125 assay, endometrial aspiration, and transvaginal ultrasound. Prophylactic hysterectomy and oophorectomy may be considered, especially in women who have completed their families (i.e., who are done with childbearing). Similarly, consideration should be given for increased cancer surveillance in family members in proven or suspected HNPCC families who do not wish to undergo germline testing.

Chapter Summary

» Colorectal cancer occurs when cells that line the colon or the rectum become abnormal and grow in an out-of-control manner.

» The risk of colon cancer in a first-degree relative of an affected individual can increase an individual's lifetime risk of colon cancer anywhere from 2-fold to 4.3-fold.

» The genetic causes of two hereditary colorectal cancer syndromes—familial adenomatous polyposis and hereditary nonpolyposis colorectal cancer—have been identified.

» If attenuated familial adenomatous polyposis is suspected within a family, it is important that family members be screened with colonoscopy rather than flexible sigmoidoscopy because polyps are not evenly distributed throughout the colon.

Chapter Review Questions

1. _____ are usually benign growths that protrude from a mucous membrane in the colon and rectum.
2. Gardner syndrome is a phenotypic variant of _____ _____.
3. When discussing sporadic versus hereditary colorectal cancer, it is important to know that _____ is more common.
4. Hereditary nonpolyposis colorectal cancer is also known as _____.
5. If genetic testing documents a gene mutation associated with hereditary nonpolyposis colorectal cancer, affected relatives should be screened with colonoscopy every _____ years beginning at age 25.

Bibliography

Aarnio, M., Mecklin, J-P., Aaltonen, L. A., Nyström-Lahti, M., & Järvinen, H. J. (1995). Life-time risk of different cancers in hereditary non-polyposis colorectal cancer (HNPCC) syndrome. *International Journal of Cancer, 64*, 430–433.

Colon polyps. (n.d.). *MayoClinic.com*. Retrieved from http://www.mayoclinic.com /health/colon-polyps/DS00511/DSECTION=risk-factors

Levin, B., Lieberman, D. A., McFarland, B., Smith, R. A., Brooks, D., Andrews, K.S., . . . Winawer, S. J. (2008). Screening and surveillance for the early detection of colorectal cancer and adenomatous polyps, 2008: A joint guideline from the American Cancer Society, the U.S. Multi-Society Task Force on Colorectal Cancer, and the American College of Radiology. *CA: A Cancer Journal for Clinicians, 58*, 130–160.

McQuaid, K. R. (2007). Alimentary tract. In S. J. McPhee, M. A. Papadakis, & L. M. Tierney, Jr. (Eds.), *Current medical diagnosis and treatment* (46th ed., pp. 648–658). New York, NY: McGraw-Hill.

National Cancer Institute. (n.d.). *Colon and rectal cancer.* Retrieved from http://www .cancer.gov/cancertopics/types/colon-and-rectal

Pagon, R. A. (2005). Genetic testing: When to test, when to refer. *American Family Physician, 72*, 33–34. Retrieved from https://www.aafp.org/afp/2005/0701/p33.html

‹ Describe hematology associated with chronic myelogenous leukemia.
‹ Detail signs and symptoms associated with chronic myelogenous leukemia.
‹ Define the Philadelphia chromosome.
‹ Provide an overview of current treatments and factors associated with recovery from chronic myelogenous leukemia.

KEY TERMS

Blast cells
Blast crisis
Chronic myelogenous
leukemia (CML)
Fluorescence in situ
hybridization (FISH)

Granulocyte
Human leukocyte antigen
(HLA)
Myelofibrosis
Oncogene
Philadelphia chromosome

Polycythemia vera
Polymerase chain reaction
(PCR)
Proto-oncogene
Thrombocythemia

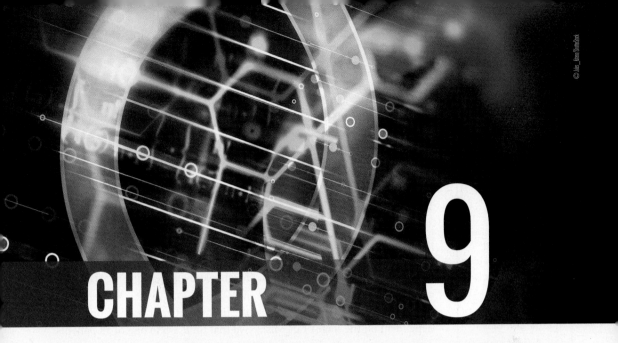

CHAPTER 9

Chronic Myelogenous Leukemia

Leukemia is the term used to describe a cancer in blood cells that are produced in the bone marrow. Specifically, leukemia of the granulocytic cell line in the bone marrow may be either acute or chronic. **Chronic myelogenous leukemia (CML)** is categorized as a myeloproliferative disorder (overproduction) that is usually insidious in onset, progressing slowly over many months to years.

Under normal circumstances, the granulocytic cell line is derived from a single pluripotent stem cell. This single stem cell differentiates into red blood cells, platelets, or white blood cells, including the **granulocytes**. Neutrophils, basophils, and eosinophils are all categorized as granulocytes. In CML, there is uncontrolled production of the granulocytic cell line, resulting in abnormally elevated amounts of both mature and immature granulocytes in both the peripheral blood and the bone marrow. Although the cells produced are usually morphologically normal, they may or may not be functional. The majority of the abnormal cells produced in CML are neutrophils, though the basophilic and eosinophilic cell lines are also slightly affected. The greater the tumor burden of these abnormal cells, the less marrow space and resources exist for healthy, fully functioning white blood cells, red blood cells, and platelets. This situation results in decreased numbers of healthy blood cells, leading to infections, anemias, and bleeding. Other myeloproliferative disorders include **polycythemia vera**, **myelofibrosis**, and essential **thrombocythemia**.

Early in the course of CML, the patient may be asymptomatic. However, as the disease progresses, it can accelerate into a blast crisis similar to an acute leukemia. In this stage, the patient will present extremely ill with a variety of infections, anemia, bleeding episodes, and other complications directly proportional to the tumor burden.

Major Phenotypic Features

The overall incidence of CML in the United States is 1 to 2 cases per 100,000 population, which represents approximately 4,000 to 10,000 cases annually. The median age at presentation is 55 years, and CML occurs slightly more frequently in men than in women. The only known predisposing risk factor is exposure to ionizing radiation.

Signs and symptoms displayed at the time of patient presentation are dependent on the stage of the disease at that time. Up to half of all patients are asymptomatic on diagnosis, with the disease being suspected because of abnormally elevated total white blood cell (WBC) count during routine peripheral blood complete blood count testing. In CML, the peripheral blood total WBC count is usually greater than 100,000 cells/μL (the normal range is 4,500–10,000 cells/μL), with a plethora of granulocytes found on the peripheral blood smear. Fatigue, night sweats, fever, and unintentional weight loss are the most common symptoms of patients who are symptomatic because of CML (**Box 9-1**). Patients may also complain of abdominal fullness related to splenomegaly. In these cases, the spleen is enlarged (often markedly so) on physical examination, and palpable sternal tenderness may be a sign of marrow overexpansion.

BOX 9-1	Signs and Symptoms Associated with Chronic Myelogenous Leukemia

Fatigue
Unexplained weight loss
Fever
Night sweats
Left upper quadrant abdominal pain or discomfort
Bleeding episodes
Early satiety
Tenderness over the lower sternum

Data from General Information About Chronic Myelogenous Leukemia. Chronic Myelogenous Leukemia Treatment (PDQ®). National Cancer Institute. U.S. National Institutes of Health. Available at http://www.cancer.gov/types/leukemia/hp/cml-treatment-pdq#section/_6. Accessed February 10, 2017.

Genetics of Chronic Myelogenous Leukemia

Chronic myelogenous leukemia is characterized by a chromosomal abnormality referred to as the **Philadelphia chromosome** t(9;22) (q34;q11), which involves a reciprocal translocation between the long arms of chromosomes 9 and 22. This translocation results in a novel product, the *BCR-ABL* fusion gene. The portion of chromosome 9 that is translocated contains the **proto-oncogene** *Abelson*, or *ABL*. The *ABL* gene normally encodes for a tightly regulated protein called tyrosine kinase, which is involved in cell growth, cell division, maturation, and apoptosis (cell death), and responds to signals in the cell to activate. When the *ABL* gene is received at a specific site on chromosome 22 referred to as the break point cluster region (*BCR*), the resulting fusion gene, *BCR/ABL*, produces a novel protein that possesses active, unregulated tyrosine kinase activity, which promotes unlimited cell growth and division. This abnormal enzyme leads to overproduction of abnormal granulocytes and an underproduction of normal granulocytes, red blood cells, and sometimes platelets. The mutation is not heritable, and exposure to ionizing radiation is the only known risk factor. No clear correlation with exposure to cytotoxic drugs has been found, and no evidence suggests a viral etiology for this mutation.

The classic Philadelphia chromosome is detectable in 90–95% of patients with the clinical and laboratory features of CML. The remaining 5–10% of patients may have variant or cryptic translocations that still encode the *BCR/ABL* fusion gene but cannot be identified by routine cytogenetic analysis (e.g., karyotype). These patients require molecular detection methods, such as fluorescence in situ hybridization (FISH) and polymerase chain reaction (PCR), to identify the *BCR/ABL* fusion gene. Patients who lack the classic translocation that characterizes the Philadelphia chromosome are referred to as having Philadelphia chromosome-negative CML, which is associated with a poorer prognosis than Philadelphia chromosome-positive CML. Evidence that the *BCR/ABL* fusion gene is pathogenic is provided by transgenic mouse models in which introduction of the gene almost invariably leads to leukemia.

Routine cytogenetic analysis is performed via karyotype and is needed in all cases at diagnosis. This type of testing requires bone marrow biopsy and aspiration, which will identify not only the presence of the Philadelphia chromosome but also the existence of other chromosomal abnormalities. The Philadelphia chromosome is usually more readily apparent in marrow metaphases than in peripheral blood metaphases.

Fluorescence in situ hybridization (FISH) is used to identify the presence of the *BCR/ABL* fusion gene, even if the Philadelphia chromosome cannot be identified by routine cytogenetic analysis. Another advantage of FISH is

KEY TERMS

Polycythemia vera: a chronic form of polycythemia of unknown cause characterized by bone marrow hyperplasia, an increase in both blood volume and the number of red cells, redness or cyanosis of the skin, and splenomegaly.

Myelofibrosis: fibrosis of the bone marrow associated with myeloid metaplasia of the spleen and other organs.

Thrombocythemia: a primary form of thrombocytopenia, in contrast to secondary forms that are associated with metastatic neoplasms, tuberculosis, and leukemia involving the bone marrow, or occurring as the result of direct suppression of bone marrow by the use of chemical agents.

Philadelphia chromosome: an abnormal chromosome, formed by a rearrangement of chromosomes 9 and 22, that is associated with chronic myelogenous leukemia.

Proto-oncogene: a gene in the normal human genome that appears to have a role in normal cellular physiology and is involved in regulation of normal cell growth or proliferation; as a result of somatic mutations, these genes may become oncogenic.

Fluorescence in situ hybridization (FISH): an analytic technique in which a nucleic acid labeled with a fluorescent dye is hybridized to suitably prepared cells or histological sections; it is then used to look for specific transcription or localization of genes to specific chromosomes.

Polymerase chain reaction (PCR): repeated cycles of DNA denaturation, renaturation with primer oligonucleotide sequences, and replication, resulting in exponential growth in the number of copies of the DNA sequence located between the primers.

that it can be performed with peripheral blood. However, it does not provide information on other chromosomal abnormalities.

Quantitative **polymerase chain reaction (PCR)** is also done at diagnosis to obtain a baseline measure of the *BCR/ABL* transcript levels before the start of therapy. Qualitative PCR may also be performed at diagnosis to identify the *BCR-ABL* fusion mRNA transcript type if the Philadelphia chromosome is not readily identified by karyotype.

Phases of Chronic Myelogenous Leukemia

Three general disease phases exist: chronic phase, accelerated phase, and blast crisis. In the earliest stage, termed the chronic phase, the patient typically has less than 10% **blast cells** in both blood and bone marrow samples. Most patients are diagnosed in this phase, which lasts between 2 and 4 years. The accelerated phase, as outlined by the World Health Organization, is characterized by a blast count of 10–19% of the cells in the peripheral blood or bone marrow. Platelet counts either decline or are greatly elevated in this stage, and other cytogenetic abnormalities appear. In the final or blastic phase of CML, 20% or more of the cells in the blood or bone marrow are blast cells; this usually occurs within 6–8 months. **Blast crisis** describes the cellular criteria of the blast phase, accompanied by fatigue, fever, and splenomegaly. Blast crisis closely resembles acute leukemia, and the median survival at this point is often less than 4 months.

Treatment

Imatinib mesylate (marketed under the trade name Gleevec) is a prototypic example of targeted molecular therapy for cancer. This drug inhibits the activity of the defective gene in CML: the *BCR/ABL* **oncogene**. This activity against the oncogene keeps the number of blast cells low by inducing apoptosis in cells with the abnormal oncogene. As a result, it is possible to ameliorate the disease progression of CML in the early phases. Imatinib mesylate also has few side effects and has shown a high response rate in most patients. Evaluation of response to treatment of CML includes the following: (1) hematologic response, assessed by the regression of WBC count, differential, and platelet count, (2) cytogenetic response, assessed by analyzing marrow cell metaphases for the presence of the Philadelphia chromosome (**Table 9-1**), and (3) molecular response, assessed by quantitative PCR of the peripheral blood. The molecular response is measured in the amount of log reduction in the *BCR/ABL* transcript level, which ranges from >2-log reduction to >4.4-log reduction.

TABLE 9-1	Hematologic and Cytogenetic Response Criteria in Chronic Myelogenous Leukemia

Diagnostic Method	Response	Criteria
Hematologic	Complete	White blood cell count < 10 × 10^9/L, normal morphology; normal hemoglobin and platelet counts
Cytogenetic		Percentage of bone marrow metaphases with Philadelphia chromosome
	Complete	0
	Major	< 35%
	Minor	36–65%
	Minimal	66–95%
	None	> 95%

Data from Baccarani, M., Cortes, J., Pane, F., Niederwieser, D., Saglio, G., Apperley J., . . . Hehlmann, R. (2009). Chronic myeloid leukemia: An update of concepts and management recommendations of European LeukemiaNet. *Journal of Clinical Oncology, 27*, 6041–6051; Baccarani, M., Deininger, M. W., Rosti, G., Hochhaus, A., Soverini, S., Apperley, J. F., . . . Hehlmann, R. (2013). European LeukemiaNet recommendations for the management of chronic myeloid leukemia. *Blood, 122*, 872–874.

KEY TERMS

Blast cells: a very immature precursor cell (e.g., erythroblast, lymphoblast).

Blast crisis: in a patient with chronic myelogenous leukemia, a disease stage characterized by high burden of blasts in the peripheral blood and/or bone marrow; it carries a clinically poor prognosis.

Oncogene: a gene that has the potential to cause cancer.

The current goal of therapy for CML is to achieve an optimal molecular response, with at least a 3-log reduction in the *BCR/ABL* level. Patients who achieve this level of molecular response have an excellent prognosis, with an increased overall survival rate and very few relapses after 3–4 years of follow-up. Patients with suboptimal molecular responses are best treated by switching from imatinib mesylate to an alternative tyrosine kinase inhibitor such as dasatinib or nilotinib. Randomized trials performed with patients in newly diagnosed chronic phase have demonstrated that agents such as dasatinib and nilotinib achieve earlier and more complete responses than imatinib, though increased overall survival has not been proved.

The only proven curative therapy for CML is allogeneic (from a donor) hematopoietic stem cell transplantation. However, this approach is not

KEY TERM

Human leukocyte antigen (HLA): system designation for the gene products of at least four linked loci (A, B, C, and D) and a number of subloci on the sixth human chromosome that have been shown to have a strong influence on human allotransplantation, transfusions in refractory patients, and certain disease associations. More than 50 alleles are recognized, most of which are found at loci HLA-A and HLA-B; they are passed on through autosomal dominant inheritance.

without significant risk. Following allogeneic transplantation, immune cells transplanted with the stem cells or developing from them can react against the patient, causing graft-versus-host disease, a condition in which the donor tissue attacks the recipient tissue. Alternatively, if the immunosuppressive preparative regimen used to treat the patient before transplant is inadequate, immunocompetent cells of the patient may lead to graft rejection. The risks of these complications are greatly influenced by the degree of matching between donor and recipient for antigens encoded by genes of the major histocompatibility complex. In addition to this, the patient is at significant risk of succumbing to infection while immunosuppressed.

The best results (50–85% long-term remission rate) are obtained in patients who are younger than 50 years of age and transplanted in chronic phase within 1 year after diagnosis from **human leukocyte antigen (HLA)**–matched siblings. Allogeneic transplantation is reserved for patients in whom disease is not well controlled, in whom disease progresses after initial control, or for those who have accelerated or blast phase disease.

Chemotherapeutic agents can be used as a supportive option while waiting to confirm diagnosis of CML or in patients with systemic symptoms. Hydroxyurea is a ribonucleotide reductase inhibitor that induces rapid disease control by disrupting the growth of the cancer cells. Initial management of patients with chemotherapy is currently reserved for rapid lowering of WBCs to avoid cerebrovascular events or death from leukostasis, reduction of symptoms, and reversal of symptomatic splenomegaly.

Relapsed CML is characterized by any evidence of progression of disease from a stable remission. Signs of progression may include any of the following: (1) increasing myeloid or blast cells in the peripheral blood or bone marrow, (2) cytogenetic positivity when previously cytogenetic negative, and (3) FISH positivity for *BCR/ABL* translocation when previously FISH was negative.

Blast crisis CML portends a poor prognosis because the treatments that are effective in chronic-phase CML are generally ineffective in the more severe, acute phase of disease.

Prognosis

Before the introduction of imatinib mesylate therapy in 2001, death was expected in 10% of patients with CML within 2 years and in approximately 20% yearly thereafter; the median survival time was approximately 4 years. Today, more than 90% of patients remain alive and without disease progression at 6 years with the use of tyrosine kinase inhibitors and other molecular targeted agents. Although allogeneic hematopoietic stem cell transplantation is the only proven curative option for CML, the disease can be controlled long-term by oral agents. Factors affecting the patient's prognosis include patient age, phase of CML, amount of blasts seen in the blood or bone marrow, cytogenetics, and the presence of comorbid diseases.

Chapter Summary

» Leukemia is a cancer that starts in blood cells in the bone marrow and causes large numbers of immature blood cells to be produced and enter the bloodstream.

» In chronic myelogenous leukemia, too many blood stem cells develop into abnormal granulocytes.

» A chromosomal abnormality referred to as the Philadelphia chromosome, which involves a reciprocal translocation between the long arms of chromosomes 9 and 22, is associated with chronic myelogenous leukemia.

» The only proven curative therapy for chronic myelogenous leukemia is allogeneic hematopoietic stem cell transplantation.

Chapter Review Questions

1. The peripheral blood cell profile in patients affected by chronic myelogenous leukemia shows an increased number of _____ and their immature precursors.
2. Patients with CML usually present with fatigue, night sweats, and fever related to the _____ caused by overproduction of white blood cells.
3. The fusion gene _____ produces a novel protein that differs from the normal gene transcript in that it possesses active, unregulated tyrosine kinase activity.
4. When fatigue, fever, and an enlarged spleen occur during the blastic phase of CML, this situation is called _____ _____ and represents acute leukemia.
5. _____ specifically inhibits the tyrosine kinase activity of the *BCR/ABL* oncogene.

Bibliography

Arber, D. A., Orazi, A., Hasserjian, R., Thiele, J., Borowitz, M. J., Le Beau, M. M., . . . Vardima, J. W. (2016). The 2016 revision to the World Health Organization classification of myeloid neoplasms and acute leukemia. *Blood, 127*, 2391–2405.

Baccarani, M., Cortes, J., Pane, F., Niederwieser, D., Saglio, G., Apperley, J., . . . Hehlmann, R. (2009). Chronic myeloid leukemia: An update of concepts and management recommendations of European LeukemiaNet. *Journal of Clinical Oncology, 27*, 6041–6051.

Baccarani, M., Deininger, M. W., Rosti, G., Hochhaus, A., Soverini, S., Apperley, J. F., . . . Hehlmann, R. (2013). European LeukemiaNet recommendations for the management of chronic myeloid leukemia: 2013. *Blood, 122,* 872–874.

Biggs, J. C., Szer, J., Crilley, P., Atkinson, K., Downs, K., Dodds, A., . . . Copelan, E. A. (1992). Treatment of chronic myeloid leukemia with allogeneic bone marrow transplantation after preparation with BuCy2. *Blood, 80,* 1352–1357.

Chen, Y., Wang, H., Kantarjian, H., & Cortes, J. (2013). Trends in chronic myeloid leukemia incidence and survival in the United States from 1975 to 2009. *Leukemia & Lymphoma, 54,* 1411–1417.

Cortes, J., & Kantarjian, H. (2012). How I treat newly diagnosed chronic phase CML. *Blood, 120,* 1390–1397.

Cortes, J. E., Saglio, G., Kantarjian, H. M., Baccarani, M., Mayer, J., Boqué, C., . . . Hochhaus, A. (2016). Final 5-year study results of DASISION: The dasatinib versus imatinib study in treatment-naïve chronic myeloid leukemia patients trial. *Journal of Clinical Oncology, 34,* 2333–2340.

Cortes, J. E., Talpaz, M., O'Brien, S., Faderl, S., Garcia-Manero, G., Ferrajoli, A., . . . Kantarjian, H. M. (2006). Staging of chronic myeloid leukemia in the imatinib era: An evaluation of the World Health Organization proposal. *Cancer, 106,* 1306–1315.

Cross, N. C., White, H. E., Muller, M. C., Saglio, G., & Hochhaus, A. (2012). Standardized definitions of molecular response in chronic myeloid leukemia. *Leukemia, 26,* 2172–2175.

Faderl, S., Talpaz, M., Estrov, Z., O'Brien, S., Kurzrock, R., & Kantarjian, H. M. (1999). The biology of chronic myeloid leukemia. *New England Journal of Medicine, 341,* 164–172.

Gratwohl, A., Hermans, J., Neiderwieser, D., Frassoni, F., Arcese, W., Gahrton, G., . . . Bosi, A. (1993). Bone marrow transplantation for chronic myeloid leukemia: Long-term results. Chronic Leukemia Working Party of the European Group for Bone Marrow Transplantation. *Bone Marrow Transplantation, 12,* 509–516.

Gurion, R., Gafter-Gvili, A., Vidal, L., Leader, A., Ram, R., Shacham-Abulafia, A., . . . Raanani, P. (2013). Has the time for first-line treatment with second generation tyrosine kinase inhibitors in patients with chronic myelogenous leukemia already come? Systematic review and meta-analysis. *Haematologica, 98,* 95–102.

Kantarjian, H. M., Cortes, J., Guilhot, F., Hochhaus, A., Baccarani, M., & Lokey, L. (2007). Diagnosis and management of chronic myeloid leukemia: A survey of American and European practice patterns. *Cancer, 109,* 1365–1375.

McGlave, P. (1990). Bone marrow transplants in chronic myelogenous leukemia: An overview of determinants of survival. *Seminars in Hematology, 27,* 23–30.

National Cancer Institute. (2018). *Chronic myelogenous leukemia treatment (PDQ®).* Retrieved from http://www.cancer.gov/types/leukemia/hp/cml-treatment-pdq

Saglio, G., Kim, D. W., Issaragrisil, S., le Coutre, P., Etienne, G., Lobo, C., . . . Kantarjian, H. M. (2010). Nilotinib versus imatinib for newly diagnosed chronic myeloid leukemia. *New England Journal of Medicine, 362,* 2251–2259.

Savage, D. G., Szydlo, R. M., & Goldman, J. M. (1997). Clinical features at diagnosis in 430 patients with chronic myeloid leukaemia seen at a referral centre over a 16-year period. *British Journal of Haematology, 96,* 111–116.

Seigel, R. L., Miller, K. D., & Jemal, A. (2017). Cancer statistics. *CA: A Cancer Journal for Clinicians, 67,* 7–30.

Swerdlow, S. H., Campo, E., Harris, N. L., Jaffe, E. S., Pileri, S. A., Stein, H., . . . Vardiman, J. W. (2008). *World Health Organization classification of tumours of haematopoietic and lymphoid tissues.* Lyon, France: IARC Press.

< Describe the etiology and various forms of hemophilia.
< Detail phenotypic features, symptoms, and physical examination findings associated with hemophilia.
< Discuss variable expressivity of genes.
< Identify bleeding disorders associated with hemophilia.
< Review current diagnosis, treatment, and surveillance recommendations for hemophilia.

KEY TERMS

Acquired hemophilia
Acquired von Willebrand's disease
Autoantibody
Bleeding diathesis
Carrier
Cephalohematoma
Clotting factor
Coagulation
De novo mutations
Deletion
Desmopressin acetate
Disseminated intravascular coagulation

Factor assay
Factor deficiency
Factor inhibitors
Factor replacement therapy
Hemarthroses
Hematoma
Hemophilia
Hemophilia A
Hemophilia B
Hemophilia B Leyden
Hemophilia C
Hemophilia treatment centers

Hemostasis
Menorrhagia
Mild hemophilia
Missense mutation
Moderate hemophilia
Proband
Severe hemophilia
Spontaneous bleeding
Thrombocytopenia
Variable expressivity
Von Willebrand's disease
X-linked recessive

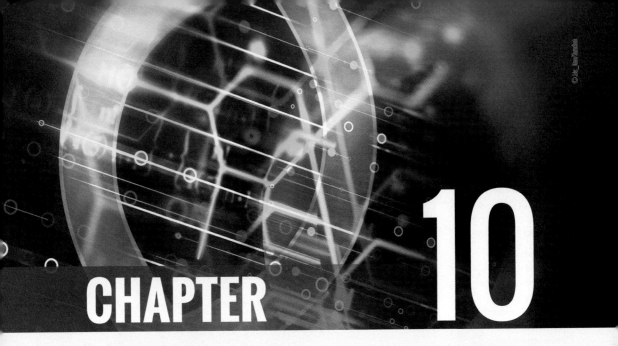

CHAPTER 10

Hemophilia

Hemophilia is a bleeding disorder caused by mutations in the *F8* or *F9* gene. Both of these genes are responsible for encoding the coagulation protein factor VIII and factor IX, which play key roles in the blood clotting cascade (**Figure 10-1**). An *F8* mutation resulting in a factor VIII deficiency manifests as **hemophilia A**, or "classic" hemophilia. An *F9* mutation causes a factor IX deficiency and is designated as **hemophilia B**, or "Christmas disease." Both *F8* and *F9* mutations are inherited in an **X-linked recessive** pattern, with mostly males being affected. Both types of hemophilia occur worldwide across all races. Approximately 1 in 4,000 males are affected with hemophilia A, whereas hemophilia B is not as common and has an incidence of approximately 1 in 20,000 males.

Clinically, these two disorders are indistinguishable from each other. Both types of hemophilia present with spontaneous bleeding into the joints (**hemarthroses**), bleeding into muscles, and variable degrees of prolonged or abnormal bleeding in other soft tissues. Postoperative and traumatic bleeding may occur depending on the severity of the disease. Hemophilia is classified as mild, moderate, or severe based on the amount of normal coagulation factor activity (**Table 10-1**). Initial laboratory findings include a *prolonged or elevated* activated partial thromboplastin time (APTT) with a *normal* prothrombin time (PT), *normal* bleeding time, and *normal* fibrinogen levels. The diagnosis is made by specific factor assays, which test for the levels of the suspected deficient factor.

Genetics of Hemophilia

Under normal circumstances, the *F8* gene provides instructions for making factor VIII. In hemophilia A, various mutations in *F8* cause the production of abnormal factor VIII proteins, which cannot carry out their expected functions. Depending on the specific mutation, the levels of normally functioning or active protein will vary; clinical manifestations are directly related to the amount of normal protein activity (Table 10-1).

KEY TERMS

Hemophilia: a bleeding disorder in which a specific clotting factor protein—namely, factor VIII or IX—is missing or does not function normally.

Hemophilia A: a deficiency or absence of factor VIII; also called "classic" hemophilia. It is the most common severe bleeding disorder.

Hemophilia B: a deficiency or absence of factor IX; also called "Christmas disease" after the first family identified with the condition.

X-linked recessive: recessive inheritance pattern of alleles at loci on the X chromosome that do not undergo crossing over during male meiosis.

Hemarthroses: bleeding into joints.

FIGURE 10-1 Coagulation cascade.

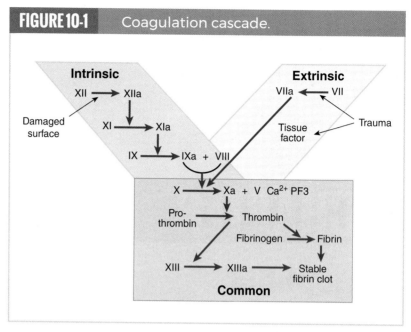

Reproduced with permission of Gordon M. Kirby, Ontario Veterinary College at the University of Guelph, Ontario, Canada.

TABLE 10-1 Classification of Hemophilia A and B by Normal Coagulation Factor Activity (Factor VIII and Factor IX) and Associated Clinical Findings

Classification	Percent Normal Factor Activity*	Associated Clinical Findings
Severe	< 1%	Spontaneous joint and muscle bleeding; posttrauma and postoperative bleeding
Moderate	1–5%	Bleeding in joints and muscles due to minor trauma; postoperative bleeding
Mild	5–40%	Postoperative and mild trauma bleeding

*Reference range for normal clotting activity is 50–150%.
Data from the National Center for Biotechnology Information. U.S. National Library of Medicine. National Institutes of Health. Adapted from https://www.hemophilia.org/Bleeding-Disorders/Types-of-Bleeding-Disorders/Hemophilia-A

The *F9* gene provides the instructions for making protein factor IX. In hemophilia B, various mutations in *F9* cause production of abnormal factor IX proteins, which results in clinical manifestations similar to hemophilia A.

Both factor VIII and factor IX are integral components of the intrinsic coagulation pathway (Figure 10-1). These two proteins work in conjunction with other components of the blood to promote clotting and stop bleeding (**hemostasis**). Hemostasis also involves the action of platelets at the site of injury and the formation of a fibrin clot in a process known as **coagulation**. Coagulation is the chemical reaction that occurs among the various coagulation factors that results in a stable fibrin clot. When an injury occurs, blood clots form, which seal off damaged blood vessels, thereby preventing further blood loss. In hemophilia, the coagulation factors are altered and are unable to mediate reactions in the coagulation cascade (Figure 10-1). As a result, clots do not form properly in response to an injury, and abnormal bleeding occurs.

The genes for hemophilia are located on the X chromosome and both hemophilia A and hemophilia B are transmitted in an X-linked recessive pattern. As we know, the sex chromosomes X and Y are distributed as XX in females and XY in males. Because males have only one X chromosome, only one mutated gene causes disease expression in them. In contrast, females have two X chromosomes, so the mutation must be present in both copies of the gene to cause the disorder in them. Therefore, males are affected by X-linked recessive disorders with greater frequency than females.

In X-linked recessive inheritance, females with one altered copy of the gene in each cell are considered **carriers**. A carrier female can pass the altered gene to her children but generally does not express the disease (or phenotype) herself. Some carrier females do manifest a mild disease expression. Because males pass only the Y chromosome on to their male offspring, hemophilia is not inherited from father to son.

Diagnosis

Because hemophilia slows the blood clotting process, affected persons often present with prolonged bleeding after injury, surgery, or tooth extraction. The severity of symptoms is often variable (Table 10-1)—a phenomenon referred to as **variable expressivity**. In **severe hemophilia**, heavy bleeding can occur without any obvious trauma—a situation called **spontaneous bleeding**. Individuals with this type of hemophilia are usually diagnosed shortly after birth. Serious complications can result from bleeding into the weight-bearing joints and muscles and into the brain or internal organs. The joints most commonly affected are the knees, ankles, and elbows. Blood irritates the synovial lining of the affected joint and can lead to limited movement of the joint. Gastrointestinal bleeding is the most frequent cause of internal bleeding. Mild head trauma can also cause unusual bleeding and lead to a collection of blood under the skull, known as a **cephalohematoma**.

KEY TERMS

Hemostasis: the process by which the body stops bleeding.

Coagulation: the chemical reaction mediated by coagulation factor proteins that results in a stable fibrin clot.

Carrier: a person (usually female) who can pass an altered gene to her children but generally does not express the disease herself.

Variable expressivity: variation in which the disease symptoms are present.

Severe hemophilia: a categorical term used to describe someone with a factor VIII or IX level that is less than 1% of normal blood levels.

Spontaneous bleeding: heavy bleeding without history of trauma.

Cephalohematoma: a collection of blood under the skull due to an effusion of blood, usually as a result of trauma.

KEY TERMS

Moderate hemophilia: a categorical term used to describe someone with a factor VIII or IX level ranging between 1% and 5% of normal blood levels.

Hematoma: bleeding into soft tissue, such as muscle or visceral organs.

Mild hemophilia: a categorical term used to describe someone with a factor VIII or IX level ranging between 5% and 25% of normal blood levels.

Menorrhagia: excessive bleeding during the time of menses, in terms of duration, volume, or both.

De novo mutations: mutations that are not inherited, but rather appear first in the affected individual.

Factor assay: a specialized lab test used to determine the level of circulating factor VIII or IX.

Desmopressin acetate: a synthetic hormone that increases factor VIII levels.

Moderate hemophilia may also present with hemarthroses or deep-tissue **hematomas** due to minor trauma or as postoperative bleeding. Persons with moderate hemophilia are typically diagnosed before 6 years of age. **Mild hemophilia** does not involve spontaneous bleeding and may become apparent only when abnormal bleeding occurs following surgery or a serious injury. Persons with mild hemophilia are frequently diagnosed later in life.

Other findings that vary with degree of severity of hemophilia include the propensity for excessive bleeding during menses (**menorrhagia**). Unexplained gastrointestinal or genitourinary bleeding may also occur. Prolonged nosebleeds that are recurrent over time, are bilateral, and are not elicited by trauma are often present. Prolonged oozing or bleeding after initial cessation of bleeding due to tooth extraction, buccal mucosa injury, or circumcision is also common.

Although a positive family history is helpful in making the diagnosis of hemophilia, it is important to note that approximately 25% of hemophiliacs do not present with a known family history. This may be attributed to very mild clinical manifestations or **de novo mutations** of the *F8* or *F9* gene. De novo mutations are alterations in the germ cell that occur for the first time in one family member.

Genetic Testing and Counseling

All individuals with a suspected bleeding disorder should undergo coagulation screening consisting of an APTT measurement, a PT measurement, a bleeding time measurement, and a platelet count.

The APTT measurement evaluates the intrinsic pathway of the coagulation cascade (Figure 10-1) and is the best individual screening test for coagulation disorders. It is most sensitive in patients with a clinical history of bleeding, such as in moderate to severe hemophilia; it is less sensitive in those persons without clinical manifestations, as in mild hemophilia. The APTT test is also clinically useful to monitor heparin therapy and to detect clotting inhibitors. The PT measurement evaluates the extrinsic pathway of the coagulation cascade and is clinically useful in monitoring long-term anticoagulant therapy with warfarin (Coumadin) as well as in evaluation of liver function and extrinsic factor disorders.

Neither PT nor APTT can differentiate between factor deficiencies or the presence of specific factor inhibitors such as antifactor VIII (antifactors will be discussed further later in this text). It is also important to note that low to normal clotting activity in these screening tests does not completely rule out the presence of hemophilia A. For these reasons, specific coagulation **factor assays** must be performed. Any person with a lifelong history of bleeding should have these coagulation factor assays performed, regardless of the results of the screening tests. Estrogens, oral contraceptives, epinephrine, **desmopressin acetate**, and vigorous exercise can all increase the levels of factors VIII and IX. Decreases in circulating factor VIII and IX may be due to in vivo consumption, such as occurs in **disseminated intravascular coagulation.**

The platelet count is most often a component of the complete blood count but may also be ordered as a single test. It is useful to rule out bleeding disorders due to quantitative platelet disorders or **thrombocytopenia**. By comparison, the bleeding time is the best screening test for platelet function disorders. It is prolonged in **von Willebrand's disease** and in qualitative platelet disorders.

Once a specific **factor deficiency** is confirmed, attempts to identify specific mutations should be made. This effort begins with targeted mutation analysis for the two most common mutations (gene inversions) detected in the majority of severe hemophiliacs. Mutations in mild to moderate disease tend to be **missense mutations**, whereas **deletions** are associated with more severe disease that responds poorly to therapy. Specific mutations in each category correlate with severity of disease and response to **factor replacement therapy**.

Because of the X-linked inheritance pattern of hemophilia A and B, the carrier status of the mother determines the risk of transmitting the faulty genes to the siblings of the affected person. The identified affected person is known as the **proband**. Females who are carriers have a 50% chance per pregnancy of passing along the *F8* mutation. As mentioned earlier, males who inherit the mutation will be affected, whereas females who inherit the mutation will be carriers. Affected males will transmit the mutation to all their daughters but to none of their sons. For families who have some members with hemophilia already identified, it is important to construct an accurate pedigree because this information will be helpful when counseling other family members.

Management and Treatment

The recommended initial evaluation for patients newly diagnosed with hemophilia A or B should include identification of the specific mutation, a personal history of bleeding, family history of bleeding, a thorough musculoskeletal evaluation, associated disease screenings, and baseline laboratory tests to detect abnormal bleeding times. Identification of the specific mutations can aid in predicting the severity of disease, the development of factor inhibitors, and related immune tolerance, resulting in no response to the treatment. A history of personal and familial bleeding tendencies can also predict the severity of the disease. A complete examination of joints and muscles contributes to the estimation of disease severity given that hemarthroses and deep-tissue hematomas tend to occur more frequently with increasing disease severity. Screening for hepatitis A, hepatitis B, hepatitis C, and HIV is recommended for individuals who received blood or blood products such as **clotting factor** concentrates before 1985.

Referral to **hemophilia treatment centers** has been shown to be beneficial to patients with hemophilia, as evidenced by the lower mortality rates for those enrolled in such programs versus those who are not enrolled. These centers constitute a group of federally funded hospitals that specialize in

KEY TERMS

Disseminated intravascular coagulation: a condition of altered coagulation that results in consumption of clotting factors and platelets and yields a clinical presentation characterized by both excessive clotting and excessive bleeding.

Thrombocytopenia: a condition in which an abnormally small number of platelets appear in the circulating blood.

Von Willebrand's disease: a bleeding disorder in which von Willebrand factor, a blood protein, is either missing or does not function properly. It is the most common congenital bleeding disorder in the United States.

Factor deficiency: any of several rare disorders characterized by the complete absence or an abnormally low level of clotting factor in the blood.

coagulation disorders; care is delivered by teams that include a hematologist, nurse, social worker, and physical therapist who work together to deliver comprehensive care by providing education, genetic counseling, and laboratory testing to patients and families. Centers may be located through the National Hemophilia Foundation (www.hemophilia.org).

Young children with hemophilia require assessment every 6–12 months. For persons receiving factor VIII concentrates, it is recommended that they initially be assessed at 3- to 6-month intervals and then annually once therapy is well established. Any individual with a milder form of hemophilia needs periodic assessment every 2–3 years. Screening is also recommended before any type of invasive surgery.

Treatment of bleeding manifestations for severe disease includes intravenous infusions of factor VIII concentrate (Bioclate) within an hour of the onset of bleeding. Patients can be trained to administer these intravenous products at home. Nasal desmopressin or factor VIII concentrate may be used in mild to moderate disease. Prevention of bleeding episodes and complications should focus on reducing the risk of injury and precipitating events. For children, these guidelines include restrictions on specific physical activities such as contact sports. However, it is important to recommend regular exercise to strengthen muscles to protect and stabilize joints. Chronic joint disease may also be ameliorated by early recognition of hemarthroses. Other circumstances to be avoided before treatment include elective surgeries such as circumcision, intramuscular injections, dental procedures, and ingestion of aspirin or products containing aspirin. Regularly scheduled factor VIII infusions are another way to help prevent acute bleeding episodes; however, these can be very costly for patients.

Two major complications associated with factor replacement therapy are transfusion-transmitted infection and development of factor antibodies/transfusion reaction. Hemophiliacs treated before 1986 are at increased risk for the development of bloodborne infections—in particular, hepatitis A, hepatitis B, hepatitis C, and HIV. These infections have been associated with factor replacement therapy in patients who received human-derived blood products before viral testing and protein purification became a routine part of development of blood products. Fortunately, the incidence of transfusion-related infection has decreased with the development of recombinant factor concentrates and greater ability to eradicate viruses from the plasma-derived products. Recombinant factor concentrates do not contain any human-derived proteins.

Antibodies that develop in patients in response to factor replacement therapy are known as **factor inhibitors**; this happens during a transfusion reaction to the factor replacement. The risk of developing these antibodies is greatest during the initial treatment for hemophilia, when the body recognizes the factor infusion as "foreign" and mounts an immune response. Recently, gene therapy clinical trials for hemophilia A and B were discontinued. In these trials, patients were not able to achieve factor expression in quantities great enough to ameliorate disease symptoms. Complications also developed in several patients.

Blood Product Transfusions

It is critical to monitor the patient very closely during any transfusion infusion, especially during the first 15 minutes. The majority of transfusion reactions occur within the first 15 minutes of therapy. After correct identification of the patient (name, date, blood bank number, blood type, and so on) by two witnesses is performed, vital signs must be taken before the transfusion has started and again after 15 minutes, 1 hour, and 2 hours. Another set of vital signs must be taken 30 minutes after the transfusion has been completed. Any blood transfusion should be no shorter in duration than 2 hours if packed red blood cells (PRBCs) or 30 minutes if factor replacement. A 20-gauge or bigger IV should be used for ease of transfusion along with the proper filtered tubing. If a patient will transfuse factor replacement at home, it is important to teach him or her that *only* normal saline can be transfused and diluted with blood products (not Lactated Ringer's Solution [LR], Dextrose 5% in Water [D5W], etc.); otherwise, clotting and hemolysis will occur. The patient should also be taught that it is not appropriate to infuse any other medications through the same IV tubing as the blood product transfusion.

If a transfusion reaction is suspected—fever/chills, pruritus, flank pain, hematuria, sudden chest pain or shortness of breath, tachycardia, headache, hypotension, increased pallor/cyanosis—the infusion should be immediately stopped. Once the transfusion is stopped, stabilization of the patient should occur (oxygen, fluids, diuretics, diphenhydramine, steroids, etc.), and then the blood should be sent to the blood bank for analysis.

Associated Syndromes

Hemophilia B Leyden is a rare variant of hemophilia B inherited in an X-linked pattern. This bleeding disorder is characterized by an altered developmental expression of blood coagulation factor IX and is associated with a variety of single-point mutations in the *F9* gene. Affected individuals experience episodes of excessive bleeding in childhood but have few bleeding problems after puberty.

Rarely, hemophilia may be acquired instead of inherited. **Acquired hemophilia** presents with the same clinical manifestations of inherited hemophilia but usually first appears in adulthood. This condition is caused by the production of **autoantibody**, which inactivates coagulation factor VIII (acquired hemophilia A) or IX (acquired hemophilia B). The production of autoantibody has been associated with pregnancy, immune system disorders, cancer, and allergic reactions to certain drugs. In many cases, the etiology is not discovered.

KEY TERMS

Hemophilia treatment centers: a group of federally funded hospitals that specialize in treating patients with coagulation disorders.

Factor inhibitors: antibodies that develop in patients in response to factor replacement therapy.

Hemophilia B Leyden: a rare variant of hemophilia B inherited in an X-linked pattern.

Acquired hemophilia: production of autoantibody that inactivates coagulation factors (VIII or IX) and results in the same clinical bleeding diathesis as occurs in inherited hemophilias.

Autoantibody: a protein that attacks the body's own tissues.

Von Willebrand's disease is a bleeding disorder associated with low factor VIII activity in which von Willebrand factor (vWF), a blood protein, is either missing or does not function properly. The primary role of the Von Willebrand protein is to bind to other proteins (such as Factor VIII) in the clotting cascade. It is integral for platelet adhesion to wound sites. This mutation is most frequently inherited in an autosomal dominant pattern with variable penetrance, although three rare subtypes show autosomal recessive inheritance patterns. Because it can be inherited by both men and women equally, von Willebrand's disease is the most common heritable bleeding disorder.

Acquired von Willebrand's disease usually develops late in life and is caused by the development of antibodies that attack and destroy vWF. **Bleeding diatheses** that present with a prolonged APTT (with or without clinical manifestations) may be differentiated based on follow-up testing. Because of the complexity of these conditions and the increased risk of bleeding associated with them, referral to a hematologist is recommended whenever they are suspected.

Factor XI deficiency—also known as plasma thromboplastin antecedent (PTA) deficiency or **hemophilia C**—is second only to von Willebrand's disease among bleeding disorders affecting females. The incidence of factor XI deficiency is 1 in 100,000. This disease follows an autosomal recessive pattern of inheritance and occurs more frequently among members of some ethnic groups. For example, in Ashkenazi Jews, the incidence is approximately 1 in 10,000. Several genetic changes are known to be associated with factor XI deficiency, each of which induces a variable effect on bleeding. Factor XI deficiency is usually diagnosed after injury-related bleeding. Symptoms are typically mild, and almost half of all patients are completely asymptomatic. Affected individuals do not experience spontaneous bleeding or hemarthroses but may have bruising, nosebleeds, blood in their urine, and prolonged bleeding after childbirth. Most affected persons do not require treatment.

Chapter Summary

» Hemophilia A ("classic hemophilia") is a bleeding disorder caused by mutations in the *F8* gene, which encodes for factor VIII.

» Hemophilia B ("Christmas disease") is a bleeding disorder caused by mutations in the *F9* gene, which encodes for factor IX.

» *F8* and *F9* gene mutations are inherited in an X-linked recessive pattern, with only males affected by the resulting hemophilia; females are carriers of the mutations but rarely develop the disease itself.

» Hemophiliacs frequently present with spontaneous bleeding into joints (hemarthroses) and muscles (hematomas) and experience variable degrees of prolonged or abnormal bleeding.

» Screening tests for hemophilia include prolonged activated partial thromboplastin time with normal prothrombin time, normal bleeding time, and normal fibrinogen levels.

» Diagnosis of hemophilia is made by specific factor assays.

» Evaluation of a person with newly diagnosed hemophilia A or B should include identification of the specific mutation, a personal history of bleeding, family history of bleeding, a thorough musculoskeletal evaluation, associated disease screenings, and baseline laboratory tests.

» Factor VIII concentrate and nasal desmopressin are used to treat bleeding episodes and for maintenance therapy.

Chapter Review Questions

1. Hemophilia is a bleeding disorder caused by mutations in the _____ or _____ genes.

2. Generally, in an X-linked recessive pattern of inheritance, only _____ are affected.

3. A person with severe hemophilia often presents with _____ _____, _____, and _____.

4. Screening test results consistent with hemophilia that warrant further evaluation include _____, _____, _____, _____, and _____.

5. Treatment for severe and moderate hemophilia includes _____.

Bibliography

Bolton-Maggs, P. H., & Pasi, K. J. (2003). Haemophilias A and B. *Lancet, 361,* 1801–1809.

Comprehensive medical care: HTCs. (n.d.). Retrieved from https://www.hemophilia .org/Researchers-Healthcare-Providers/Comprehensive-Medical-Care-Hemophilia -Treatment-Centers

Hemophilia. (n.d.). *Genetics home reference.* Retrieved from https://ghr.nlm.nih.gov /condition/hemophilia

Konkle, B. A., Huston, H., & Nakaya Fletcher, S. (2017, June). Hemophilia A. Retrieved from https://www.ncbi.nlm.nih.gov/books/NBK1404/

Konkle, B. A., Huston, H., & Nakaya Fletcher, S. (2017, June). Hemophilia B. Retrieved from https://www.ncbi.nlm.nih.gov/books/NBK1495/

Pierce, G. F., Lillicrap, D., Pipe, S. W., & Vandendriessche, T. (2007). Gene therapy, bioengineered clotting factors and novel technologies for hemophilia treatment. *Journal of Thrombosis and Haemostasis, 5,* 901–906.

‹ Describe the etiology and various forms of sickle cell disease.
‹ Detail the symptoms associated with sickle cell disease.
‹ Discuss novel property mutations, heterozygote advantage, and ethnic variation of allelic frequency.
‹ Review the current treatment recommendations for sickle cell disease.

KEY TERMS

Anemia
Ethnic variation of allelic frequency
Hemoglobin C disease

Hemoglobin SC disease
Heterozygote advantage
Novel property mutation
Point mutation

Sickle cell trait
Target cell

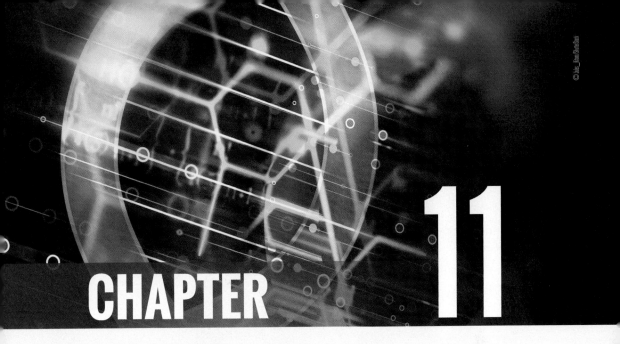

CHAPTER 11

Sickle Cell Disease

Sickle cell disease results from a **point mutation** in the *hemoglobin beta* (*HBB*) gene that causes a single change in the amino acid sequence and results in substitution of valine for glutamine in the β subunit of hemoglobin. This change confers a new property on hemoglobin but does not alter how this protein binds to oxygen in the blood. Such a change in a gene is known as a **novel property mutation**. The change in the amino acid sequence alters the solubility of the protein in blood, especially when it is deoxygenated, or the pH of the blood is reduced.

Normal adult hemoglobin is designated hemoglobin A (HbA), whereas adult sickle hemoglobin is designated as hemoglobin S (HbS). Hemoglobin exists in the blood as a tetramer of paired alpha chains and paired non-alpha chains. Normal hemoglobin contains 2 HbA chains. A sickle cell carrier has one chain of HbA and one chain of HbS (heterozygous), while an individual with sickle cell disease (SCD) has 2 chains of HbS (homozygous). The carrier state for HbS is correlated with lower rates of mortality among those who are typically of African and Mediterranean descent because the HbS allele decreases the risk of infection by malarial parasites endemic in those areas. This property is referred to as **heterozygote advantage**.

Sickle cell disease is inherited in an autosomal recessive pattern. Because recessive inheritance requires that both alleles be present for disease expression, both defective genes (SS) are needed for sickle cell disease to occur. When offspring inherit one recessive allele (S) and one normal allele (A), they become unaffected carriers (AS) (**Figure 11-1**). This heterozygous expression of HbS is known as **sickle cell trait**.

When red cells deoxygenate, the HbS chains are transformed into rigid polymers, which results in rigid, crescent-shaped red blood cells. These "sickled" cells are unable to flow freely through small vessels, which results in pain and ultimately vaso-occlusive infarctions in multiple organ systems. Pain,

FIGURE 11-1 Inheritance pattern of hemoglobin S.

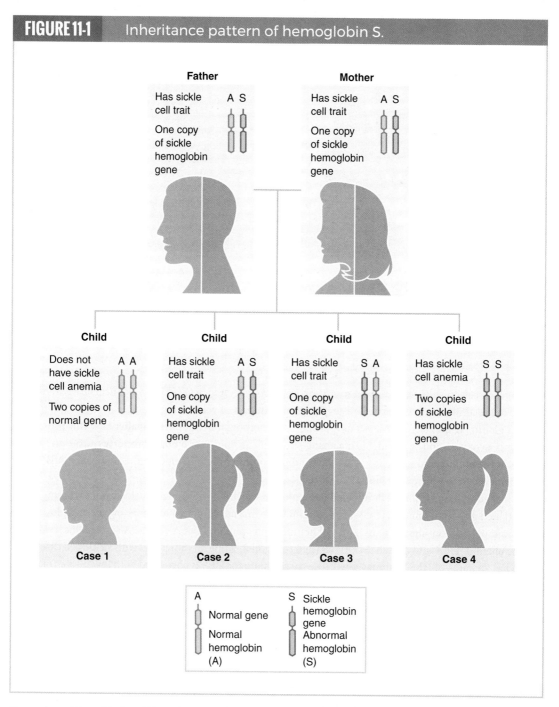

Reproduced from National Heart, Lung, and Blood Institute, Disease and Conditions Index. Available at https://www.nhlbi.nih.gov/health/health-topics/topics/sca/causes. Accessed January 31, 2017.

infections, and bone infarctions are hallmark clinical presentations of sickle cell disease, along with varying degrees of **anemia**. The vascular endothelium, white blood cells, inflammatory process, and coagulation cascade are also adversely affected.

Epidemiology

The overall prevalence of sickle cell disease in the United States is approximately 1 in 100,000 and varies by ethnic origin. Among African Americans, the incidence is about 1 in 365, whereas in Hispanic Americans the incidence is 1 in 16,300. The sickle cell mutation is also more common among persons whose ancestry is geographically connected to sub-Saharan Africa, Cuba, South America, Central America, Saudi Arabia, India, and the Mediterranean regions—a phenomenon known as **ethnic variation of allelic frequency**. An estimated 2 million Americans carry the sickle cell trait.

Phenotypic Features

The abnormal hemoglobin of sickle cell disease (SS) is detectable at birth. Consequently, all states in the United States now require newborn screening for HbS. Affected individuals who test negative on newborn screening or who bypass screening usually present with the disease within the first 2 years of life. Commonly, presenting symptoms in babies start around 5 months of age as fetal hemoglobin levels drop and are replaced by rising levels of hemoglobin S. Symptoms include failure to thrive, pain, anemia, splenomegaly, multiple chronic infections, and swelling of the extremities resulting from vaso-occlusion. Patients who present much more acutely—that is, "in crisis"—may have severe abdominal pain, stroke, acute chest syndrome, renal necrosis, leg ulcers, priapism (a painful persistent erection), or loss of vision due to a massive vaso-occlusive infarction.

The clinical manifestations of sickle cell disease are related directly or indirectly to hemolysis and vaso-occlusion. Hemolysis contributes to chronic anemia and subsequent jaundice. Rapid red blood cell destruction increases bilirubin and can lead to cholelithiasis; it also predisposes affected patients to aplastic crisis. Vaso-occlusion can cause tissue ischemia distal to the obstruction and result in tissue death. The brain, lungs, kidneys, and glans penis are frequently affected by this kind of vaso-occlusive disease.

The spleen is particularly susceptible to ischemia, with frequent episodes of splenomegaly being noted in patients with **hemoglobin SC disease**, whereas HbSS patients will undergo splenic auto-infarction during childhood. Hemoglobin SC disease occurs in people who have one copy of the gene for sickle cell disease and one copy of the gene for **hemoglobin C disease**. Symptoms associated with HbSC disease are similar to those of sickle cell disease but tend to be milder in some patients. A notable clinical differentiation between hemoglobin

KEY TERMS

Point mutation: the alteration of a single nucleotide to a different nucleotide.

Novel property mutation: a mutation that confers a new property on the protein product.

Heterozygote advantage: a mutated allele at the same locus as a normal allele that confers the advantage of protection against a disease and increases survival.

Sickle cell trait: the heterozygous state of the gene for hemoglobin S in sickle cell anemia.

Anemia: any condition in which the number of red blood cells per cubic millimeter (mm^3), the amount of hemoglobin in 100 mL of blood, and/or the volume of packed red blood cells per 100 mL of blood are less than normal.

Ethnic variation of allelic frequency: a situation in which frequency of mutated alleles is higher among certain ethnic groups than others.

TABLE 11-1	Typical Laboratory Findings in Sickle Cell Disease					
Genotype	**Hb (g/dL)†**	**HbS (%)**	**HbA (%)**	**HbA2 (%)**	**HbF (%)**	**HbC (%)**
SS	6–9	>90	0	<3.5	<10	0
Sβ⁰-thalassemia	7–9	>80	0	>3.5	<20	0
Sβ⁺-thalassemia	9–12	>60	10–30	>3.5	<20	0
SC	9–14	50	0	<3.5	<1.0	45

Hb: hemoglobin; HbS: sickle hemoglobin; HbA: normal adult hemoglobin; HbA2: minor variant of adult hemoglobin; HbF: fetal hemoglobin; HbC: hemoglobin variant that causes manifestations of SCD when paired with HbS.
†The hemoglobin values in this exhibit apply in the absence of a blood transfusion in the last 4 months, are not absolute, and are applicable to adults and children only (not newborns).
Reproduced from National Heart, Lung, and Blood Institute. (2014). *Evidence-based management of sickle cell disease: Expert panel report, 2014* (p. 2). Retrieved from https://www.nhlbi.nih.gov/health-pro/guidelines/sickle-cell-disease-guidelines

KEY TERMS

Hemoglobin SC disease: a type of hemoglobin-related disease that occurs in people who have one copy of the gene for sickle cell disease and one copy of the gene for hemoglobin C disease.

Hemoglobin C disease: a type of hemoglobin-related disease characterized by episodes of abdominal and joint pain, an enlarged spleen, and mild jaundice, but no severe crises. This disease occurs mostly in African Americans, who may show few symptoms of its presence.

SS and hemoglobin SC disease is that SC patients tend to have higher hemoglobin levels (9–14 g/dL) than SS patients (6.0–9.0 g/dL) (**Table 11-1**).

Painful swelling of the hands and feet may be the earliest manifestation of sickle cell disease in infants and young children. This is known as dactylitis. Acute chest syndrome occurs when vascular occlusion and inflammation affect the small vessels of the bronchial tree. Although the signs and symptoms of acute chest syndrome vary among patients, infiltrates may or may not be identified on chest x-ray, and patients may present with pain, respiratory illness, fever, and shortness of breath. Treatment of acute chest syndrome should be based on presenting clinical symptoms, given that accurate chest x-ray diagnosis will lag behind the clinical picture in many cases. The leading cause of death among adult patients with sickle cell disease is acute chest syndrome. Infection and fat emboli are also thought to play a role in bringing about this syndrome.

An acutely enlarged spleen with a hemoglobin level at least 2 g/dL below baseline is indicative of splenic sequestration of red blood cells. Low platelet count, abdominal pain, nausea, and vomiting may also be present. This presentation occurs most frequently in young children with sickle cell disease and may include a febrile illness.

When vessels in the brain become occluded, patients with sickle cell disease may present with acute stroke-like symptoms such as headache, hemiparesis, seizures, impaired speech, palsies involving cranial nerves, or mental status changes. The age range associated with stroke risk is bimodal—namely, children between the ages of 2 and 9 years and older adults are at greatest risk.

In the absence of a stroke, smaller infarctions may lead to gradual cognitive changes in persons with sickle cell disease.

Priapism is a frequent occurrence in males with sickle cell disease and may cause permanent tissue damage and impotence if not treated. Other problems associated with reduced blood supply include avascular necrosis of the femoral and/or humeral head, renal failure, cardiomyopathies, delayed growth, and superficial ulcers of the lower extremities. Even though patients with sickle cell trait do not usually have clinical symptoms, under some circumstances, a change in environmental conditions may lead to episodes of ischemia in these individuals. For example, exposures to high altitudes (such as in mountain hiking or flying in an unpressurized aircraft) and prolonged severe physical exertion can result in symptoms similar to those of sickle cell disease due to severe anoxia.

Clinical Diagnosis and Testing

Sickle cell disease is suspected when a young child presents with painful swelling of the hands and feet, a condition that is also known as "hand–foot syndrome," or dactylitis. Patients may also present with symptoms of anemia, infection, splenomegaly, or acute chest syndrome. Family history is helpful in establishing a working diagnosis.

The complete blood count (CBC) typically demonstrates a normocytic anemia with **target cells**. When hypoxemia is present, sickled cells are also reported. This finding should prompt the clinician to screen for HbS by using a solubility test. This test causes any HbS that is present to precipitate, but it does not differentiate between sickle cell disease and sickle cell trait because HbS is present in both states. Any screening test that is positive for HbS or other significant hemoglobinopathies in a newborn must be confirmed by 6 weeks of age. The presence of large quantities of HbS using hemoglobin electrophoresis is considered diagnostic for sickle cell disease. Similarly, electrophoresis is used to confirm sickle cell trait by identifying the presence of HbS, albeit in lower quantities than are present in sickle cell disease. Because of the high mortality rate associated with undiagnosed sickle cell disease in infants and young children, newborn screenings are now required for all infants born in a U.S. state or territory.

Other Sickle Cell Disorders

Sickle cell disease exists in many forms, but HbSS is the most common type, followed by HbSC. Nonsickling beta hemoglobin disorders such as thalassemia can coexist with a sickle cell disease mutation to cause clinically significant disease; these variants of sickle cell disease expression are known as sickle beta-plus thalassemia (HbSβ$^{+ \text{THAL}}$) and sickle beta-zero thalassemia (HbSβ$^{0 \text{THAL}}$) (**Table 11-2**).

> **KEY TERM**
>
> **Target cell:** an erythrocyte with a dark center surrounded by a light band that is encircled by a darker ring; thus, it resembles a shooting target.

TABLE 11-2	Hemoglobin Distribution in Sickle Cell Syndromes

Genotype	Clinical Diagnosis (Phenotype)	HbA[1]	HbS[2]	HbA2[3]	HbF[4]
AA	Normal	97–99%	0	1–2%	<1%
AS	Sickle trait	60%	40%	1–2%	<1%
SS	Sickle cell anemia	0	86–98%	1–3%	5–15%
Sβ⁰-thalassemia*	Sickle β-thalassemia	0	70–80%	3–5%	10–20%
Sβ⁺-thalassemia†	Sickle β-thalassemia	10–20%	60–75%	3–5%	10–20%
AS, α-thalassemia‡	Sickle trait	70–75%	25–30%	1–2%	<1%

1. HbA: hemoglobin A (adult).
2. HbS: hemoglobin S (sickle).
3. HbA2: hemoglobin A2 (adult 2).
4. HbF: hemoglobin F (fetal).
*Sβ⁰ THAL: sickle beta-zero thalassemia.
†Sβ⁺ THAL: sickle beta-plus thalassemia.
‡α-thalassemia: alpha thalassemia.
Reproduced from Papadakis, M. A., & McPhee, S. J. (2014). *Current medical diagnosis & treatment* (53rd ed., p. 487). Copyright © The McGraw-Hill Companies, Inc. All rights reserved.

Management and Treatment

Management of sickle cell disease primarily focuses on prevention of crises and management of symptoms. Patients should be counseled to avoid precipitating activities that might lead to sickle cell crisis, such as dehydration, physical stress, infection, change in altitude, and prolonged exposure to extreme temperatures of heat or cold. Symptoms associated with crises are addressed specifically, and a pain management plan should be developed for this possibility, which may involve the use of opiates and other analgesics. Broad-spectrum antibiotics are indicated when the patient presents with fever. It is important that affected individuals stay current on immunizations (i.e., influenza, pneumonia). Furthermore, patients should be counseled to seek immediate medical attention for signs and symptoms of crises so as to prevent complications.

Surveillance is individualized, but laboratory tests routinely include annual CBC, reticulocyte count, iron status, liver enzymes, bilirubin, blood urea nitrogen, creatinine, and urinalysis. Doppler studies of the brain to detect areas of decreased or increased flow, chest x-rays, pulmonary function testing, gallbladder ultrasound, and echocardiogram may be indicated depending upon the patient's status and age. Red cell transfusions of sickle negative and leukoreduced blood by simple or exchange transfusion can benefit at-risk patients by decreasing their risk of stroke or recurrent cerebrovascular accident (CVA), pulmonary hypertension, and painful crises. Conversely, repeated transfusions will result in iron overload, so iron and ferritin levels must be monitored closely and reduced before iron accumulates and causes permanent organ damage. Liver biopsy with iron dry-weight quantitation or liver MRI will provide the most accurate picture of the total body iron burden. Repeated or prolonged transfusion regimens can also result in allo-immunization, or the exposure to foreign antigens in the red blood cell unit. This condition results in circulating antibodies in the patient, making it more difficult to ensure future compatibility with donor red blood cell units.

Hydroxyurea is and has been the most commonly prescribed therapy for sickle cell disease since it was approved for use in this patient population in 1998. It works by multiple mechanisms. First, it improves red blood cell survival by inducing production of fetal hemoglobin (HgF) that is resistant to sickling. Second, it lowers the white blood cell count and arrests inflammatory processes. Third, it metabolizes into nitric oxide, which acts as a vasodilator to help improve blood flow and reduce the risk of stroke. The use of hydroxyurea has been shown to reduce the number of painful episodes, acute chest syndrome, and transfusions as well as to improve overall survival among persons with sickle cell disease. Multiple U.S. and international clinical trials have been under way, searching for additional ways to help this patient population with reducing crisis pain. A recently completed phase 2 study is promising, showing that monthly infusions of crizanlizumab (P-selectin antibody) significantly reduced the rates of sickle-related pain crisis in study patients. This is an exciting new route that needs additional study.

Allogeneic transplant is the only available curative treatment for sickle cell disease, but few patients have a suitable donor available. When a suitable donor is available, stem cell transplant has been reported to produce a disease-free survival rate as high as 85%, with the best outcomes reported in pediatric patients.

Genetic Counseling

When counseling high-risk individuals, it is important to consider other beta-chain disorders that may contribute to sickle cell disease. The carrier states for hemoglobinopathies other than HbS may be unknown in those persons who have never been screened for these abnormalities. The optimal time for counseling is during preconception family planning. When patients present after conception, early testing is important. Prenatal diagnosis for those at increased risk is possible through amniocentesis. However, because there is wide variation in clinical presentations among affected individuals, it is impossible to predict the extent or outcome of sickle cell disease.

Chapter Summary

» Sickle cell disease is caused by a mutation in the hemoglobin beta (HBB) gene, leading to a single change in amino acid sequence.

» Sickle cell disease typically presents in early childhood in the United States, identified through required newborn screening.

» The diagnosis of sickle cell disease is made from hemoglobin electrophoresis and other confirmatory testing after a positive screening test.

» Sickle cell trait is usually clinically silent, but it may produce symptoms when exacerbated by hypoxia.

» Mortality in sickle cell disease is related to the number and severity of crises; crises may lead to stroke, acute chest syndrome, complications of anemia, and infections.

» Surveillance guidelines are individualized depending on the patient's age and disease status.

» Hydroxyurea improves overall survival and reduces symptoms.

Chapter Review Questions

1. When the offspring inherit one affected recessive allele (S) and one normal allele (A), they become unaffected carriers (AS) and are said to have _____.

2. The mutation that causes sickle cell disease is more common among persons whose ancestry is connected to the following geographic regions: _____, _____, _____, _____, _____, _____, and _____.

3. The chance of two parents with sickle cell trait (HbAS) having a child with sickle cell disease (HbSS) is _____; this is described as a(n) _____ pattern of inheritance.

4. Clinical findings that raise suspicion for sickle cell disease in a young child include _____, _____, _____ and _____.

5. A mutation that confers a new property on the protein is called a _____ mutation.

Bibliography

Ashley-Koch, A., Yang, Q., & Olney, R.S. (2000). Sickle hemoglobin (HbS) allele and sickle cell disease: A HuGE Review. *American Journal of Epidemiology, 151*(9), 839–845.

Ataga, K. I., Kutlar, A., Kanter, J., Liles, D., Cancado, R., Friedrisch, J., . . . Rother, R. P. (2017). Crizanlizumab for the prevention of pain crisis in sickle cell disease. *New England Journal of Medicine, 376*, 429–439.

Bender, M. A. (2017, August). Sickle cell disease. Retrieved from https://www.ncbi.nlm.nih.gov/books/NBK1377/

Braunstein, E. M. (2010). Hemoglobin C, S-C, and E diseases. *Merck Manual.* https://www.merckmanuals.com/home/blood-disorders/anemia/hemoglobin-c,-s-c,-and-e-diseases

Centers for Disease Control and Prevention. (2016). *Sickle cell disease (SCD).* Retrieved from https://www.cdc.gov/ncbddd/sicklecell/data.html

Charache, S., Terrin, M. L., Moore, R. D., Dover, G. J., Barton, F. B., Eckert, S. V., . . . Bonds, D. R. (1995). Effect of hydroxyurea on the frequency of painful crisis in sickle cell anemia. *New England Journal of Medicine, 332*, 1317–1322. Retrieved from http://www.nejm.org/doi/full/10.1056/NEJM199505183322001#t=article

Hemoglobin S. (n.d.). In *Stedman's online medical dictionary*. Retrieved from http://www.stedmansonline.com

Jorde, L. B., Carey, J. C., Bamshad, M. J., & White, R. L. (2006). *Medical genetics* (3rd ed.). Philadelphia, PA: Mosby.

Linker, C. A. (2006). Blood. In L. M. Tierney, Jr., S. J. McPhee, & M. A. Papadakis (Eds.), *Current medical diagnosis and treatment* (45th ed., pp. 481–535). New York, NY: McGraw-Hill.

National Heart, Lung, and Blood Institute. (2014). *Evidence-based management of sickle cell disease: Expert panel report, 2014.* Retrieved from https://www.nhlbi.nih.gov/health-pro/guidelines/sickle-cell-disease-guidelines

Newborn Screening ACT Sheet [FS]: Sickle Cell Anemia (HbSS Disease or HbS/Beta Zero Thalassemia). (2012). Retrieved from http://www.acmg.net/PDFLibrary/Sickle-Cell-Anemia-HBss.pdf

Sickle cell disease. (n.d.). Retrieved from http://www.hematology.org/Patients/Anemia/Sickle-Cell.aspx

Sickle cell disease. (n.d.). Retrieved from https://www.nhlbi.nih.gov/health-topics/sickle-cell-disease

Tietz, N. W. (1995). *Clinical guide to laboratory tests* (3rd ed.). Philadelphia, PA: W.B. Saunders.

‹ Describe etiology and forms of hemochromatosis.
‹ Detail phenotypic features, symptoms, and physical examination findings associated with hemochromatosis.
‹ Discuss sex-influenced phenotype, variable expressivity, and penetrance.
‹ Review current treatment and surveillance recommendations for hemochromatosis.

KEY TERMS

Acute-phase reactant
Cardiomyopathy
Carrier
Chelating agent
Cirrhosis
Compound heterozygote
Hepatic ultrasound
Hepatitis
Hepatoma

Hepatomegaly
Hereditary hemochromatosis
Penetrance
Point mutation
Polymerase chain reaction (PCR)
Serum ferritin levels
Serum iron levels

Sex-influenced phenotype
Synergistic hepatotoxic effects
Therapeutic phlebotomy
Total iron-binding capacity (TIBC)
Transferrin
Transferrin saturation levels
Variable expressivity

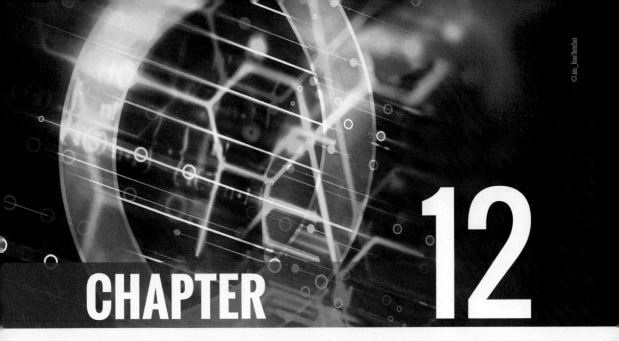

CHAPTER 12

Hemochromatosis

Hereditary hemochromatosis (type 1 HH) is an autosomal recessive disorder that is most commonly caused by a single mutation in the *HFE* gene. This mutation causes increased intestinal absorption of iron and results in increased iron deposits in body tissues such as those found in the liver, pancreas, skin, heart, and other organs—a phenomenon referred to as HFE-associated hereditary hemochromatosis (HFE-HH). In the United States, approximately 1 in 200 Caucasian persons are homozygous for the *HFE* mutation, while another 1 in 10 are heterozygous. Thus HFE-HH is the most common single-gene disorder among Caucasians in the United States. Male patients with HH manifest with symptoms of the disease approximately 10 times more frequently than females. Heterozygotes for recessive disorders are known as **carriers**.

Phenotypic Features

Although the clinical manifestations of HH are related to total body iron levels, the disease begins with increased serum iron concentration. Because persons with HH absorb excess iron over a period of years, clinical evidence of disease does not typically present until the affected individual is 40 years of age or older. The average body stores approximately 4 g of total iron in various forms. In symptomatic individuals with HH, total body iron increases at a rate of approximately 1 g per year, and levels may be over 10 times what is required for proper body functioning.

Accumulation of iron over time results in tissue injury and ultimate progression to **cirrhosis** of the liver and other organ failure. Cirrhosis is a degenerative liver disease characterized by formation of

KEY TERMS

Hereditary hemochromatosis: an autosomal recessive disorder usually caused by a single mutation in the *HFE* gene, which causes increased intestinal absorption of iron and results in increased iron storage in body tissues.

Carrier: a term used to describe heterozygotes in recessive disorders who do not express disease characteristics themselves but can pass the mutation on to their offspring.

Cirrhosis: a degenerative disease of the liver characterized by formation of fibrous tissue and scarring, resulting in the inhibition of normal cellular function.

Hepatomegaly: enlargement of the liver.

Penetrance: the proportion of individuals carrying a particular mutation who express an associated, observable trait.

scarring, fibrous tissue, and nodules along with abnormal cellular function. Although asymptomatic disease is common, the most common findings present at the time of diagnosis include fatigue, abnormal liver function tests, diabetes, and hyperpigmentation of the skin. Hyperpigmentation in HH results from a combination of iron deposits in the skin and increased melanin (skin pigment). In the past, hemochromatosis was referred to as "bronze diabetes" because of the common occurrence of insulin resistance and darkened skin coloration. Less common findings include an enlarged liver (**hepatomegaly**), abdominal pain, heart murmurs, conduction disturbances noted on electrocardiogram, hypothyroidism, hypogonadism (e.g., impotence in males) and arthritis.

Expression of disease symptoms varies among individuals with the same genetic mutation, with these variations reflecting differences in **penetrance** and **variable expressivity**. Penetrance describes the proportion of individuals carrying a particular mutation who express an associated, observable trait. It indicates the likelihood that symptoms will develop in the presence of a mutation. Variable expressivity describes the wide variation in types of symptoms and severity of symptoms observed when disease expression is present. However, disease expression can be accelerated by conditions causing decreased liver function, such as alcohol abuse and **hepatitis**. Many manifestations of HH resolve after treatment; others are nonreversible (**Table 12-1**).

TABLE 12-1	Clinical Presentation of Hereditary Hemochromatosis	
Reversible Manifestations		**Permanent Manifestations**
Abdominal pain		Arthritis
Abnormal liver function tests		Cirrhosis
Arrhythmia		Diabetes mellitus
Cardiomyopathy (unless severe)		Hepatocellular carcinoma
Hepatomegaly		Hypogonadism (if older than 40)
Infection		Hypothyroidism
Liver damage without cirrhosis		
Skin hyperpigmentation		

Phenotypic expression of HH is found in both men and women but is clinically expressed at a much greater frequency in men. The lower incidence of clinical expression in women is attributed to regular iron loss through the blood loss associated with menstruation. This difference in disease expression by gender is an example of a **sex-influenced phenotype**.

Genetics of HFE-Associated Hemochromatosis

The *HFE* gene associated with type 1 HH is located on the short arm of chromosome 6. Mutations caused by a single amino acid substitution are known as **point mutations**; the two most common point mutations in the *HFE* gene are designated as C282Y and H63D. Although iron overload may occur with any *HFE* mutation, the greatest risk is conferred with being homozygous for the C282Y mutation.

Over 80% of patients with HH are homozygous for the C282Y mutation, whereas only 1% are homozygous for the H63D mutation. Interestingly, up to 10% of HH cases are **compound heterozygotes**, having a combination of two mutations that may include C282Y, H63D, or other less common mutations.

Diagnosis

Because symptoms are often absent until late in the disease course, the diagnosis of HH relies principally on laboratory studies. These include findings of elevated **transferrin** saturation and serum ferritin concentrations. As mentioned in the phenotypic features section, abnormal serum liver enzymes may be identified, which indicate hepatic damage but are not specific to HH. Other findings suggestive of HH on history or physical examination should be considered, though they do not replace thoughtful laboratory testing in reaching a diagnosis of HH.

Under normal circumstances, 70% of iron in the body is present as hemoglobin in red blood cells. The remaining iron exists in the iron storage protein ferritin, as free iron, and as intracellular deposits known as hemosiderin. Intracellular deposits of hemosiderin damage the native tissues and are responsible for most of the manifestations of HH. Although most iron is obtained from the diet (i.e., through consumption of red meat), only 10% of all iron ingested in a typical Western diet is absorbed from the small intestine into the bloodstream. In the blood, iron is bound to the protein transferrin and then transported to the bone marrow, where it can be incorporated into hemoglobin molecules. Surplus iron can also be stored as ferritin in the liver, spleen, bone marrow, and muscles.

KEY TERMS

Variable expressivity: variation in disease symptoms among persons with the same mutation.

Hepatitis: inflammation of the liver causing impaired function as a result of toxins (e.g., alcohol, iron, drugs), autoimmune disorders, or infectious agents (viruses).

Sex-influenced phenotype: a phenotype expressed in both males and females but with different frequencies in the two sexes.

Point mutation: the alteration of a single nucleotide to a different nucleotide.

Compound heterozygote: an individual who carries two different mutant alleles for the same gene.

Transferrin: the globulin protein that transports iron to the bone marrow.

TABLE 12-2	Summary of Expected Serum Iron Values in Hereditary Hemochromatosis	
Assay	**Assay Explanation**	**Result**
Serum iron	Free iron in serum	Normal to increased
Serum ferritin	Iron storage protein	Increased
Total iron-binding capacity	Transferrin available to bind iron	Normal to decreased
Serum transferrin saturation	Transferrin bound to iron in serum	Increased

Tietz, N. W. (1995). *Clinical guide to laboratory tests* (3rd ed.). Philadelphia, PA: W. B. Saunders.

KEY TERMS

Serum iron levels: a measure of the amount of unbound iron that has been transported to the blood.

Serum ferritin levels: a measure that estimates the amount of iron stored in the body.

Total iron-binding capacity (TIBC): a measure of all proteins available to bind iron and an indirect measure of transferrin levels.

Transferrin saturation levels: the portion of transferrin bound to iron. This value is found by dividing the serum iron by the total iron-binding capacity.

Laboratory studies for HH typically include **serum iron levels, serum ferritin levels, total iron binding capacity (TIBC)**, and **transferrin saturation levels** (**Table 12-2**). Serum iron identifies the amount of free iron that was recently absorbed from the diet but before it has become bound to transferrin. Normal serum iron levels are often detected in HH because of storage of the majority of iron in other forms. The amount of stored iron in the body is estimated by the serum level of ferritin, the protein that stores iron. The TIBC is a measure of all proteins that are available to bind iron. It indirectly measures the amount of transferrin present, whereas transferrin saturation represents the portion of transferrin bound to iron. Transferrin saturation is determined by dividing serum iron by the TIBC:

$$\text{Transferrin saturation (\%)} = \frac{\text{Serum iron level} \times 100\%}{\text{TIBC}}$$

Approximately 80% of all persons with an *HFE* mutation will have a fasting transferrin saturation above the normal maximum of 45% (females) to 50% (males), with higher values often observed in males. Transferrin saturation rates are not related to age, however, and they do not correlate with disease symptomology or severity. Because this value is directly correlated with the iron burden, serum transferrin saturation has a high sensitivity and specificity for HH: A threshold transferrin saturation of 45% is sensitive for detecting HH. Elevated transferrin saturation levels are typically the earliest phenotypic manifestation of HH, preceding clinical manifestations of the disease.

Serum ferritin levels increase progressively over time in individuals with HH. Elevated serum ferritin levels are sensitive predictors of disease but are not specific to HH because any inflammatory process may elevate serum ferritin. Thus, this biomarker is referred to as an **acute-phase reactant**. Serum ferritin tends to increase or decrease in the same direction as iron stores and provides a rough estimate of total body iron.

When both transferrin saturation and serum ferritin are elevated, these findings have a higher combined sensitivity and specificity in supporting the diagnosis of HH than using either value alone. Importantly, cirrhosis (which may be caused by HH) is an independent risk factor for the development of hepatocellular carcinoma. Although liver biopsy can be performed to confirm a diagnosis of HH or to diagnose cirrhosis and/or hepatocellular carcinoma, imaging and genetic testing have largely replaced it. When imaging of the liver is desired, **hepatic ultrasound** is typically performed; magnetic resonance imaging (MRI) is the most sensitive technique. Both imaging techniques can detect solid tumors or cystic changes in the liver. Ultrasonography is recommended for patients with cirrhosis (including from HH) because of the increased risk of hepatic cancers such as primary hepatocellular carcinoma (also known as **hepatoma**).

Genetic Testing and Counseling

The wide availability of *HFE* gene testing has largely eliminated the need for liver biopsy. It identifies the C282Y and H63D mutations and can determine if an individual is homozygous, is heterozygous, or has normal *HFE* alleles. This testing is performed by **polymerase chain reaction (PCR)** using a whole blood sample, which makes it relatively affordable compared to other genetic tests. This technique is very useful for screening family members of an affected person.

Although most parents of HH-affected individuals are heterozygous for the *HFE* mutation and do not develop the disease themselves, the iron studies detailed previously may also be used to screen for disease expression. However, it is important to note that carriers may have abnormal test results. Each sibling of an affected person has a 25% chance of being affected and a 50% risk of being a carrier. Because the disease does not become manifest until later in adult life, identifying those persons at risk for iron overload may help to reduce complications and improve overall survival. These factors make it reasonable to screen all adult patients with any family history of iron overload or signs and symptoms of HH. Once an individual is diagnosed with HH, all adult family members should be assessed for evidence of iron overload. Pediatric screening is not recommended.

Management and Treatment

Therapeutic phlebotomy, which involves the removal of a portion of the affected individual's blood, is the treatment of choice for iron overload in symptomatic patients, as well as asymptomatic patients with a serum ferritin

---

KEY TERMS

Acute-phase reactant: any substance that can be elevated in inflammatory processes.

Hepatic ultrasound: an imaging study of the liver used to detect the presence of tissue changes such as tumors, abscesses, and cysts.

Hepatoma: the most common type of nonmetastatic liver cancer; also known as primary hepatocellular carcinoma.

Polymerase chain reaction (PCR): repeated cycles of DNA denaturation, renaturation with primer oligonucleotide sequences, and replication, resulting in exponential growth in the number of copies of the DNA sequence located between the primers.

Therapeutic phlebotomy: removal of a portion of the blood volume to alleviate symptoms.

KEY TERMS

Chelating agent: a drug that binds to a substance in the body, rendering it unable to be used and/or less harmful to the body.

Synergistic hepatotoxic effects: toxic effects that work together such that the total toxic effect is greater than the sum of the two (or more) single effects.

greater than 1,000 μg/L or an elevated fasting transferrin saturation. This intervention is a simple, effective, and inexpensive method to reduce the iron burden in patients with HH.

Therapeutic phlebotomy is routinely initiated when clinical symptoms of HH are present, with 400–500 mL of blood being removed on each occasion. In most patients, this volume of whole blood effectively removes 160–200 mg of iron. Most specialists recommend weekly phlebotomy until the serum ferritin level reaches approximately 50 μg/L and the transferrin saturation is less than 50%. Continued measurement of serum ferritin levels should be performed to monitor the therapeutic effects of phlebotomy. Men often require the removal of two to four times more blood volume than women to achieve the desired results. Once these target levels are achieved, maintenance phlebotomy may be performed four times annually in men and twice annually in women to prevent the reaccumulation of iron. Serum ferritin levels should be reassessed at these same follow-up intervals. **Chelating agents** are drugs that bind to iron and prevent its use or deposition in the body. These are rarely needed in patients with HH because of the efficacy of phlebotomy but may be considered in special cases.

Liver transplant is the only treatment for HH patients with end-stage liver disease. Historically, posttransplant survival in this patient population has been poor, but this has greatly improved in recent years.

Dietary management should involve avoidance of iron-containing supplements and limited intake of foods that are high in iron, such as red meat. Consumption of excessive amounts of vitamin C should also be avoided—this water-soluble vitamin increases absorption of dietary iron. Patients with impaired hepatic function should avoid drinking alcohol because iron and alcohol have **synergistic hepatotoxic effects**.

Associated Syndromes

Primary iron overload syndromes are defined by an increased absorption of iron from a normal diet. Most are types of HH that are unrelated to mutations in the *HFE* gene. For example, type 2 HH results from mutations in the *HJV*, or *HAMP* gene. Although this disease has characteristics that are similar to those of HFE-HH, its clinical manifestations are often more severe and appear at an earlier age. TFR2-related HH (type 3 HH) is caused by mutations in the *TFR2* gene; incidence of this disease is higher in certain Italian populations. Like type 2 HH, type 3 HH presents at an earlier age but is not as severe as type 2. Both type 1 and type 2 HH are inherited in an autosomal recessive pattern. Ferroportin-related iron overload (type 4 HH) is caused by mutations in the *SLC40A1* gene and is inherited in an autosomal dominant pattern. African (Bantu) iron overload is a predisposition to iron overload that is exacerbated by excessive intake of iron. Neonatal hemochromatosis is a severe iron overload syndrome that begins in utero and is often fatal. To date, no specific mutations or inheritance patterns have been identified for neonatal hemochromatosis.

Secondary iron overload syndromes include conditions or diseases that result in specific tissue damage and iron overload from increased iron intake. Culprits include iron that is either ingested in dietary forms or absorbed from iron cookware, as well as other sources of iron such as intramuscular supplements or blood transfusions. Persons at risk for secondary iron overload syndromes include individuals with alcoholic liver disease, viral hepatitis, porphyria cutanea tarda, rheumatoid arthritis, sickle cell disease, thalassemia, and other chronic anemias that require transfusion therapy.

> **KEY TERM**
>
> **Cardiomyopathy:** a disease of the myocardium (heart muscle) that has variable etiologies and clinical presentations.

Chapter Summary

» Hereditary hemochromatosis is most often caused by point mutations in the *HFE* gene and is inherited in an autosomal recessive pattern.

» HFE-associated hereditary hemochromatosis is relatively common, affecting 1 in every 200 Caucasian persons in the United States.

» Males with HH are more likely to manifest with symptoms of the disease compared with females. This is largely due to regular blood loss during menstruation.

» The mutations responsible for HH result in increased iron absorption and are characterized by increased iron storage in body tissues such as the liver, pancreas, skin, and heart.

» Hemochromatosis frequently presents with nonspecific symptoms such as abdominal pain, fatigue, and arthralgias.

» Factors that may raise clinical suspicion for advanced-stage iron overload include hepatomegaly, hepatic cirrhosis, hepatocellular carcinoma, diabetes mellitus, **cardiomyopathy**, hypogonadism, arthritis, and hyperpigmented skin.

» Serum ferritin and transferrin saturation have the greatest sensitivity and specificity as biomarkers for hereditary hemochromatosis.

» Persons with cirrhosis (which may be caused by HH) are at increased risk for developing hepatocellular carcinoma.

» Therapeutic phlebotomy is the treatment of choice for iron overload.

Chapter Review Questions

1. Most hereditary hemochromatosis (HH) is associated with an HFE mutation and is inherited in a _____ pattern with a disease incidence of _____ in the United States.

2. The most common findings at the time of diagnosis in patients with HH are _____, _____, _____, and _____.

3. Laboratory testing provides evidence of iron overload and would demonstrate elevated levels of _____ and _____ _____.

4. Organs that may be harmed in the setting of iron overload (as in HH) include the _____, _____, _____, and _____.

5. _____ is the standard treatment for patients with HH that have symptoms or markedly elevated iron stores.

Bibliography

Acton, R. T., Barton, J. C., Passmore, L. V., Adams, P. C., Speechly, M. R., Dawkins, F. W., . . . Castro, O. (2006). Relationship of serum ferritin, transferring saturation, and *HFE* mutations and self-reported diabetes in the Hemochromatosis and Iron Overload Screening (HEIRS) study. *Diabetes Care, 29*(9), 2084–2089.

Adams, P. C., Reboussin, D. M., Barton, J. C., McLaren, C. R., Eckfeldt, J. H., McLaren, G. D., . . . Sholinsky, P. (2005). Hemochromatosis and iron-overload screening in a racially diverse population. *New England Journal of Medicine, 352,* 1769–1778.

Brandhagen, D. J., Fairbanks, V. F., & Baldus, W. (2002). Recognition and management of hereditary hemochromatosis. *American Family Physician, 65*(5), 853–860.

Imperatore, G., Pinsky, L. E., Motulsky, A., & Reyes, M. (2003). Hereditary hemochromatosis: Perspectives of public health, medical genetics, and primary care. *Genetics in Medicine, 5*(1), 1–8.

Iron Studies. (n.d.). In *Stedman's online medical dictionary.* Retrieved from http://www.stedmansonline.com

Morrison, E. D., Brandhagen, D. J., Phatak, P. D., Barton, J. C., Krawitt, E. L., El-Serag, H. B., . . . Kowdley, K. V. (2003). Serum ferritin level predicts advanced hepatic fibrosis among U.S. patients with phenotypic hemochromatosis. *Annals of Internal Medicine, 138,* 627–633.

Schmitt, B., Golub, R. M., & Green, R. (2005). Screening primary care patients for hereditary hemochromatosis with transferrin saturation and serum ferritin level: Systematic review for the American College of Physicians. *Annals of Internal Medicine, 143,* 522–536.

Scrier, S. L., & Bacon, B. R. (2018a). Approach to the patient with suspected iron overload. *UpToDate.* Retrieved from https://www.uptodate.com/contents/approach-to-the-patient-with-suspected-iron-overload

Scrier, S. L., & Bacon, B. R. (2018b). Clinical manifestations and diagnosis of hereditary hemochromatosis. *UpToDate.* Retrieved from https://www.uptodate.com/contents/clinical-manifestations-and-diagnosis-of-hereditary-hemochromatosis

Scrier, S. L., & Bacon, B. R. (2018c). Genetics of hereditary hemochromatosis. *UpToDate*. Retrieved from https://www.uptodate.com/contents/genetics-of -hereditary-hemochromatosis

Scrier, S. L., & Bacon, B. R. (2018d). Management of patients with hereditary hemochromatosis. *UpToDate*. Retrieved from https://www.uptodate.com/contents /management-of-patients-with-hereditary-hemochromatosis

Scrier, S. L., & Bacon, B. R. (2018e). Screening for hereditary hemochromatosis. *UpToDate*. Retrieved from https://www.uptodate.com/contents/screening-for -hereditary-hemochromatosis

Seckington, R., & Powell, L. (2015, September). *HFE*-associated hereditary hemochromatosis. Retrieved from https://www.ncbi.nlm.nih.gov/books/NBK1440/

Tietz, N. W. (1995). *Clinical guide to laboratory tests* (3rd ed.). Philadelphia, PA: W. B. Saunders.

CHAPTER OBJECTIVES

‹ Describe the etiology and various forms of cystic fibrosis.
‹ Describe related disorders, such as congenital absence of vas deferens.
‹ Detail phenotypic features, symptoms, and physical examination findings associated with cystic fibrosis.
‹ Discuss variable expressivity, environmental modifiers, and genetic modifiers.
‹ Review current surveillance and treatment recommendations for cystic fibrosis.

KEY TERMS

Azoospermia
Biliary cirrhosis
Cor pulmonale

Cystic fibrosis-related diabetes mellitus
Meconium ileus

Portal hypertension
Steatorrhea
Varices

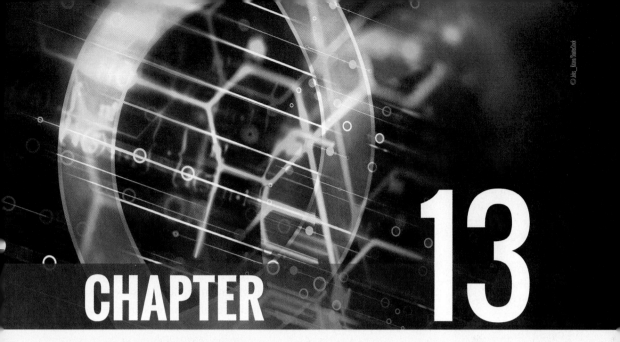

CHAPTER 13

Cystic Fibrosis

Cystic fibrosis (CF) is a disorder affecting the *cystic fibrosis transmembrane conductance regulator* (*CFTR*) gene, which controls the chloride channels and is regulated by cyclic adenosine monophosphate. These chloride channels are present on epithelial cells in multiple organ systems. Although the most common cause of morbidity associated with CF is pulmonary disease, dysfunction of the exocrine pancreas, intestines, male genitourinary tract, hepatobiliary system, and exocrine glands are also common features of this disease. A mutation in the *CFTR* gene has been shown to cause this disease.

Inheritance of CF follows an autosomal recessive pattern; thus, two copies of the mutated gene are required to cause disease. Among Caucasians in the United States, CF is the most common lethal inherited disorder. The disease incidence is 1 in 3,200 live births; the frequency of carriers in the U.S. population is approximately 1 in 25. CF is more common in persons of Northern European descent and occurs in lower frequencies among other ethnic populations.

Phenotypic Features

CF is a diagnosis most commonly made in early childhood, usually during the first year of life. In approximately 5% of cases, patients who are mildly symptomatic have been diagnosed as adults. Failure to thrive and/or poor growth rate is a common finding in children. It may be due to malabsorption associated with pancreatic insufficiency, increased caloric expenditure due to chronic infection, or both. The majority of patients with CF suffer from chronic pulmonary infections. In patients with CF, the pulmonary system is unable to mount a successful defense against the most common pathogens. This leads to sinusitis in the upper airways and bronchitis in the bronchial tree. The most commonly isolated pathogens in chronic sinus infection and pneumonia are *Staphylococcus aureus* and *Pseudomonas aeruginosa*. Concomitant fungal infections with *Aspergillus fumigates* occur in approximately 10% of CF patients. In the upper airways of persons with CF, nasal polyps, nosebleeds, and chronic sinus infections that are resistant to first-line antibiotics are common.

In the lower airways of CF patients, thick mucous production and neutrophilic inflammation build up to cause airway obstruction. High concentration of DNA in airway secretions (due to chronic airway inflammation and autolysis of neutrophils) increases sputum viscosity. Clinically, this process manifests as a chronic cough with or without sputum production and dyspnea on exertion. After the acute illness subsides, chronic bronchitis persists because of structural changes that have occurred in the airway. Eventually, the functional lung parenchyma is replaced with nonfunctional tissues such as cysts, abscesses, and fibrosis. This effect increases alveolar resistance and results in high blood pressure in the pulmonary artery and the right side of the heart. A sustained high pressure will eventually lead to right-sided heart failure, known as **cor pulmonale**.

During periods of acute infection, hemoptysis (coughing up blood) is a common presenting feature of CF. The chronic inflammation, structural changes, and increased pressure associated with this disease all contribute to damage in the vascular beds. The goal of patients with CF in acute exacerbations is to prevent them from getting intubated. Either chronic blood loss or multiple episodes of massive hemoptysis can result in iron-deficiency anemia. Patients who retain mucus (especially in the upper lobes) get chest x-rays. The physical exam may indicate digital clubbing and increased anterior-posterior diameter. Pulmonary function tests (PFTs) often show a mixed obstructive and restrictive pattern, along with respiratory acidosis. The primary cause of death in those with CF is respiratory failure.

Pancreatic involvement and gastrointestinal malabsorption are also commonly associated with CF. The pancreas is affected when thickened secretions obstruct the pancreatic ducts, which can lead to inflammation and pancreatitis. Some patients will maintain sufficient pancreatic function with mild inflammation, whereas others will lose total pancreatic function. Chronic obstruction of the pancreatic ducts may eventually cause the pancreatic tissues to become fibrotic, resulting in pancreatic insufficiency and decreased or absent digestive enzyme (e.g., amylase, lipase) production. Clinically, this phenomenon is manifested as dietary fats being excreted in the stool (**steatorrhea**) rather than being digested and absorbed. The inability to digest or absorb nutrients in turn leads to a decline in growth rate, disorders of blood coagulation, skin rashes, and anemia. Pancreatic insufficiency and malabsorption may be the only symptoms associated with CF in some patients, with approximately 10% of patients developing only pancreatic insufficiency without pulmonary disease.

Although the exocrine pancreas is most often affected by CF-related changes, the endocrine pancreas may also become involved. Both insulin secretion and the number of islet cells are reduced when pancreatic fibrosis occurs. Additionally, peripheral insulin resistance has been observed in some patients. When this condition occurs, it is referred to as **cystic fibrosis-related diabetes mellitus**. Although it may present as early as adolescence, its incidence is typically increased in adulthood.

Hepatobiliary disease has a similar pathology to pancreatic disease in patients with CF, in that obstruction of the biliary tract due to thickened mucus can lead to congestion of the liver or **biliary cirrhosis**. As damage to the liver progresses, the patient may experience **portal hypertension** and develop **varices**. Liver disease is the second-leading cause of mortality (after pulmonary disease) in patients with CF.

Meconium ileus affects approximately 20% of newborns with CF. This type of intestinal obstruction (ileus) is caused by the presence of unusually thick fetal waste products (meconium). Under normal circumstances, pancreatic enzymes, such as trypsin, are able to break down the meconium, allowing it to be passed in the feces of the newborn. In the absence of this enzymatic activity (characteristic of CF), the dense meconium is retained in the fetal intestines.

Almost all CF-affected males are infertile because of the absence of spermatozoa (**azoospermia**). This results from the congenital absence of the vas deferens or other supportive structures. Congenital absence of the vas deferens can also occur as the only feature of a *CFTR* mutation in men without pulmonary or gastrointestinal symptoms. Females with CF are generally ovulatory but may experience difficulty becoming pregnant if they have abnormal cervical mucus.

Overall, there is a wide variation among affected individuals in terms of the constellation of symptoms, age at presentation, organ system manifestation, severity, and progression of CF. As a result, CF may initially be misdiagnosed as celiac disease, pancreatitis, asthma, or chronic bronchitis. Physical findings are not consistent among affected family members, but rather depend on the severity of *CFTR* mutations, modifier genes, and environmental factors.

Genetics

The *CFTR* gene is the only known gene associated with CF; to date, more than 1,000 different mutations in this gene have been identified. The *CFTR* gene is located on chromosome 7. Normally, this gene carries instructions for an integral membrane protein that regulates chloride channels in epithelial cells. Under normal physiological conditions, chloride is excreted while excess sodium uptake is inhibited. This process maintains the appropriate water balance in secretions. However, in *CFTR* mutations this process is disrupted. In

KEY TERMS

Portal hypertension: elevation of pressure in the hepatic portal circulation due to cirrhosis or other fibrotic changes in liver tissue. When pressure exceeds 10 mm Hg, collateral circulation may develop to maintain venous return from structures drained by the portal vein; engorgement of collateral veins can lead to esophageal varices and, less often, caput medusae.

Varices: an enlarged and tortuous vein, artery, or lymphatic vessel.

Meconium ileus: obstruction of the intestines due to retention of a dark green waste product (meconium) that is normally passed shortly after a child's birth.

Azoospermia: the absence of spermatozoa in the semen.

the lungs, this disruption causes defective chloride transport across the membrane (the primary defect) and enhanced sodium absorption (the secondary defect). These changes in ion transport lead to a net increase in water absorption, thinning of the airway surface liquid, and decreased ciliary clearance. In turn, the ability of bacteria to adhere to airway surfaces, proliferate, and resist phagocytosis is enhanced by these changes.

Deletions, nonsense mutations, frameshift mutations, and splice site mutations of the *CFTR* gene result in the complete absence of a functional *CFTR* and represent the majority of CF mutations. However, missense mutations appear to only partially alter the function of *CFTR*. The amount of functional *CFTR* seems to determine the clinical presentation and course of disease (**Table 13-1**). Missense mutations often present later in life and may be associated with a milder disease course. It is this variety of mutations in the *CFTR* gene that is responsible for the variable clinical phenotypes.

The *CFTR* mutations leading to CF also vary widely among affected kindred and are often scattered across the gene (genetic heterogeneity). Mutations can result in qualitative defects (affecting protein function) or quantitative defects (affecting the amount of functional protein present) of the protein. Within families, variable expressivity of the symptoms is observed. Some affected individuals have multiple or severe symptoms, whereas others exhibit fewer or milder symptoms. It is important to note that the degree of

TABLE 13-1	Relationship between the Amount of Functional *CFTR* Gene Produced and Phenotypic Expression from *CFTR* Mutations	

Percentage of Normal *CFTR* Function	Manifestations of Cystic Fibrosis
<1%	Classic disease
<4.5%	Progressive pulmonary disease
<5%	Clinically demonstrable sweat abnormality
<10%	Congenital absence of the vas deferens (male infertility)
10–49%	No known abnormality
50–100%	No known abnormality (asymptomatic carriers)

CFTR: cystic fibrosis transmembrane conductance regulator
Data from www.cysticfibrosismedicine.com.

severity in one affected individual does not dictate the degree of severity in the offspring of that individual.

CF is inherited in an autosomal recessive pattern. For Caucasians without a family history of CF, the risk of being a carrier of a *CFTR* mutation is 1 in 25. The risk of a couple having a child with the disease is approximately 1 in 2,500. For couples who have one child affected by CF, the risk of CF appearing in future offspring is 1 in 4. Therefore, the risk of inheriting the *CFTR* mutation in two alleles and developing the disease is 25% if both parents are carriers.

Diagnosis

The diagnosis of CF may be established in individuals with at least one phenotypic feature and a mutation in *CFTR* as evidenced by one of the following: (1) presence of two mutations in the *CFTR* gene; (2) two abnormal quantitative sweat chloride tests (by the quantitative pilocarpine iontophoresis method); or (3) two transepithelial nasal potential difference measurements. The detection rate for *CFTR* mutations varies depending on the test method employed and the ethnicity of the patient. The quantitative pilocarpine iontophoresis for sweat chloride (commonly referred to as the sweat chloride test) is considered the primary test for the diagnosis of CF. This assay reportedly has an accuracy of 90%. Molecular genetic testing is indicated when confirming a positive sweat chloride test, when sweat chloride testing is inconclusive, or when sweat chloride testing is unavailable. In the rare instance that both sweat chloride testing and mutation testing are either not available or inconclusive, transepithelial nasal potential difference measurements may be used to diagnose CF.

In some special circumstances, the molecular testing method may be used as the first diagnostic study. For example, this technique may be employed for prenatal testing in a high-risk pregnancy, diagnosis in a fetus demonstrating an echogenic bowel on ultrasound, and assessment of a symptomatic newborn or another individual who does not produce adequate volumes of sweat. It is also indicated as the initial test for siblings of an affected proband.

Diagnosis of CF can be made even without phenotypic expression by using newborn screenings and prenatal testing of the amniotic fluid. *CFTR* mutation testing can be performed using the blood of newborns as well as amniotic fluid taken from their mothers. Sweat chloride testing and transepithelial nasal potential difference are also appropriate screening tests for newborns. In many cases, newborn screening is performed using the immunoreactive trypsinogen assay, which is part of a screening panel routinely applied to blood specimens shortly after birth.

CF should always be kept in the back of your mind when a patient fails to respond to conventional respiratory therapy.

Genetic Testing and Counseling

Because all *CFTR* mutations are inherited in an autosomal recessive pattern, the siblings of an affected proband have a 1 in 4 chance of being affected by CF disease and a 1 in 2 chance of being a carrier of a CF-related mutation. Carriers are generally asymptomatic. Most affected individuals with two mutated alleles become symptomatic early in life, so very few parents are initially tested and diagnosed as a result of positive newborn screening. The American College of Medical Geneticists recommends that carrier screening for CF be offered to all Caucasians of non-Jewish descent and Ashkenazi Jews. This assessment is accomplished using a panel of 23 different known mutations that occur in high frequencies among the U.S. population.

Management, Treatment, and Surveillance

Increased overall survival and enhanced quality of life can be best achieved for those affected with CF when a comprehensive treatment plan is developed following an early diagnosis. This plan should include replacement of pancreatic enzymes and fat-soluble vitamins by dietary supplementation, use of bronchodilators to maintain patent airways, antibiotics for respiratory infections, administration of mucous-thinning agents, pain management, anti-inflammatory agents such as ibuprofen, respiratory therapy, chest physiotherapy, and even lung transplant. Attention should be focused on treating disease manifestations as well as preventing future complications.

Treatment of disease manifestations often addresses pulmonary complications by using antibiotics, anti-inflammatory agents, inhaled recombinant DNase, inhaled bronchodilators, mucolytic agents, and chest physiotherapy. Lung transplant may be possible in some patients; however, the three-year survival rate following a transplant is 55%. Sinus-related complications can be treated using anti-inflammatory agents, antibiotics, and surgical interventions. Chest physiotherapy involves external manual percussion of the chest wall, handheld devices that percuss the chest wall, or inflatable vests that vibrate the chest wall. All these modalities function to move mucus in the lungs to physically clear obstructed airways and are usually performed at least twice daily. Collectively, these treatments optimize pulmonary function by opening airways, thinning sputum, allowing secretions to be expectorated, and treating inflammatory and infectious components in as much of the pulmonary surface area as possible.

Immunizations for common pulmonary pathogens are also indicated as preventive measures, including pertussis, measles, varicella, *Haemophilus influenzae* type B, *Streptococcus pneumonia*, respiratory syncytial virus, and influenza virus. Regularly scheduled physical examinations that include PFTs, chest x-rays, and sputum cultures are important components of pulmonary surveillance. All respiratory irritants such as smoke, dust, and fumes should be strictly avoided.

Gastrointestinal complications require nutritional support and enzyme replacement therapy. Indeed, maintaining good growth rates and body weight is crucial to overall health. Patients with a low body mass index may benefit from increased caloric intake and use of high-fat supplements under the supervision of a nutritionist specializing in CF. Pancreatic insufficiency can result in low serum protein levels and secondary edema. Pancreatic enzyme and fat-soluble vitamin supplementation are mainstays of prevention. Annual screening of blood glucose levels for CF-related diabetes should be performed; if present, this disease should be managed by an endocrinologist.

Biliary cirrhosis should be suspected when hepatic enzymes (i.e., alanine transaminase, aspartate transferase) are elevated. Obstruction of the bile duct can be managed through use of oral bile acids, which dissolve and prevent gallstones. Baseline bone density should be determined in adolescence or as early as possible and repeated annually to detect evolving osteoporosis. Maintaining overall hydration status is also important because decreased total body water can exacerbate thickening of secretions and associated complications. Regular physical exercise has also been shown to improve bone health and patency of airways.

Currently, there is no cure for CF. For now, delaying respiratory tract infections and earlier lung transplantation are the most promising therapies. Newer therapies currently under investigation involve methods to bypass *CFTR* in the ion transport process and improve *CFTR* protein function.

The improved survival of women with CF is responsible for an increase in the pregnancy rates among these patients. Women with CF should receive prenatal counseling and should be managed by a team of professionals that includes a CF specialist, a dietician, and a high-risk obstetrician.

Associated Syndromes

Males without pulmonary or gastrointestinal manifestations of CF may have congenital absence of the vas deferens (CAVD), a condition that is commonly identified during evaluation for infertility. The diagnosis of *CFTR*-related CAVD may be established in males with low semen volume, low sperm count, absent or malformed vas deferens on physical examination or imaging, and at least one *CFTR* mutation. Typically, those affected with *CFTR*-related CAVD produce semen that has a volume less than 2 mL (normal 3–5 mL), pH < 7.0 (normal > 8.0), elevated citric acid concentration, elevated acid phosphatase concentration, low fructose concentration, and failure to coagulate. A low sperm count (less than 5 million sperm per milliliter of semen) may be a separate indicator or occur in conjunction with low semen volume.

Evidence of structural abnormalities of the seminal vesicles or vas deferens is typically first discovered on physical examination and confirmed by ultrasound imaging. These abnormalities occur in bilateral and unilateral patterns. Testicular function, including spermatogenesis, is typically normal. Clinical evaluation by a urologist is warranted in any of these circumstances, and disease etiology should be determined by molecular genetic testing for *CFTR* mutations.

Chapter Summary

» Cystic fibrosis involves an ion transport disorder in the epithelial cells of multiple organ systems and results in pulmonary disease, pancreatic dysfunction, hepatobiliary disorders, and exocrine dysfunction.

» Cystic fibrosis typically presents in infancy and early childhood.

» The diagnosis of cystic fibrosis is made using screening methods and specific mutation testing.

» Mortality in cystic fibrosis is generally related to pulmonary failure (e.g., pneumonia).

» Surveillance guidelines include population screening.

» Congenital absence of the vas deferens is a disorder related to mutation in the cystic fibrosis transmembrane conductance regulator gene.

Chapter Review Questions

1. Cystic fibrosis is the result of a mutation in the _____ gene.
2. The most life-threatening complication associated with cystic fibrosis is _____.
3. The chance of two carriers having offspring with cystic fibrosis is _____, which is described as a/an _____ pattern of inheritance.
4. Physical examination findings that raise clinical suspicion for cystic fibrosis in infants and young children include _____, _____, and _____.
5. Infertile males without pulmonary or gastrointestinal manifestations of cystic fibrosis may have _____.

Bibliography

Anson, D. S., Smith, G. J., & Parsons, D. W. (2006). Gene therapy for cystic fibrosis airway disease. *Current Gene Therapy, 6,* 161–179.

Bennett, C., & Peckham, D. (2002, August). *The genetics of cystic fibrosis* [online]. Leeds, England: Leeds University Teaching Hospitals. Retrieved from http://www .cfmedicine.com/cfdocs/cftext/genetics.htm

Goss, C. H., Newsom, S. A., Schildcrout, J. S., Sheppard, L., & Kaufman, J. D. (2004). Effect of ambient air pollution on pulmonary exacerbations and lung function in cystic fibrosis. *American Journal of Respiratory and Critical Care Medicine, 169,* 816–821.

Moskowitz, S. M., Chmiel, J. F., Sternen, D. L., Cheng, E., Gibson, R. L., Marshall, S. G., & Cutting, G. R. (2008). Clinical practice and genetic counseling for cystic fibrosis and *CFTR*-related disorders. *Genetics in Medicine, 10*(12), 851–868.

Nick, J. A., & Rodman, D. M. (2005). Manifestations of cystic fibrosis diagnosed in adulthood. *Current Opinion in Pulmonary Medicine, 11,* 513–518.

Ong, T., Marshall, S. G., Karczeski, B. A., Sternen, D. L., Cheng, E., & Cutting, G. R. (2017, February). Cystic fibrosis and congenital absence of the vas deferens. Retrieved from https://www.ncbi.nlm.nih.gov/books/NBK1250/

Vanscoy, L. L., Blackman, S. M., Collaco, J. M., Bowers, A., Lai, T., Naughton, K., . . . Cutting, G. R. (2007). Heritability of lung disease severity in cystic fibrosis. *American Journal Respiratory Critical Care Medicine, 175,* 1036–1043.

KEY TERMS

Callus

Coxa vara

Dentinogenesis imperfecta

Osteogenesis
   imperfecta (OI)

Rhizomelia

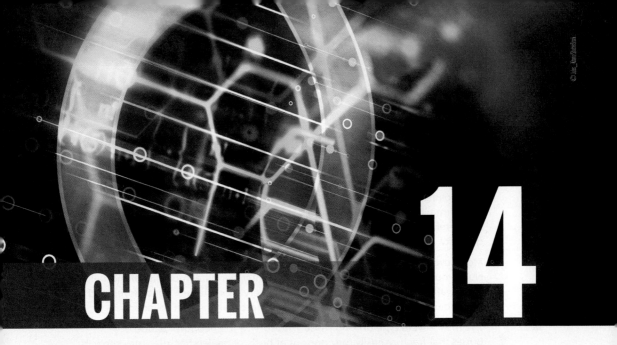

CHAPTER 14

Osteogenesis Imperfecta

Osteogenesis imperfecta (OI) is a group of genetic disorders that affect the development of bones. Specifically, mutations in the genes that are normally responsible for the coding of proteins for collagen type I are compromised, leading to the weakening of connective tissue, especially bones. Fractures may occur in any bone in the body but most commonly appear in one of the extremities. The occurrence of fractures leads to the varying conditions that are more plainly referred to as brittle bone disease. The disease is classified based on severity, with eight current forms categorized as osteogenesis imperfecta I–VIII. This classification differs from a logical progression of disease, however; type I is the mildest of the forms, type II is the most severe, and types III–VIII are varying combinations of type II and type I. Advancing genetics has played a key role in the ability to classify the various forms of the disease. OI is known to have different autosomal dominant inheritance patterns of type I collagen. These are known as OI types I, II, III, IV, and V. OI may also be inherited in a recessive manner (types VII and VIII). Types V and VI are not associated with type I collagen mutation, although their gene origin is unknown **(Table 14-1)**.

The clinical features of OI range widely; some individuals are asymptomatic and simply have a predisposition for fractures, such as those with type I disease. This is in stark contrast to other individuals, who suffer from short stature, **dentinogenesis imperfecta (DI)**, mobility impairment, or perinatal death. DI is characterized by discolored teeth, usually a gray or brown color, that easily degrade, break, or wear down. Those individuals with type II often present with fracture of no evident cause, even out of the womb. They are often plagued by respiratory difficulties and may have a short life because of their small, fragile rib cage and underdeveloped lungs. Often, those affected will have a blue or gray tint to the sclera (white portion of the eye) and progressive loss of hearing in adulthood, but normal or near normal height. Women are at markedly higher risk because they are more prone to developing fractures during

TABLE 14-1	Varying Types of Osteogenesis Imperfecta and Their Features

Type	Characteristics
I	*Most common type and mildest* Predisposed to fracture (most before puberty); normal or near normal stature; loose joints; muscle weakness; triangular face; tendency of spinal curvature; absent to minimal bone deformity; possible dentinogenesis imperfecta; possible hearing loss, often occurring in early 20s or 30s; normal collagen structure but less in quantity.
II	*Most severe form of OI* Numerous fractures and severe bone deformity; perinatal mortality or mortality shortly after birth due to respiratory issues; very short stature; underdeveloped lungs; blue-, purple-, or gray-tinted sclera; improperly formed collagen.
III	*The most severe type among those who survive the neonatal period* Bones that fracture easily may present at birth, or healed fractures may show in the womb. Other characteristics include short stature; blue, purple, or gray sclera; loose joints; poor muscle development in the arms and legs; triangular face; spinal curvature; severe bone deformity; possible respiratory problems; possible dentinogenesis imperfecta; possible hearing loss; improperly formed collagen.
IV	*Between types III and I in severity* Bones fracture easily (most often before puberty); small in stature; normal sclera; mild to moderate bone deformity; triangular face; possible tendency of spinal curvature; possible dentinogenesis imperfecta; possible hearing loss; improperly formed collagen.
V	*Similar to type IV* Dense band seen on x-rays adjacent to the growth plates on long bones; unusually large **calluses** (hypertrophic calluses) at the site of fractures or surgical procedures; calcification of the membrane between the radius and the ulna, which leads to restriction of forearm rotation; normal sclera; normal teeth with "meshlike" appearance to bone when viewed under a microscope.
VI	*Similar to type IV; extremely rare* Elevated alkaline phosphatase activity; bone has a "fish scale" appearance under a microscope.
VII	*Similar to type IV in the first documented cases* Short humerus and femur; small stature; **coxa vara**.
VIII	*Resembles lethal type II or type III OI, except infants have white or near-white sclera* Severe growth deficiency; extreme skeletal undermineralization.

pregnancy and after menopause. It can be difficult to detect OI in some women, who may be asymptomatic throughout the course of childhood and into adulthood and develop fractures only once they are postmenopausal.

OI has an incidence rate of 6–7 people per 100,000 worldwide; type I and type IV are noted as the most common forms, with an incidence rate of 4–5 per 100,000 persons. Type II has a reported incidence rate of 1 in 60,000 at birth. Very few cases of type V, VI, and VII have been reported.

Diagnosis

In general, OI is a clinical diagnosis. A practitioner who is presented with a patient who has multiple features of OI generally has sufficient information to make the diagnosis; these features include, but are not limited to, the presence of blue sclera, progressive hearing loss, short stature, bone fragility or multiple fractures, dentinogenesis imperfecta, ligamentous laxity, and/or a family history of the disease. Although pathologic fractures are a feature of OI, other causes, such as nutritional deficiencies, malignancies, or even battered child syndrome may also need to be ruled out at the time of diagnosis. Radiographic features are major findings and have a tendency to vary with age and severity of disease. One diagnostic feature is known as "codfish" vertebrae. Seen more commonly among adult patients, this is the consequence of many spinal compression fractures. Patients may show wormian bones, or "structural bones which are 6 mm by 4 mm in diameter or larger, in excess of ten in number, with a tendency to arrange in a mosaic pattern" (Steiner, Adsit, & Basel, 2013). Those with Type I OI have been shown to have a distinct mottling pattern on skull radiographs due to the small islands of irregular ossification, whereas type II is so severe that complications are commonly seen in utero or immediately postpartum. The immense fragility of the connective tissue frequently leads to incomplete bone formation, or ossification, multiple stages of rib fracturing or beading, and crumpled long bones (accordion femora). In types III and IV, the slightest physical trauma can create severe consequences such as deformity. Another common feature associated with these forms is kyphoscoliosis, which, if severe enough, may lead to impaired respiration. An ominous sign present in some patients with types III and IV is the appearance of popcorn deposits on the ends of long bones. It develops from the overabundance of mineral deposition at these sites and can lead to further complications. Type V OI is recognized by the presence of dislocated radial heads and hyperplastic callus formation. **Rhizomelia** and coxa vara are observed in patients with type VII OI.

Individuals with OI, regardless of the type (with the exception of type I), have decreased bone mineral density, usually with varying degrees of osteopenia. The specific degree, or range of degrees for specific type, can be

KEY TERMS

Osteogenesis imperfecta (OI): comes from the increasing likelihood of fracture from seemingly minor injuries or, in some cases, with no apparent cause at all.

Dentinogenesis imperfecta: characterized by discolored teeth, usually gray or brown, that easily degrade, break, or wear down.

Rhizomelia: a disproportion in the length of the proximal limb, creating a shorter than normal limb.

Callus: area of new bone that is laid down at the fracture site as part of the healing process.

Coxa vara: a deformed hip joint in which the neck of the femur is bent downward; the acute angle of the femur head is less than 120 degrees and subsequently affects the hip socket.

difficult to conclude because of the likelihood of limited exercise due to more recurrent fractures in some forms of OI, which in turn increases the degree of osteopenia. Although bone density may be detected through the use of dual energy x-ray absorptiometry (DEXA), bone density may appear to be normal because DEXA measures mineral content, as opposed to collagen content.

Genetic Testing and Counseling

As stated, OI is inherited in multiple ways. Types I, II, III, IV, and V are inherited through an autosomal dominant trait. It has been noted that patients with OI type I present with no family history of OI, suggesting either previous misdiagnosis or sporadic mutations. Sporadic mutations are present in the more lethal forms of OI as well, occurring in the germline in one of the parents.

It has been proven that mutations in the *COL1A1*, *COL1A2*, *CRTAP*, and *P3H1* genes cause OI, with *COL1A1* and *COL1A2* responsible for more than 90% of cases. These genes are those responsible for coding proteins, which assemble type 1 collagen. Type 1 collagen is immensely important because it is the most abundant protein in bone, skin, and other connective tissues responsible for giving structure and strength to the entire human body. When the gene *COL1A1* or *COL1A2* is altered, an alteration in the structure of the type 1 collagen molecule follows; mutations in either the *CRTAP* or *P3H1* gene lead to disruption in the normal folding, assembly, and secretion of collagen molecules because together they are responsible for processing collagen to its mature form. Mutations of *P3H1* generally lead to type VIII OI, in contrast to mutations of *CRTAP*, which are usually classified as type VII.

OI is associated with a defect in type I collagen synthesis in more than two-thirds of patients; this molecular defect can be detected through the incubation of skin fibroblasts with radioactive amino acids and then analyzing the proα chains by polyacrylamide gel electrophoresis (**Figure 14-1**). This process is known as biochemical testing, which is fairly reliable; it currently detects abnormalities in approximately 98% of individuals with classified OI type II, approximately 90% with OI type I, and about 84% with OI types III and IV. Molecular genetic testing of *COL1A1* and *COL1A2* detects abnormalities in more than 90% of individuals with historically classified OI types II, III, IV, and I.

Individuals who have inherited the disease through mutation must undergo DNA analysis to confirm the diagnosis. This is because these mutations actually code for the N-terminus of the helical region and do not result in the overmodified collagen, making it extremely difficult to pick up on gel electrophoresis. Instead, DNA sequencing must be implemented, requiring approximately 10,000 bases in each of the two genes. The process usually requires 100 polymerase chain reactions (PCRs), followed by an extensive screening for mutated strands. After the collagen mutation has been identified, additional

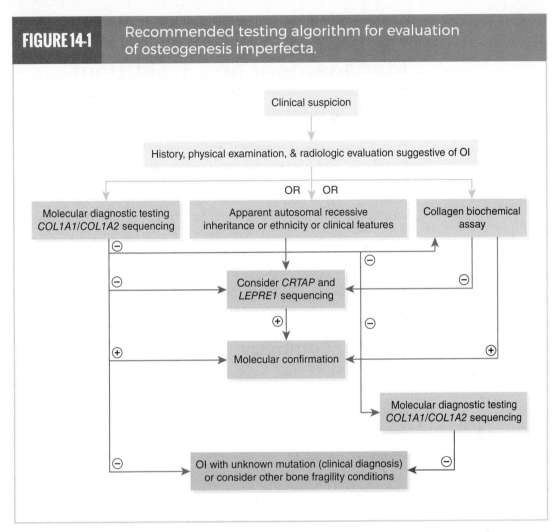

FIGURE 14-1   Recommended testing algorithm for evaluation of osteogenesis imperfecta.

family members may be screened using a much simpler PCR technique. Ultrasound examination performed in a center with experience diagnosing OI can be valuable in the prenatal diagnosis of the lethal form and most severe forms before 20 weeks' gestation; milder forms may be detected later in pregnancy if fractures or deformities occur. Prenatal testing in at-risk pregnancies may also be performed through the use of molecular genetic testing. OI also may be inherited in a recessive manner, such as in types VII and VIII. *De novo mutations* have also been reported in classic nondeforming OI; 60% of blue sclera or common variable OI with normal sclera may be attributed to *de novo mutation*, whereas 100% of perinatally lethal OI and progressively deforming OI are de novo. Children of those with the dominant form of OI have a 50% chance of developing OI themselves.

Management and Treatment

No treatment exists to prevent or delay disease expression for any of the types of OI. The primary management of OI patients remains with a multidisciplinary team of orthopedics, physical therapy, pediatric dentistry, and otology/otolaryngology specialists. The severity of the diagnosis will dictate what the child can and cannot do, such as participation in sports and other physical activities. The mainstay approach involves bracing the limbs, using orthotics to provide stabilization, promoting physical activity in appropriate environments, and providing physical and occupational therapy to maximize bone stability, improve mobility, and prevent deformities and contractures. The treatment of fractures will be significant, with intramedullary rodding as needed and casting along with short-period immobility and supplementary physical therapy after cast removal. In those with DI, dental care is aimed toward maintaining primary and permanent dentition, optimal gingival health, and overall appearance; dental visits should be scheduled twice a year.

Chapter Summary

» Osteogenesis imperfecta is a disorder characterized by collagen type II malformation that leads to bone instability.

» There are currently eight recognized types of OI, with varying criteria for each, including differences in inheritance pattern.

» Although the majority of OI patients have inherited the disease through an autosomal dominant, some are subjected to random gene mutation.

» Most providers are able to diagnose OI based on a few clinical features, such as fragile bones or multiple fractures (usually without cause or from unsubstantial force), blue sclera, varying stature size, progressive hearing loss, and possible dentition problems.

» There is currently no specific treatment for patients with OI; rather, the approach centers on management of the associated symptoms and regular health screenings in anticipation of future problems.

Chapter Review Questions

1. Discoloration of teeth that exhibit unexpected degradation, breakage or wear is known as _____.

2. Apart from the bone disorders that are characteristic of Osteogenesis imperfecta, patients may also exhibit _____, _____, and _____.

3. A derformed hip in the neck of the femur in patients with Osteogenesis imperfecta that affects the hip socket is known as _____.

4. The management approach of Osteogenesis imperfecta is focused on _____.

5. The recommended frequency of dental visits for patients with Osteogenesis imperfecta is _____.

Bibliography

Kasper, D. L., Fauci, A. S., Hauser, S. L., Longo, D. L., Jameson, J. L., & Loscalzo, J. (2015). Harrison's principles of internal medicine (19th edition). New York: McGraw Hill Education.

Osteogenesis imperfecta. (2013). *Genetics home reference.* National Library of Medicine, National Institutes of Health, U.S. Department of Health & Human Services. Retrieved from https://ghr.nlm.nih.gov/condition/osteogenesis-imperfecta

Osteogenesis imperfecta overview. (n.d.). National Institute of Arthritis and Musculoskeletal and Skin Diseases, National Institutes of Health, U.S. Department of Health and Human Services. Retrieved from https://www.niams.nih.gov/health_info/bone/osteogenesis_imperfecta/overview.asp

Steiner, R. D., Adsit, J., & Basel, D. (2013). *COL1A1/2*-related osteogenesis imperfecta. GeneReviews® [Internet]. Retrieved from https://www.ncbi.nlm.nih.gov/books/NBK1295/

‹ Describe the etiology and various forms of muscular dystrophies.
‹ Detail symptoms associated with muscular dystrophies.
‹ Discuss diagnostic criteria for muscular dystrophies.
‹ Discuss reduced penetrance.
‹ Review current surveillance and treatment recommendations for muscular dystrophies.

KEY TERMS

Atrophy
Autosomal dominant
Autosomal recessive
Biopsy

Carrier
Chromosomes
Contractures
Creatine kinase (CK)

Dystrophin
Pseudohypertrophy
X-linked recessive

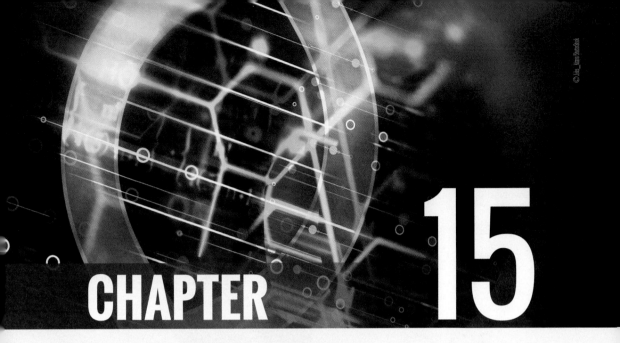

CHAPTER 15

Muscular Dystrophies

Overview

Muscular dystrophy (MD) is a collective group of more than 30 genetically inherited noninflammatory diseases that are characterized by progressive muscle wasting, or **atrophy** (Do, 2017; National Institute of Neurological Disorders and Stroke [NINDS], 2017; National Library of Medicine, 2017). The word *dystrophy* is derived from the Greek *dys*, which means "difficult" or "faulty," and *troph*, meaning "nourish." (NINDS, 2017). The condition of MD is caused by a gene mutation that affects the production of muscle proteins needed to build healthy muscle tissue (Newman, 2017). The absence of **dystrophin** in Duchenne muscular dystrophy causes the muscle tissue to lack integrity (see **Figure 15-1**) (NINDS, 2017). The disease affects the muscles with fiber degeneration but without creating central or peripheral nerve abnormalities. Muscular dystrophies affect skeletal muscles primarily in males. The skeletal muscles affected in these conditions are used in joint and cardiac movements. The two most common types are Duchenne muscular dystrophy (DMD) and Becker muscular dystrophy (BMD). The conditions on the spectrum of dystrophin-lacking diseases are also known as dystrophinopathies. The two dystrophies have similar signs and symptoms, but they are caused by different mutations within the same gene.

The main differences between the two dystrophies are age of onset, severity, and rate of progression. In males diagnosed with DMD, onset of muscle weakness is in early childhood, and it progresses rapidly. In BMD, the signs and symptoms appear with less severity and progress slower. In addition, most children demonstrate muscle weakness later in childhood or in adolescence (Darras, 2017; National Library of Medicine, 2017).

FIGURE 15-1 Absence of dystrophin in Duchenne muscular dystrophy.

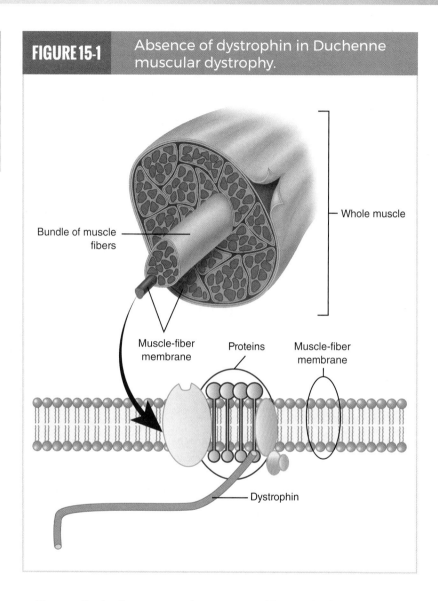

Historically, the first account of MD was noted by Sir Charles Bell in 1830. He wrote of a progressive muscle weakness evident in males. In 1836, another scientist researched two brothers who demonstrated signs and symptoms of general muscle weakness and muscle damage whereby muscle tissue was replaced with connective tissue and fat. In the 1850s, medical journals described how the boys grew weaker, were eventually unable to walk, and died at a young age. In the 1860s, a French neurologist named Guillaume Duchenne studied a group of 13 boys with varying forms of the disease. Later, it became evident that the disease may occur in both sexes and in all ages (NINDS, 2017).

Together, DMD and BMD affect 1 in 3,500 to 5,000 newborn males worldwide. In the United States, between 400 and 600 boys are born with these conditions each year (Newman, 2017; NINDS, 2017). DMD is inherited in an **X-linked recessive** pattern (see **Figure 15-2**). Because the gene that affects DMD is located on the X chromosome, the male receives the defective gene from the **carrier** mother and a Y chromosome from the father. Females receive two X **chromosomes**, so she may receive one defective gene from the

KEY TERMS

X-linked recessive: a pattern of disease inheritance in which the mother carries the affected gene on the chromosome that determines the child's sex and passes it to her son.

Carrier: an individual who doesn't have a disease but has one normal gene and one gene for a genetic disorder; therefore, the individual is capable of passing the disease to her or his children.

Chromosomes: genetic structures that contain DNA.

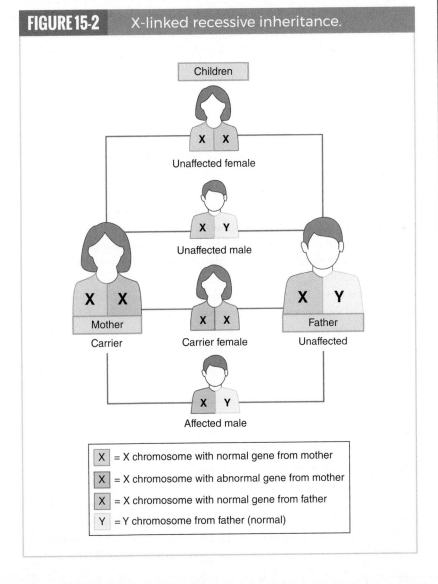

FIGURE 15-2 X-linked recessive inheritance.

X	= X chromosome with normal gene from mother
X	= X chromosome with abnormal gene from mother
X	= X chromosome with normal gene from father
Y	= Y chromosome from father (normal)

KEY TERMS

Pseudohypertrophy: increase in size of an organ or a part that is not due to an increase in size or number of the specific functional elements, but to that of some other tissue, fatty or fibrous.

Creatine kinase (CK): a protein needed for the chemical reactions that produce energy for muscle contractions; high levels in the blood indicate muscle damage.

mother's X chromosome, but most likely will receive a normal gene from the father's X chromosome. Each son born to a mother who is a carrier of the defective gene has a 50% chance of acquiring DMD. Each daughter born to a mother who carries the defective gene has a 50% chance of becoming a carrier. DMD carriers may not have any signs of DMD, but they carry the risk of acquiring cardiomyopathy. Men with DMD cannot give the defective gene to their sons because they donate the Y chromosome that does not carry the gene. The father may, however, pass the defective gene to his daughter because he donates the defective X chromosome (Muscular Dystrophy Association, 2017). Muscle weakness occurs in 2.5–20% of female carriers of a mutated dystrophin gene. Females are more likely to develop symptoms of DMD or BMD. In very rare cases, a female carrier may have a defective second X chromosome that would cause her to develop DMD or BMD exactly like a male (Darras, 2017; Muscular Dystrophy Association, 2017).

Diagnosis

There are different methods of diagnosing MD. One way is by obtaining a thorough history and physical examination. Knowing the signs and symptoms of the most common types of MD can alert the clinician about a possible diagnosis. Initial symptoms of DMD include waddling gait, pain or stiff muscles, difficulty with running and jumping, walking on toes, difficulty sitting up or standing up, and learning disabilities. Ironically, the individual's inability to jump and walk is diminished while his or her calf muscles become abnormally enlarged. The physical change is known as **pseudohypertrophy** (n.d.). The replacement of muscle tissue with fat and fibrous tissue makes the gastrocnemius-soleus complex appear larger than normal. Later signs and symptoms include inability to walk, shortening of muscles and tendons, further limiting movement, breathing problems, abnormal curvature of the spine, cardiac problems, and difficulty swallowing that can lead to causing aspiration pneumonia (Newman, 2017; NINDS, 2017). On physical examination, Gowers' sign may be evident in most children who suffer from MD. Gowers' sign is a classic sign noted when a child has proximal muscle weakness. The child requires the use of "walking up" his legs with his hands to maintain an upright posture (see **Figure 15-3**) (Darras, 2017; Jinguji, 2017).

Laboratory and other diagnostic tests can easily confirm the diagnosis. An enzyme assay examining for elevated **creatine kinase (CK)** levels is the first test considered when a muscular dystrophy diagnosis is suspected. Damaged muscles produce CK; elevated levels of CK without evidence of muscle damage could suggest muscular dystrophy (National Library of Medicine, 2017). Children begin to show signs of muscle weakness around 2–3 years of age. At that time, CK levels are 10–20 times higher than the upper level of normal

FIGURE 15-3	Gowers' sign.

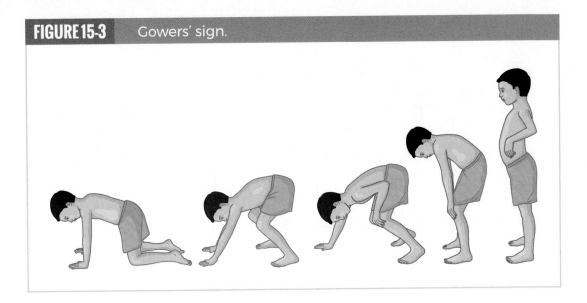

(Darras, 2017). Serum tests may demonstrate high levels of myoglobin, which indicate breakdown of skeletal and cardiac muscle tissue (NINDS, 2017). Heart monitoring, such as performing an electrocardiogram or an echocardiogram, can allow for the diagnosis of myotonic MD where notable musculature changes can be noted in the heart. In addition, changes may include resting sinus tachycardia, deep inferior-lateral Q waves, and a tall R in lead V1 due to the underlying cardiomyopathy (see **Figure 15-4**). Electromyography is a more invasive method: a needle is placed into the heart muscle to measure electrical activity. The results may demonstrate muscle disease. Lung monitoring is a testing method that may determine the functionality of the individual's lung capacity and endurance. Finally, a **biopsy** is the most definitive test to show signs of MD. A portion of the muscle is removed and examined under a microscope to find signs of the disease. Dystrophin analysis may be performed to examine the lack or absence of dystrophin in immunoblots of 100 mcg of total muscle protein (Darras, 2017). Genetic testing is used to screen for genetic mutations associated with the disease. Genetic testing is the most common method of diagnosing; muscle biopsy is rarely needed. Skeletal muscle biopsy is warranted for Western blot and immunohistochemistry studies of dystrophin if no DMD variant is identified by genetic testing (Darras, 2017; National Library of Medicine, 2017).

Understanding the characteristics among the different types of muscular dystrophy is necessary when deciding on a treatment intervention to

KEY TERM

Biopsy: a procedure in which tissue or other material is removed from the body and studied for signs of disease.

FIGURE 15-4 ECG test.

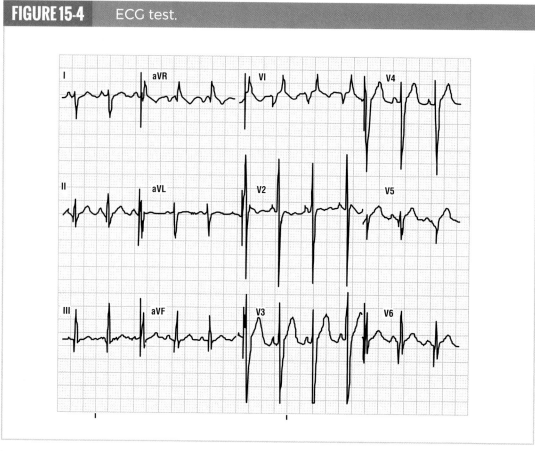

Reproduced with permission from: McKenna WJ. Inherited syndromes associated with cardiac disease. In: UpToDate, Post TW (Ed), UpToDate, Waltham, MA. (Accessed on February 2, 2018). Copyright © 2018 UpToDate, Inc. For more information visit www.uptodate.com

implement. The following groups are the most commonly diagnosed types of muscular dystrophy:

» **Duchenne muscular dystrophy**—the most common form of the disease. Symptoms normally begin in childhood, before age 3. Most children are wheelchair bound by age 12 and die of respiratory failure in their early to mid-20s. It is most common among males.

» **Becker muscular dystrophy**—similar symptoms to Duchenne but with a later onset and slower progression. Death usually occurs in the mid-40s. It is most common among males.

» **Myotonic (Steinert's disease)**—the most common adult-onset form of muscular dystrophy. The facial and neck muscles are often affected first.

Symptoms also include cataracts, sleepiness, and arrhythmia. A unique characteristic is that the individual has difficulty relaxing a group of muscles once they have contracted.

» **Congenital**—this type is evident from birth or before the age of 2. It affects both females and males. Some forms progress slowly, whereas others can move quickly and cause significant disability.

» **Emery-Dreifuss muscular dystrophy (EDMD)**—this type is characterized by joint **contractures** that begin in early childhood and slowly progressive muscle wasting and weakness. The weakness begins in a humeroperoneal distribution and later extends to the scapular and pelvic girdle muscles. Cardiac involvement may include palpitations, presyncope and syncope, poor exercise tolerance, and congestive heart failure.

» **Facioscapulohumeral (FSHD)**—most commonly seen during the teenage years, though onset can be at almost any age. The muscular weakness is initially noted in the face and shoulders. Individuals often have difficulty keeping their eyes closed while sleeping. In addition, scapular winging is noted when the individual raises his arms.

» **Limb-girdle**—usually begins in childhood or teenage years. The first effects are notable with shoulder and hip muscle wasting and weakness. Individuals with limb-girdle muscular dystrophy might have difficulty dorsiflexing their feet. The lack of movement may cause the patient to trip and fall.

» **Oculopharyngeal muscular dystrophy**—adulthood onset, usually between the ages of 40 and 70 years. Eyelids, throat, and face muscles are affected first, and as the disease progresses, the shoulder and pelvis become involved (Darras, Miller, & Urion, 2014; Newman, 2017; NINDS, 2017).

Genetic Testing and Counseling

Molecular biology advancements highlight the genetic basis underlying all MD. The defects in the genetic code for dystrophin, a 427-kd skeletal muscle protein (Dp427), result in the various manifestations commonly associated with MD. Dystrophin can also be found in cardiac smooth muscles and in the brain. The genetic defect allows for characteristics such as muscle weakness, pseudohypertrophy, cardiomyopathy, and mild intellectual disability to be evident (National Library of Medicine, 2017). Molecular genetic testing is indicated for an individual who has markedly elevated CK levels in addition to dystrophinopathy. Female carriers who demonstrate an early onset of progressive muscle wasting may also present with diseases such as 45X, 46XY, or Turner mosaic karyotypes. If a symptomatic female has markedly elevated serum CK levels, a chromosomal analysis is indicated (Darras, 2017). Often, **autosomal dominant** and **autosomal recessive** conditions do not follow Mendelian genetics, so there may be reduced or incomplete penetrance. Penetrance is defined as the percentage of individuals who demonstrate the phenotype of a disorder. Complete

KEY TERMS

Contractures: chronic shortening of a muscle or tendon that limits movement of a bony joint, such as the elbow.

Autosomal dominant: a pattern of inheritance in which a child acquires a disease by receiving a normal gene from one parent and a defective gene from the other parent.

Autosomal recessive: a pattern of inheritance in which both parents carry and pass on a defective gene to their child.

penetrance occurs in diseases where the individual's phenotype reflects the genotype of the disorder. Incomplete or reduced penetrance occurs when an individual does not exhibit the trait but carries the allele. The phenomenon of incomplete or reduced penetrance occurs in Emery-Dreifuss muscular dystrophy (Shawky, 2014).

Genetic counseling may be complex in DMD and BMD. Prenatal counseling for patients who are carriers or diagnosed with DMD is recommended. Two tests can be performed so that expectant parents can know if their child will be affected by the disease. An amniocentesis can be performed at 14–16 weeks of pregnancy. The test sample of amniotic fluid contains the same DNA as the fetus. Results arrive within 1–2 weeks. Another test is chorionic villus sampling, which involves removing a sample of the placenta to examine the DNA of the fetus. Examination results arrive within 2 weeks (Darras, 2017; Darras et al., 2014; NINDS, 2017).

It is recommended that female carriers with a known DNA deletion, duplication, or sequence variant be counseled about the disease. If a mutation is not found, a linkage analysis may be performed to detect an abnormal allele. Female carriers who are symptomatic should undergo an evaluation to rule out hypertrophic cardiomyopathy before the pregnancy. In addition, individuals should seek the services of a high-risk obstetrician once they become pregnant (Darras, 2017; Darras et al., 2014).

Associated Syndromes

Many heritable diseases affect the muscles, the nerves, or the neuromuscular junction. Inflammatory myopathy, progressive muscle weakness, and cardiomyopathy may produce symptoms that are similar to MD; the difference is that other diseases do not have the same genetic defects that are found in the group of MD diseases. When examining the possibilities of MD, the differential diagnosis should include diseases such as congenital myopathy, spinal muscular atrophy, and congenital myasthenic syndromes. Genetic testing can offer a definitive diagnosis for most types of MD (NINDS, 2017). Other differentials may include behavioral toe-walking, cerebral palsy, or heel cord contractures (Jinguji, 2017).

Management and Treatment

MD is a progressive disease, and there is no cure or specific treatment to reverse its progression (NINDS, 2017). Until treatment is found for the basic genetic defect, the disease will continue to require a variety of management and treatment interventions to optimize the individual's quality of life. Treatment mainstays are medications and physical therapy. The two most common medications are corticosteroids and cardiac medications. The role of corticosteroid therapy is to assist in muscle strength and respiratory function while slowing the progression of the disease. The downside to corticosteroids is that long-term use leads to weight gain, short stature, high blood pressure, brittle bones, and cataracts (Newman, 2017; NINDS, 2017). Because MD also affects the heart, medications such as angiotensin-converting enzyme (ACE) inhibitors and beta blockers are useful in protecting the cardiovascular system. Other medications that are commonly used to manage and treat MD are anticonvulsants, immunosuppressants, and antibiotics. Anticonvulsants are used to control seizures and relieve muscle spasms. Immunosuppressants are used to delay the progression of dying muscle cells. Antibiotics are utilized to treat respiratory infections (Newman, 2017).

Physical therapy treatment interventions are key to optimizing independence during activities of daily living. Physical and occupational therapists employ different therapeutic modalities to assist the individual's optimization of function. Therapeutic exercises, such as range of motion, strength, stretching, aerobic, and endurance training, ultimately improve the patient's overall function. The muscles and tendons shorten with lack of movement, and with time, these individuals develop contractures that limit their mobility and independence. Aerobic exercises such as swimming and walking not only allow for improved endurance but also slow the disease progression. Physical therapists, respiratory therapists, and nurses are trained to assist individuals with MD to strengthen their respiratory muscles. As the disease progresses, individuals lose respiratory muscle function and require devices that assist in oxygen delivery. In the late stages of the disease, some individuals may require the use of a ventilator to breathe on their behalf. The use of mobility aids such as canes, walkers, or wheelchairs will provide individuals who acquire muscular weakness with the assistance that they need to be more independent. Braces are used to give joints stability and to stretch out muscles and tendons. A variety of static and dynamic braces allow the individual to acquire the support and stability needed to maintain proper posture during rest, standing, or walking (Newman, 2017). Speech therapy may be warranted for individuals suffering from difficulty swallowing. Surgical intervention techniques are used in cases of extreme muscular contractures. Surgical release of tendons allows for improved mobility and decreased pain for those individuals suffering from muscular contractures. For children who begin to acquire scoliosis, spinal fusion may be indicated to properly align the vertebrae. Prevention of scoliosis using bracing, adaptive seating, and surgical intervention in children will prevent cardiopulmonary compromise due to poor postural control (NINDS, 2017).

Although there is no cure for MD, genetic research has brought science closer to one. Gene replacement therapy using the replacement of the dystrophin protein is being investigated. The problem with this therapeutic method is that the immune system can reject the new protein and its corresponding gene. Increasing the production of utrophin, a similar protein to dystrophin, may be another approach to slowing the disease's progression. Stem cell research is examining new ways to insert muscle stem cells that will produce dystrophin. Researchers are also investigating alternatives to gene therapy, such as searching for drugs that can slow or stop muscle wasting. If the muscle wasting could be delayed, the quality of life may be drastically improved for these individuals (Newman, 2017).

Prognosis

The prognosis in MD is heavily dependent on the type of MD and the rate of progression of the disease. Some types that are slowly progressing may allow the individual to have a normal life span, while the more aggressive types of MD cause loss of muscle strength that eventually leads to loss of function, loss of independence, and early death (NINDS, 2017).

Chapter Summary

» Muscular dystrophy is a collection of muscle-wasting conditions.

» Duchenne muscular dystrophy is the most common type.

» The main cause of muscular dystrophy is a defective gene located on the X chromosome that is responsible for the lack or absence of a protein called dystrophin.

» Gene therapy trials are under way to combat the disease.

» Currently, there is no cure for muscular dystrophy.

Chapter Review Questions

1. What is the main role in using corticosteroids for the treatment of an individual with Duchenne muscular dystrophy? _____.
2. Describe the main similarities and differences between Duchenne and Becker muscular dystrophies. _____.
3. What is the most common adult-onset muscular dystrophy?
   A. Becker muscular dystrophy
   B. Limb-girdle muscular dystrophy
   C. Facioscapulohumeral muscular dystrophy
   D. Myotonic muscular dystrophy
4. True or False: Muscular dystrophy can be acquired through injury.
5. Which of the following statements are true about DMD carriers?
   A. DMD carriers may not have any signs of DMD.
   B. DMD carriers have cardiomyopathy.
   C. DMD carriers are all males.
   D. DMD carriers lack the protein dystrophin.

Bibliography

Darras, B. T. (2017). Clinical features and diagnosis of Duchenne and Becker muscular dystrophy. *UpToDate*. Retrieved from https://www.uptodate.com/contents/duchenne-and-becker-muscular-dystrophy-clinical-features-and-diagnosis

Darras, B. T., Miller, D. T., & Urion, D. K. (2014). Dystrophinopathies. *GeneReviews*. Retrieved from https://www.ncbi.nlm.nih.gov/books/NBK1119/

Do, T. T. (2017, January 6). Muscular dystrophy. *Medscape*. Retrieved from http://emedicine.medscape.com/article/1259041-overview

Muscular Dystrophy Association. (2017). *Duchenne muscular dystrophy (DMD)*. Retrieved from https://www.mda.org/disease/duchenne-muscular-dystrophy/causes-inheritance

National Institute of Neurological Disorders and Stroke. (2017). *Muscular dystrophy: Hope through research*. Retrieved from https://www.ninds.nih.gov/Disorders/Patient-Caregiver-Education/Hope-Through-Research/Muscular-Dystrophy-Hope-Through-Research#3171_5

National Library of Medicine. (2017). *Duchenne and Becker muscular dystrophy*. Genetics Home Reference, National Library of Medicine. Retrieved from https://ghr.nlm.nih.gov/condition/duchenne-and-becker-muscular-dystrophy#synonyms

Newman, T. (2017). All about muscular dystrophy. *Medical News Today*. Retrieved from http://www.medicalnewstoday.com/articles/187618.php

Pseudohypertrophy. (n.d.). *Farlex partner medical dictionary*. Retrieved from http://medical-dictionary.thefreedictionary.com/pseudohypertrophy

Shawky, R. M. (2014). Reduced penetrance in human inherited disease. *Egyptian Journal of Medical Human Genetics, 15*, 103–111.

< Describe the etiology and various forms of familial thoracic aortic aneurysms and dissections.
< Detail symptoms associated with familial thoracic aortic aneurysms and dissections.
< Discuss penetrance and variable expressivity.
< Review other syndromes associated with familial thoracic aneurysms and dissections.
< Review current surveillance and treatment recommendations for familial thoracic aneurysms and dissections.

Aortic aneurysm
Aortic dissection
Iris flocculi

Livedo reticularis
Marfan syndrome
Penetrance

Thoracic aortic aneurysm
Variable expressivity

Familial Thoracic Aortic Aneurysms and Dissections

A **thoracic aortic aneurysm** is a widening or bulging of the upper portion of the aorta that may occur in the descending thoracic aorta, the ascending aorta, or the aortic arch. **Aortic dissection** is a longitudinal tear between the layers of the aorta that may progress because of the high-pressure flow inside the aorta. Familial thoracic aortic aneurysm and dissection (TAAD) is a confirmed diagnosis of thoracic aortic aneurysm in any individual with a positive family history of thoracic aortic aneurysm. This disorder is the 13th-leading cause of death in the United States, accounting for nearly 15,000 deaths annually. Approximately 20% of thoracic aortic aneurysms and dissections result from a familial predisposition.

The aorta is the largest artery in the body. Like all arteries, it is composed of three layers. The innermost layer in direct contact with blood is the intima, which is composed of endothelial cells. The middle layer, the media, is made up of smooth muscle cells and elastic tissue. The outermost layer of connective tissue is known as the adventitia.

In aortic dissection, the tear begins in the intima and progresses to the media. The increased pressure associated with this blood flow damages and tears the media, allowing more blood to fill and divide the layers. This division continues along the length of aorta toward the heart, away from the heart, or in both directions. The onset and rate of progression of the aortic dilatation vary among affected persons. However, if this condition is not identified and treated, the aorta may eventually rupture and lead to a massive hemorrhage that usually proves fatal. Unfortunately, aortic dissection is a medical emergency that can lead to sudden death, even with appropriate treatment.

Diagnosis

Familial TAAD is diagnosed based on the presence of dilation and/or dissection of the thoracic aorta and a positive family history that is not attributable to **Marfan syndrome** or other connective tissue abnormalities. The major diagnostic criteria for TAAD include the presence of dilatation and/or dissection of the ascending thoracic aorta or dissection of the descending aorta distal to the subclavian artery. Diagnosis is confirmed by measuring the dimensions of the aorta at the level of the sinuses of Valsalva and by measuring the ascending aorta using either computerized tomography (CT), magnetic resonance imaging (MRI), or transesophageal echocardiography. These dimensions are then compared with age-appropriate nomograms that have been adjusted for body surface area. The progressive enlargement of the ascending aorta can involve sinuses of Valsalva, ascending aorta, or both. When making a diagnosis of TAAD, it is also necessary to specifically exclude Marfan syndrome, Loeys-Dietz syndrome, and other connective tissue abnormalities. Both family history and genetic testing are helpful in this regard.

Although plain films (x-rays) are not the diagnostic imaging study of choice for TAAD, posterior–anterior and lateral views of the chest are often the first imaging studies ordered for the patient presenting with a chief complaint of "chest pain." Abnormal chest x-ray findings that should raise suspicion of TAAD include an enlarged aortic knob or localized bulge, widened mediastinum, extension of the aortic shadow beyond a calcified wall, and longitudinal aortic enlargement. A double density of the aorta may also be evident because the false lumen is less radiopaque than the true lumen. The loss of space between the aorta and the pulmonic artery (the aortopulmonic window) on the posterior–anterior view is also indicative of aneurysm or dissection.

Plain films of the chest are not diagnostically reliable for aortic dissection, however, and TAAD may not be excluded based on a normal chest x-ray. Echocardiography, CT, and MRI are imaging modalities that are useful in the diagnosis of TAAD and should be considered even in the absence of findings on plain films. Recent changes in the recommendations for persons with a family history of TAAD require that all first-degree relatives of the affected proband have an initial screening to measure the aortic root diameter and follow-up imaging to evaluate disease progression at regular intervals.

For an initial screening, CT is generally preferred for several reasons. For example, CT is more readily available, is noninvasive, and is more easily tolerated by the patient. MRI is often contraindicated in patients who require aortic imaging, such as in persons with implanted pacemakers or other metallic devices. Both MRI and CT measure the external aortic diameter, making either modality preferred over echocardiogram. However, the CT measures from the center of intraluminal flow to each side of the aortic wall, giving a

BOX 16-1	Aortic Dissection Bundle Questions to Assess Risk of Familial Thoracic Aortic Aneurysm and Dissection

Does the patient's family have a history of aortic dissection?
Does the patient have Marfan syndrome or a family history of Marfan syndrome?
Do physical findings suggest that the patient may have undiagnosed Marfan syndrome?

Note: A single yes answer means that aortic dissection may be the cause of the patient's pain and the diagnosis should be excluded by emergent computerized tomography scan, magnetic resonance imaging, or transesophageal echocardiogram.

Data from Best Care News. Methodist Health System. Available at http://bestcare.org/methodist -hospital/about/aortic-dissection-at-any-age-the-tyler-kahle-story/diagnosing-aortic-dissection/

more accurate representation of the true diameter. For acute dissection, CT is also a more rapid diagnostic tool. Regardless of which imaging modality is used, providers should consider specific elements when evaluating reports of TAAD, to include location of measurements, filling defects, presence of genetic syndromes, and comparison of any prior images.

When screening patients of any age for the chief complaint of "chest pain," it is strongly suggested that the aortic dissection bundle questions be included in the initial patient history (**Box 16-1**). These questions can help identify patients at risk for TAAD based on personal and family history by prompting the clinician to include TAAD in the differential diagnosis for chest pain. Electrocardiogram (ECG) findings may be normal or show non-specific changes, such as left ventricular hypertrophy or blocks. If the patient has previously undergone ECG, it may be helpful to compare new findings with baseline studies. Sinus tachycardia is the most common abnormal ECG finding.

The primary manifestation of TAAD may be (1) dilatation of the aorta at the level of the ascending aorta or at the level of the sinuses of Valsalva, (2) dissection of the ascending aorta, or (3) both. Affected individuals typically have progressive enlargement of the ascending aorta, leading to either an aortic dissection involving the ascending aorta (type A dissection) or rupture (**Figure 16-1**). Dissections may also begin in the arch or distal to the arch and propagate distally (type B dissection).

Clinical features of aortic aneurysms and dissection include severe pain in the anterior chest, posterior chest, or both. Pain may also be referred to either shoulder but is most commonly noted in the left shoulder. When the tear involves the abdominal aorta, abdominal pain may be the predominant feature. Dissections can also cause other signs and symptoms, including "the four Ps": pallor, pulselessness, paresthesias, and paralysis. When blood fills the dissection, it is not available in the general circulation, resulting in loss

FIGURE 16-1	Stanford and DeBakey classification systems for thoracic aortic dissection.

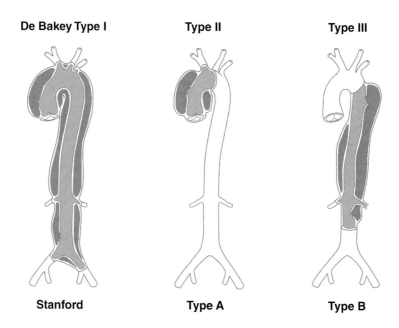

De Bakey
Type I: Originates in the ascending aorta, propagates at least to the aortic arch, and often beyond it distally.
Type II: Originates in and is confined to the ascending aorta.
Type III: Originates in the descending aorta and extends distally down the aorta or, rarely, retrograde into the aortic arch and ascending aorta.

Stanford
Type A: All dissections involving the ascending aorta, regardless of the site of origin.
Type B: All dissections not involving the ascending aorta.

of perfusion to extremities and vital organs. This shunting can contribute to pulse deficits—a major physical examination finding in TAAD. Paresthesias are another manifestation of decreased peripheral perfusion. Paralysis results from nerve compression by the enlarging aneurysmal sac. This constellation of signs and symptoms is frequently misdiagnosed as a cerebrovascular accident, or "stroke." Younger persons presenting with TAAD are most likely to be misdiagnosed with pulmonary causes of chest pain such as pleurisy, bronchitis, or pneumonia.

In families with TAAD, one individual in the family may present with an **aortic aneurysm** at a young age, whereas another individual may present at an elderly age—a phenomenon known as **variable expressivity**. Notably, the mean age of presentation of individuals with familial TAAD is younger than that of individuals with nonfamilial TAAD, but generally older than the mean age of presentation of individuals who have Marfan syndrome. Aortic dissection is exceedingly rare in persons younger than the age of 16, but aortic dilatation may be present in childhood.

Members of some families with TAAD have been observed to have an increase in inguinal hernias and scoliosis. The propensity for arterial dilatation results in aneurysms in other locations along the aorta, as well as cerebral aneurysms. A minority of these families have an increased incidence of bicuspid aortic valve.

The pathological basis for weakening of the aortic wall in familial TAAD is cystic medial necrosis. In this process, the middle layer (media) of the aorta loses smooth muscle fibers and hence elasticity. These cells are replaced with mucoid material, which is less elastic and weakens the walls of the aorta.

Genetic Testing and Counseling

Four genes—*TGFBR2*, *TGFBR1*, *MYH11*, and *ACTA2*—found at either of two loci (*FAA1* and *TAAD1*) are known to be associated with TAAD. Molecular genetic testing for all four associated genes at these two loci is available.

TAAD1 mutations and *ACTA2* mutations account for the majority of mutations in TAAD families, and all mutations appear to be inherited in an autosomal dominant manner. The majority of those individuals who are diagnosed with TAAD also have an affected parent. Siblings of the proband are at increased risk depending on the status of the parents. For this reason, it is important to evaluate both parents and all siblings of those individuals positively or presumptively diagnosed with TAAD. Parents, siblings, and offspring of a proband have a 50% risk of having TAAD.

Affected persons with *TGFBR2* mutations may experience aortic dissection at aortic dilatation of 5.0 cm, which is well below the average threshold of 6.0 cm. These individuals frequently present with aortic disease and have an increased risk for aneurysms and dissection of other vessels such as cerebral arteries.

Penetrance is indicated by the proportion of individuals carrying a particular mutation who also express an associated, observable trait. Persons with mutation of the *FAA1* gene show full penetrance of aortic dilation and dissection, whereas individuals with *TAAD1* mutations show decreased penetrance (especially among women). Mutations in *MYH11* have been associated with patent ductus arteriosus. **Livedo reticularis** and **iris flocculi** are physical findings associated with families demonstrating mutations of the *ACTA2* gene. Iris flocculi are an ocular abnormality found in persons with familial TAAD (**Figure 16-2**). Livedo reticularis manifests as a purplish skin discoloration in a lacy pattern caused by constriction of deep dermal capillaries (**Figure 16-3**).

KEY TERMS

Aortic aneurysm: an abnormal dilation of the aorta at the level of the ascending aorta or the sinuses of Valsalva (descending aorta).

Variable expressivity: variation in disease symptoms among persons with the same mutation.

Penetrance: the proportion of individuals carrying a particular mutation who express an associated, observable trait.

Livedo reticularis: a purplish skin discoloration in a lacy pattern caused by constriction of deep dermal capillaries.

Iris flocculi: an ocular abnormality found in persons with familial thoracic aortic aneurysms and dissections that is highly associated with *ACTA2* mutations.

| **FIGURE 16-2** | Iris flocculi at the pupillary margin as observed by high-powered slit lamp. |

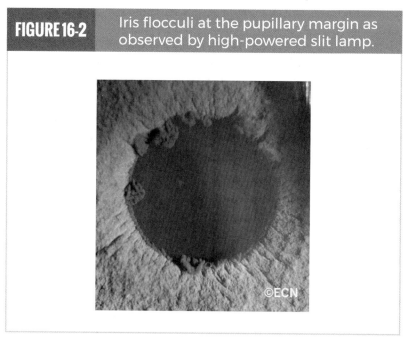

Courtesy of Dr. Paul Finger. www.eyecancer.com.

| **FIGURE 16-3** | Example of livedo reticularis. |

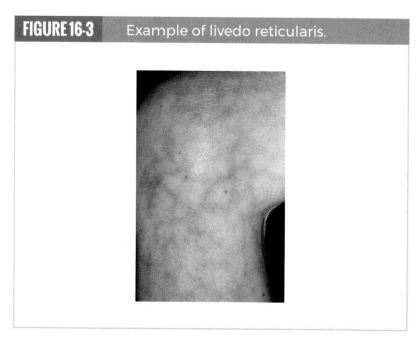

© Dr. P. Marazzi/Science Source.

Management and Treatment

Initial evaluations that are recommended for TAAD include echocardiography of the aorta and aortic valve and cerebrovascular imaging to identify any other aneurysms. Physical examination for inguinal hernias and scoliosis should be performed with appropriate follow-up testing for any abnormal findings. Ocular examination, to exclude lens displacement (ectopia lentis) due to Marfan syndrome, is also indicated.

Control of hypertension is essential in managing TAAD. For example, beta-adrenergic blocking agents are commonly used to reduce hemodynamic stress when aortic dilatation is present. Surgical repair of asymptomatic thoracic aortic aneurysms is indicated to prevent future dissection or rupture. Criteria for prophylactic repair include dilation that increases at a rate of 1.0 cm annually and the presence of aortic regurgitation. For TAAD associated with *TGFBR2* mutations and in persons with a bicuspid aortic valve, the threshold undertaking for such repair is reached when the ascending aorta is 5.0 cm in diameter. For other individuals, the threshold for prophylactic repair is an ascending aortic diameter of 5.0–5.5 cm. Any individuals with a family history of dissection or rupture without prior evidence of aortic root enlargement should undergo earlier repair.

Just as in Marfan syndrome, pregnancy represents a special circumstance for women with TAAD. During pregnancy, labor, delivery, and the postpartum period, the aortic root may enlarge at an increased rate because of the changing hemodynamics associated with pregnancy. Dissection and rupture are more common during this time, so close monitoring of these patients is recommended. Women with TAAD should receive care from a high-risk obstetrician and a cardiologist during their pregnancy.

Surveillance measures for stable individuals should include annual examinations and echocardiogram to monitor the status of the aorta. More frequent exams and imaging studies are indicated for those persons with larger aortic dimensions or rapid rates of dilatation. Individuals who require closer surveillance include those with an aortic root diameter greater than 4.5 cm, those whose aortic growth rate exceeds 0.5 cm annually, and those with evidence of aortic regurgitation.

All first-degree relatives of affected individuals should be assessed annually by echocardiogram to evaluate the ascending aorta. It is recommended that the entire aorta be imaged every 4–5 years by CT or MRI angiography, with this surveillance beginning at 6–7 years of age. All previously undiagnosed individuals who are found to have abnormalities by this screening should have their first-degree relatives screened as well. Furthermore, any sons of women who are first-degree relatives of an affected individual should be screened regardless of the mother's echocardiogram results because decreased penetrance is common in women. Avoidance of isometric exercises (weight lifting), rapid deceleration (motor vehicle accidents), and contact sports is recommended because these activities may contribute to accelerated dilatation, dissection, and rupture.

Associated Syndromes

Marfan syndrome is primarily associated with *FBN1* mutations but may also be seen in conjunction with *TGFBR2* mutations, similar to TAAD. Marfan syndrome is inherited in an autosomal dominant pattern (see Chapter 15).

Loeys-Dietz syndrome is caused by mutations in the *TGFBR1* and *TGFBR2* genes. It is characterized by aneurysms, arterial dissections and tortuosities, craniofacial abnormalities, and skeletal abnormalities. The mode of inheritance for this syndrome is also autosomal dominant.

Chapter Summary

» Familial thoracic aortic aneurysm and dissection is caused by connective tissue defects that result in a loss of smooth muscle fibers and elasticity, thereby weakening the aorta and other arteries.

» Familial thoracic aortic aneurysm and dissection typically presents at an earlier age than sporadic thoracic aneurysm.

» Familial thoracic aortic aneurysm and dissection is diagnosed based on the presence of dilation and/or dissection of the thoracic aorta and a positive family history that is not attributable to Marfan syndrome or other connective tissue abnormalities.

» The aortic dissection bundle questions should be included in the initial history for all patients complaining of chest pain regardless of age.

» The most common presenting complaint with familial thoracic aortic aneurysm and dissection is ripping or tearing chest pain that may be associated with pallor, pulse deficits, paresthesias, and paralysis.

» Surveillance guidelines for first-degree relatives include annual imaging of the aorta beginning in childhood.

» Pregnancy presents a special surveillance consideration because women with familial thoracic aortic aneurysm and dissection are at increased risk for aortic dissection and rupture.

Chapter Review Questions

1. The majority of familial thoracic aortic aneurysms and dissections are the result of mutations in the _____ and _____ genes.

2. The most life-threatening complication associated with thoracic aortic aneurysms and dissections is _____.

3. The chance of an affected individual having offspring with familial thoracic aortic aneurysm and dissection is _____, which is described as a/an _____ pattern of inheritance.

4. Signs and symptoms that raise clinical suspicion for familial thoracic aortic aneurysms and dissections include _____, _____, _____, and _____.

5. Initial recommended evaluations for familial thoracic aortic aneurysms and dissections include _____ of the aorta and aortic valve and _____ to identify any other aneurysms.

Bibliography

Albornoz, G., Coady, M. A., Roberts, M., Davies, R. R., Tranquilli, M., Rizzo, J. A., & Elefteriades, J. A. (2006). Familial thoracic aortic aneurysm and dissections: Incidence, modes of inheritance, and phenotypic patterns. *Annals of Thoracic Surgery, 82*, 1400–1406.

Biddinger, A., Rocklin, M., Coselli, J., & Milewicz, D. M. (1997). Familial thoracic aortic dilations and dissections: A case control study. *Journal of Vascular Surgery, 25*, 506–511.

Hasham, S. N., Guo, D. C., & Milewicz, D. M. (2002). Genetic basis of thoracic aortic aneurysms and dissections. *Current Opinions in Cardiology, 17*, 677–683.

Hasham, S. N., Lewin, M. R., Tran, V. T., Pannu, H., Muilenburg, A., Willing, M., & Milewicz, D. M. (2004). Nonsyndromic genetic predisposition to aortic dissection: A newly recognized, diagnosable, and preventable occurrence in families. *Annals of Emergency Medicine, 43*, 79–82.

Hiratzka, L. F., Bakris, G. L., Beckman, J. A., Bersin, R. M., Carr, V. F., Casey, D. E., . . . Society for Vascular Medicine. (2010). 2010 ACCF/AHA/AATS/ACR/ASA/SCA/SCAI/SIR/STS/SVM guidelines for diagnosis and management of patients with thoracic aortic disease: Executive summary. *Circulation, 121*, 1544–1579.

Milewicz, D. M., Chen, H., Park, E. S., Petty, E. M., Zaghi, H., Shashidhar, G., . . . Patel, V. (1998). Reduced penetrance and variable expressivity of familial thoracic aortic aneurysms/dissections. *American Journal of Cardiology, 82*, 474–479.

Milewicz, D. M., & Regalado, E. (2003). Heritable thoracic aortic disease overview. *GeneReviews*. Retrieved from https://www.ncbi.nlm.nih.gov/books/NBK1120/

Nienaber, C. A., & Eagle, K. A. (2003). Aortic dissection: New frontiers in diagnosis and management: Part I: From etiology to diagnostic strategies. *Circulation, 108*, 628–635.

Singh, K. K., Rommel, K., Mishra, A., Karck, M., Haverich, A., Schmidtke, J., & Arslan-Kirchner, M. (2006). *TGFBR1* and *TGFBR2* mutations in patients with features of Marfan syndrome and Loeys-Dietz syndrome. *Human Mutations, 27*, 770–777.

< Describe the etiology and various forms of familial hypercholesterolemia.
< Detail symptoms associated with familial hypercholesterolemia.
< Discuss allelic variants, loss-of-function mutations, and gain-of-function mutations.
< Review current screening and treatment recommendations for familial hypercholesterolemia.

Allelic variant	Cholesterol	Low-density lipoprotein
Angina	Founder effect	Myocardial infarction
Arcus corneus	Gain-of-function mutation	Xanthomas
Atherosclerosis	Loss-of-function mutation	Xanthelasmata

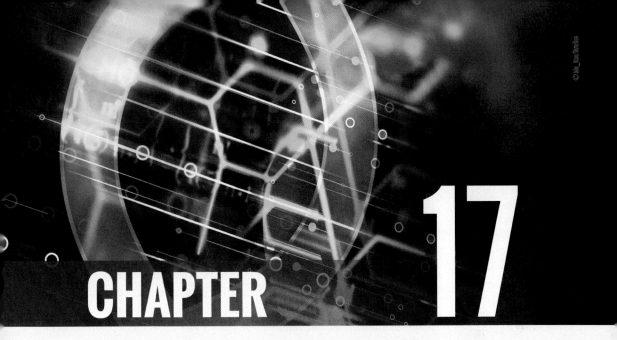

CHAPTER 17

Familial Hypercholesterolemia

Hypercholesterolemia is defined as a fasting total blood **cholesterol** level of more than 240 mg/dL. More than 34 million American adults have elevated blood cholesterol levels, although the inherited forms of hypercholesterolemia are less common. The most widely inherited form of high cholesterol, called familial hypercholesterolemia (FH), affects approximately 1 in every 500 people. FH is characterized by increased levels of total serum cholesterol (TC) with increased **low-density lipoprotein** cholesterol (LDL-C), tendinous xanthomata, and premature symptoms of coronary heart disease. This clinical phenotype may be inherited in either an autosomal dominant pattern or an autosomal recessive pattern, depending on the specific mutation. In all cases, the phenotype is associated with premature death. Persons with FH usually have higher levels of TC compared with the general population. A higher frequency of FH is noted to occur among certain populations, such as South Africans, French Canadians, Lebanese, Ashkenazi Jews, Asian Indians, and Finns. These populations are responsible for the random genetic mutation that occurs as a result of its proliferation from only a few parent colonizers—a phenomenon known as the **founder effect**.

Genetics

The low-density lipoprotein receptor (LDLR) protein is encoded on the *LDLR* gene. This receptor binds to LDL particles that function as carriers for cholesterol in the blood. Under normal circumstances, these receptors function to eliminate LDL from the blood, thereby regulating TC levels. However, in FH, the cell surface receptors for LDL may be defective or absent, resulting in unregulated synthesis of LDL-C. When LDL receptors are absent or have diminished ability to function, excess cholesterol accumulates in the body and is deposited in tissues in abnormal amounts. The skin, tendons, and arteries are the tissues that are most commonly affected by this problem.

When the *LDLR* gene is absent, the phenotype has even more severe effects compared with the phenotype expressed for *LDLR* gene defects. To date, more than 1,000 different defects, known as **allelic variants**, have been identified in the *LDLR* gene. When this defect exists in the homozygous state (two affected genes), **atherosclerosis** develops in early childhood, and serum cholesterol levels may reach be as high as 8 times the upper limits of normal. Affected individuals may require liver transplantation to decrease hepatic lipid production and ameliorate the disease process.

The homozygous form of FH is relatively rare (1 in 1 million) and is detectable at birth. The heterozygous manifestation (only one affected gene) of the disease presents clinically with serum LDL-C levels that are 2 times the upper limits of normal. Atherosclerotic disease begins to develop in the third and fourth decades of life in these individuals. The incidence of heterozygous FH is approximately 1 in 500, making it roughly 2,000 times more common than the homozygous expression.

Environmental Risk Factors

High blood cholesterol levels in the general population typically result from a combination of genetic and environmental risk factors. Lifestyle choices, including diet, exercise, and tobacco smoking, strongly influence the amount of cholesterol in the blood. Other factors that affect cholesterol levels include a person's gender, age, and chronic health problems such as diabetes and obesity. The extent to which these environmental risk factors increase morbidity and mortality specific to FH is not known.

Physical Examination Findings

Cholesterol is a fatty substance that is produced in the liver and can also be obtained from animal-based foods such as eggs, meat, and dairy products. Not all cholesterol is necessarily bad. In fact, cholesterol is an integral part of cellular membranes and certain steroid hormones, and it aids in the digestion of dietary fats. Nevertheless, it has been well documented that high blood cholesterol levels contribute to the development of atherosclerosis and are a risk factor for heart attack and stroke.

When present in excess amounts in the blood, cholesterol is deposited onto the walls of blood vessels, such as the coronary arteries that supply blood to the heart. These deposits are known as plaques. Development of atherosclerosis begins with an injury to the endothelium of the vessel wall; inflammation, infection, smoking, and elevated LDL-C, for example, can all cause the initial injury. Once injured, LDL-C enters the vessel wall, and the LDL-C particles become oxidized and recruit blood monocytes to the site of injury. The monocytes phagocytize the LDL-C particles, which results in the microscopic appearance of "foamy," lipid-laden macrophages known as foam cells.

Eventually, as the disease progresses, the heavy burden of lipids in individual cells causes cellular death, leaving behind cholesterol crystals in the plaque. The plaque can either cause obstruction of the lumen of the vessel (occlusion) or rupture. When the vessel is 70% obstructed, ischemic symptoms may develop, such as **angina**—chest pain that is associated with exercise or physical activity and is relieved by rest. When the plaque ruptures, it becomes a circulating thrombus that may completely occlude smaller vessels, such as the coronary arteries that provide blood to the myocardium. When blood flow is blocked to the distal tissues, cell death—otherwise known as **myocardial infarction**, or heart attack—occurs. This permanent damage may be fatal if it is extensive enough to prevent normal cardiac function.

Cholesterol deposits that accumulate in tendons cause abnormal growths known as tendon **xanthomas**. Most commonly, these growths involve the Achilles tendon as well as tendons in the hands and fingers. Similar deposits in the skin result in xanthomas and **xanthelasmata**, which are yellowish cholesterol deposits under the skin or under the eyelids, respectively. Cholesterol may also be deposited at the peripheral border of the cornea, resulting in **arcus corneus**. This generally occurs before the age of 45.

Related Disorders

In addition to the *LDLR* mutation, mutations in some other genes have also been shown to cause hypercholesterolemia. Mutations in the *APOB*, *LDLRAP1*, and *PCSK9* genes result in increased blood cholesterol and are not uncommon.

Various *APOB* gene mutations result in a type of inherited hypercholesterolemia known as familial defective apolipoprotein B-100. Each of these mutations changes a single amino acid in a critical region of the gene, which inhibits normal binding of LDL-C particles to cell surface receptors. Consequently, fewer LDL-C particles are removed from the blood, and circulating cholesterol levels increase ("Hypercholesterolemia," 2010).

LDLARP1 mutations are linked to an autosomal recessive inheritance pattern of hypercholesterolemia. A variety of mutations in this gene have been shown to either diminish the amount of protein synthesized or lead to production of an abnormal protein. Although the receptors maintain their ability to bind LDL-C particles, they are not able to transport them across the cell membrane, thus allowing the cholesterol particles to accumulate in the blood.

The *PCSK9* gene encodes instructions for the protein that determines the number of LDL receptors. This protein breaks down LDL receptors before they reach the cell surface, thereby controlling cholesterol levels. A **gain-of-function mutation** in *PCSK9* enhances the normal activity of the protein. In this case, there is increased destruction of LDL-C receptors, which in turn

KEY TERMS

Angina: chest pain that is precipitated by exertion and relieved by rest; it is caused by inadequate oxygen delivery to the heart muscles.

Myocardial infarction: death of the heart muscle, caused by occlusion of the coronary vessels.

Xanthomas: a cutaneous manifestation of lipid accumulation in the large foam cells that presents clinically as small eruptions with distinct morphologies along tendons such as the Achilles tendon.

Xanthelasmata: sharply demarcated yellowish collections of cholesterol in foam cells observed underneath the skin, and especially on the eyelids.

Arcus corneus: a corneal disease caused by deposits of phospholipids and cholesterol in the corneal stroma and anterior sclera surrounding the iris of the eye.

results in increased circulating LDL-C levels. Other gene mutations may result in diminished normal activity. In such a case, more LDL receptors would reach the cell surface and be able to bind more LDL-C, thereby reducing the amount of circulating LDL cholesterol in the blood. Such a mutation leading to decreased normal activity is known as a **loss-of function mutation**. In any case, hypercholesterolemia results when the LDLRs are unable to effectively remove cholesterol from the blood.

Environmental and Other Factors

The interaction between genes and environmental factors as demonstrated in FH is unclear. Increased age, obesity, diabetes, lipid levels, and smoking are all strong predictors of risk independent of mutation status. When stratifying risk, modifiable lifestyle changes should be considered in early intervention and prevention strategies.

Factors that may cause an increase in TC include hypothyroidism, nephrotic syndrome, chronic renal insufficiency, liver disease, menopause, and Cushing's disease. In addition, drugs that may increase TC levels include anabolic steroids, oral contraceptives, diuretics, and some α-blockers. It is prudent to rule out secondary causes of abnormal lipid results before initiating lipid-lowering pharmacotherapy.

Testing

Today, routine screening tools for hypercholesterolemia include family history, pedigree, and a fasting lipid profile. Mutation testing is currently not commonly performed, but its use is projected to grow among families in whom early coronary heart disease is prevalent. Cascade screening is recommended as a means of identifying those at risk for hypercholesterolemia by using systematic family tracing. Obviously, it is important for the clinician to have an understanding of the most up-to-date cholesterol screening guidelines for various patient populations (**Table 17-1**). Adults with other coronary risk factors or equivalents such as peripheral artery disease, aortic aneurysm, carotid artery disease, or diabetes should be screened and monitored more closely.

Children and adolescents should be screened regardless of family history. If there is no family history, universal screening is recommended once between 9 and 11 and between 17 and 21. For those with a positive family history, screening should begin at age 2. Their risk is stratified using established cholesterol level criteria for children between the ages of 2 and 19. Special consideration should also be given to other high-risk populations, such as persons on antiretroviral therapy used in HIV infection, patients with liver disease, and postmenopausal females. As yet, no screening criteria have been established for these populations.

TABLE 17-1	Atherosclerotic Cardiovascular Disease Risk Categories and LDL-C Treatment Goals

			Treatment Goals		
	Risk Category	Risk Factors/10-Year Risk	LDL-C (mg/dL)	Non-HDL-C (mg/dL)	apoB (mg/dL)
Extreme Risk	AACE	‹ Progressive ASCVD after achieving an LDL-C <70 mg/dL ‹ Established clinical cardiovascular disease in patients with DM, CKD ¾, or HeFH ‹ History of premature ASCVD (<55 male, <65 female)	<55	<80	<70
	EAS	No recommendation made	-	-	-
Very High Risk	AACE	‹ Established or recent hospitalization for ACS, coronary, carotid, or peripheral vascular disease, 10-year risk >20% ‹ Diabetes or CKD ¾ with 1 or more risk factor(s) ‹ HeFH	<70	<100	<80
	EAS	‹ Established ASCVD ‹ Severe CKD (GFR <30) ‹ DM with target organ damage or major risk factor	<70	<100	<80
High Risk	AACE	‹ >2 risk factors and 10-year risk 10–20% ‹ Diabetes or CKD ¾ with no other risk factors	<100	<130	<90
	EAS	‹ Diabetes, moderate CKD (GFR 30-50), 10-year risk 5-10%, familial hypercholesterolemia	<100	<130	<100
Moderate Risk	AACE	<2 risk factors and 10-year risk <10%	<100	<130	<90
	EAS	10-year risk 1–5%	<115	-	-
Low Risk	AACE	No risk factors	<130	<160	NR
	EAS	10-year risk <1%	<115	-	-

Reproduced from Baer, J. AACE and EAS Lipid Guidelines. (2017). Retrieved from http://www.acc.org/latest-in-cardiology/articles/2017/08/11/08/35/aace-and-eas-lipid-guidelines

Another consideration is how lipids are analyzed and reported by clinical laboratories. For example, TC level alone is not valuable unless fractionated values for high-density lipoprotein cholesterol (HDL-C) and LDL-C are also available. Unlike other parameters, there is no established "reference range" for blood lipids. Instead, risk is stratified by desired levels and is expressed as "acceptable," "borderline," or "high" depending on TC and LDL-C levels (Table 17-1).

Finally, it is important to understand the relationship of the various lipid fractions to coronary risk. Three different lipoproteins carry cholesterol and are classified based on their density and composition: (1) very-low-density lipoprotein cholesterol (VLDL-C), which is the greatest measure of triglycerides (TG); (2) LDL-C; and (3) HDL-C. The TC measure roughly translates into the sum of these components. The majority of clinical laboratories directly analyze TC, total TG, and HDL-C, whereas LDL-C levels are calculated using the following equation:

$$LDL\text{-}C = TC - HDL\text{-}C - TG/5$$

The American Heart Association recommends that at least three fasting lipid profiles be performed as baseline testing before initiating lipid-lowering therapy. When hyperlipidemia of any type is confirmed by this method, a phenotype may be determined according to the Fredrickson classification (**Table 17-2**). This classification serves as an aid in selecting appropriate pharmacotherapeutic agents. The family history and pedigree should include

TABLE 17-2	Lipoprotein Phenotyping (Frederickson Classification) of Lipid Disorders				
Type	Appearance	Elevated Particles	Associated Clinical Disorders	Serum TC	Serum TG
I	Creamy top	Chylomicrons	Primary to familial lipoprotein lipase deficiency, apolipoprotein C-II deficiency Secondary to uncontrolled diabetes, systemic lupus erythematosus, dysgammaglobulinemia	→	↓↓

Type	Appearance	Elevated Particles	Associated Clinical Disorders	Serum TC	Serum TG
IIa	Clear	LDL	Primary to familial hypercholesterolemia, polygenic hypercholesterolemia, familial combined hyperlipidemia Secondary to nephrotic syndrome, dysgammaglobulinemia, hypothyroidism	↑↑	→
IIb	Clear	LDL, VLDL	Primary to familial combined hyperlipidemia, familial hypercholesterolemia, hyper-pre-β-lipoproteinemia Secondary to nephrotic syndrome, dysgammaglobulinemia, hypothyroidism	↑↑	↑
III	Turbid	IDL	Primary to dysbetalipoproteinemia, apolipoprotein E3 deficiency Secondary to uncontrolled diabetes, hypothyroidism, dysgammaglobulinemia, alcohol excess	↑	↑
IV	Turbid	VLDL	Primary to familial hypertriglyceridemia, familial combined hyperlipidemia, sporadic hypertriglyceridemia Secondary to uncontrolled diabetes, nephrotic syndrome, dysgammaglobulinemia, chronic renal failure, alcoholism	→↑	↑↑

TABLE 17-2	Lipoprotein Phenotyping (Frederickson Classification) of Lipid Disorders *(Continued)*

Type	Appearance	Elevated Particles	Associated Clinical Disorders	Serum TC	Serum TG
V	Creamy top, turbid bottom	Chylomicrons	Primary to familial monogenic hypertriglyceridemia, apolipoprotein C-II deficiency Secondary to uncontrolled diabetes, nephrotic syndrome, dysgammaglobulinemia, alcoholism	↑	↑↑

IDL: intermediate-density lipoprotein; LDL: low-density lipoprotein; TC: total cholesterol; TG: triglycerides; VLDL: very-low-density lipoprotein; ↑ = increased; ↑↑ = greatly increased; → = normal; →↑ = normal or increased.
Data from Tietz, N. W. (1995). *Clinical guide to laboratory tests* (3rd ed.). Philadelphia, PA: W. B. Saunders.

TABLE 17-3	Major Risk Factors That Modify Low-Density Lipoprotein Cholesterol*

Cigarette smoking
Hypertension (blood pressure >140/90 mm Hg or on antihypertensive medication)
Low level of HDL cholesterol (<40 mg/dL)[†]
Family history of premature CHD (CHD in male first-degree relative <55 years; CHD in female first-degree relative <65 years)
Age (men >45 years; women >55 years)

CHD: coronary heart disease; HDL: high-density lipoprotein.
*Diabetes is regarded as a coronary heart disease risk equivalent.
[†]HDL cholesterol >60 mg/dL counts as a "negative" risk factor; its presence removes one risk factor from the total count.
Data from National Cholesterol Education Program. Third Report of the Expert Panel on Detection, Evaluation, and Treatment of High Blood Cholesterol in Adults (Adult Treatment Panel III). ATP III At-A-Glance: Quick Desk Reference. Retrieved from http://www.nhlbi.nih.gov/guidelines/cholesterol.

identification of kindred with known cardiovascular disease, smoking history, hypertension, age at diagnosis, presence of diabetes or other major illness, gender, longevity, and cause of death (**Table 17-3**).

Management and Surveillance

The current target goal for LDL-C is less than 100 mg/dL. Pharmacotherapy is beneficial in FH heterozygotes, using either lipid-lowering statins or statin/bile resin combination therapies (**Table 17-4**). In adults, the goal of therapy

TABLE 17-4	Low-Density Lipoprotein and Non-High-Density Lipoprotein Cholesterol Goals and Thresholds for Therapeutic Lifestyle Changes and Drug Therapy in Different Risk Categories			
Risk Category	**LDL Level at LDL Goal (mg/dL)**	**LDL Level at Which to Initiate Lifestyle Changes (mg/dL)**	**LDL Level at Which to Consider Drug Therapy (mg/dL)**	**Non-HDL Goal (mg/dL)***
CHD or CHD risk equivalents: diabetes mellitus, atherosclerotic disease (CAD or stroke), or multiple risk factors (10-year risk >20%)	<100	>100	≥130 (100–129; drug optional)[†]	<130
2+ risk factors: HDL <40 mg/dL, strong family history, age >45 years, and smoking (10-year risk >20%)	<130	≥130	10-year risk 10% to 20% ≥130 10-year risk <10%: ≥160	<160
0–1 risk factor[‡]	<160	≥160	≥190 (160 to 189: LDL-lowering drug optional)	<190

CAD: coronary artery disease; CHD: coronary heart disease; HDL: high-density lipoprotein; LDL: low-density lipoprotein.

*Non-HDL cholesterol: (total cholesterol – HDL). When LDL cannot be measured because the triglyceride level >200 mg/dL, non-HDL cholesterol may be used as a secondary goal. The non-HDL cholesterol goal is 30 mg/dL higher than the LDL cholesterol goal.

[†]Some authorities recommend use of LDL-lowering drugs in this category if an LDL cholesterol level <100 mg/dL cannot be achieved by therapeutic lifestyle changes (dietary and exercise intervention). Others prefer use of drugs that primarily modify triglycerides and HDL (e.g., nicotine acid or fibrates). Clinical judgment also may suggest deferring drug therapy in this subcategory.

[‡]Almost all people with zero or one risk factor have a 10-year risk less than 10%; thus, 10-year risk assessment in people with zero or one risk factor is not necessary.

Reproduced from U.S. Department of Health and Human Services. National Guideline Clearinghouse. *Prevention of Secondary Disease: Lipid Screening and Cardiovascular Risk.* Retrieved from www.guideline.gov/summary/summary.aspx?doc_id=10963.

is a greater than or equal to 50% decrease in LDL-C. The therapy of choice is statin therapy. In pregnancy statins, ezetimibe and niacin are contraindicated, however, the standard of care is to use Bile acid sequestrants for this population. In children, the current target goal is 50% reduction of the overall LDL-C or an LDL-C <130mg/dL. The recommendations for children are to begin low fat diets at 1 year of age for kids at high-risk and begin pharmacologic therapy at age 10 if diet was not successful. The American Academy of Pediatrics recommends beginning medications in children under the age of 8 years old if the LDL >500mg/dL. Pravastatin is currrently FDA approved for children 8 and older. Lovastatin, simvastatin, fluvastatin, atorvastatin, and rosuvastatin are currently FDA approved in children 10 and older. Statins remain the most effective agents for lowering LDL-C by inhibition of the enzyme that is responsible for endogenous hepatic cholesterol production—namely, 3-hydroxy-3-methylglutaryl-coenzyme A reductase (HMG-CoA reductase).

Inhibition of HMG-CoA reductase lowers intracellular cholesterol levels, which causes an up-regulation of LDLRs. As a result, LDL-C clearance from the circulation is increased. As a group, the statins are generally well tolerated and have been well documented to lower cholesterol by as much as 25–50% below baseline. Statin doses required to attain an approximate 30–40% reduction in LDL-C levels have also been well established. Furthermore, the reduction of LDL-C in adults is directly proportional to a reduction of coronary events. For example, a sustained 5% reduction in LDL-C is equivalent to a 5% reduction in coronary events.

In some cases, statin treatment will cause an increase in liver enzymes (AST, ALT), so these enzyme levels need to be monitored for any abnormal elevation during treatment. Another adverse effect is muscle pain (especially in the lower legs); patients need to be educated to report such muscle pain because there have been reported associations between statin use and rhabdomyolysis.

Cholesterol absorption inhibitors (e.g., ezetimibe) block intestinal absorption of cholesterol from the diet. This class of drugs has been shown to reduce LDL-C by 15–20% and is frequently used in conjunction with statins to reach target goals. Few side effects and relative safety yield a good compliance rate with these medications.

Bile-acid-binding resins (e.g., colesevelam, colestipol) work by binding the cholesterol in bile acids in the intestines. Once bound, the cholesterol is not absorbed into the systemic circulation. The average cholesterol-lowering effects achieved are between 10% and 20% of baseline. However, gastrointestinal side effects such as constipation, cramping, and bloating are common reasons for patient noncompliance.

Niacin produces a secondary reduction in LDL-C but primarily functions to lower triglycerides (VLDL-C) and increase HDL-C. The LDL-C response occurs best at higher doses of the drug. Unfortunately, the adverse effects associated with niacin—such as pruritis, flushing, gout exacerbation, and peptic ulcer disease—contribute to decreased patient compliance. To reduce flushing, patients are advised to take a 325 mg aspirin 30 minutes before taking niacin and to take the medication with food (e.g., applesauce). Fibric acid derivatives also reduce synthesis of triglycerides (VLDL-C) and have been shown to reduce LDL-C between 10% and 15%, with some increase in HDL-C being noted as well. Although an increased risk of hepatitis and myositis has been reported in some patients who take these medications, the most common adverse reactions include elevated liver transaminases.

Recommended lifestyle changes for patients with dyslipidemia include smoking cessation, dietary changes (i.e., decrease consumption of fatty/fried foods, increase consumption of fruits and vegetables), weight loss, increased exercise, and management of diabetes mellitus and hypertension. The reduction of inflammation in the presence of chronic inflammatory diseases or infection is also beneficial. Dietary changes are a critical component of therapy for heterozygous FH because they can reduce many risk factors and lower LDL-C levels. Increased consumption of dietary fiber is thought to help lower LDL-C by binding the fiber with cholesterol in bile acids, thereby preventing the cholesterol from being absorbed in the gastrointestinal tract. Increased intake of monounsaturated fats such as olive oil may also reduce LDL-C oxidation. Although increased physical activity primarily increases HDL-C and lowers serum triglycerides, it has also been shown to lower LDL-C levels. Although many of these recommendations seem obvious for all patients—not just those with FH—in our current society, it is very difficult for patients to adhere to them. Thus, noncompliance is the greatest barrier to any of these suggested therapeutic lifestyle changes.

For healthcare providers, it is important to maintain a good working relationship with FH patients. This includes routine follow-up visits at least every 6 months. Given that most of the pharmacotherapeutic treatments for hyperlipidemia affect the liver, it is important to monitor not only fasting lipid profiles but also liver transaminases at least annually once desired blood cholesterol levels are achieved. Adjustments in medication doses may be necessary over the course of treatment, with each case being treated individually.

Chapter Summary

» Familial hypercholesterolemia (FH) is characterized by increased levels of total serum cholesterol (hypercholesterolemia) with increased low-density lipoprotein cholesterol (LDL-C), tendinous xanthomata, and premature symptoms of coronary heart disease.

» Hypercholesterolemia is defined as a fasting total blood cholesterol level of more than 240 mg/dL.

» The LDL-C target goal is less than 100 mg/dL.

» Diagnostic tools for FH are not standardized but often include a positive family history, clinical history of atherosclerotic disease, physical examination findings, blood cholesterol levels, and genetic testing for the *LDLR* gene.

» Several pharmacotherapeutic options are available to treat FH.

» Patients with FH should address modifiable risk factors such as poor dietary habits and smoking.

» Early diagnosis of FH can reduce the morbidity and mortality associated with this disease.

Chapter Review Questions

1. Familial hypercholesterolemia can result from a mutation in any of four genes: _____, _____, _____, or _____.
2. Familial hypercholesterolemia is characterized by increased levels of _____ and _____ and the physical examination findings of _____ and _____.
3. The target goal for LDL-C levels is _____.
4. The reduction of _____ in adults is directly proportional to the reduction of coronary events.
5. Thyroid abnormalities such as _____ are an important secondary cause of hypercholesterolemia.

Bibliography

American Heart Association. (n.d.). Retrieved from http://www.americanheart.org

Austin, M. A., Hutter, C. M., Zimmern, R. L., & Humphries, S. E. (2004). Familial hypercholesterolemia and coronary heart disease: A HuGE association review. *American Journal of Epidemiology, 160*, 421–429.

Austin, M. A., Hutter C. M., Zimmern R. L., & Humphries, S. E. (2004). Genetic causes of monogenic heterozygous familial hypercholesterolemia: A HuGE prevalence review. *American Journal of Epidemiology, 160*, 407–420.

Daniels, S. R., & Greer, F. R. (2008). Lipid screening and cardiovascular health in childhood. *Pediatrics, 122*, 198–208.

Goldstein, J. L., Hobbs, H. H., & Brown, M. S. (2001). Familial hypercholesterolemia. In C. R. Scriver, A. L. Beaudet, W. S. Sly, D. Valle, B. Childs, K. W. Kinzler, & B. Vogelstein (Eds.), *The metabolic and molecular basis of inherited disease* (8th ed., pp. 2863–2914). New York, NY: McGraw-Hill.

Gotto, A., & Pownall, H. (2003). *Manual of lipid disorders* (3rd ed.). Philadelphia, PA: Lippincott, Williams and Wilkins.

Grundy, S. M., Cleeman, J. I., Merz, N. B., Brewer, H. B., Jr., Clark, L. T., Hunninghake, D. B. . . . American Heart Association. (2004). Implications of recent clinical trials for the National Cholesterol Education Program Adult Treatment Panel III Guidelines. *Circulation, 110,* 227–239.

Hypercholesterolemia. (2018). In *Genetics Home Reference*. Retrieved from https:// ghr.nlm.nih.gov/condition/hypercholesterolemia

Leigh, S. E., Foster, A. H., Whittall, R. A., Hubbart, B. S., & Humphries, S. E. (2008). Update and analysis of the University College London low density lipoprotein receptor familial hypercholesterolemia database. *Annals of Human Genetics, 72,* 485–498.

National Library of Medicine. (n.d.). *Genetics Home Reference*. Retrieved from http:// ghr.nlm.nih.gov/

Tietz, N. W. (1995). *Clinical guide to laboratory tests* (3rd ed.) Philadelphia, PA: W. B. Saunders.

Youngblom, E., Pariani, M., & Knowles, J. W. (2016, December). Familial hypercholesterolemia. Retrieved from https://www.ncbi.nlm.nih.gov/books /NBK174884/

‹ Describe the etiology and various forms of hereditary cardiomyopathies.
‹ Detail symptoms associated with hereditary cardiomyopathies.
‹ Discuss diagnostic criteria for hereditary cardiomyopathies.
‹ Discuss reduced penetrance.
‹ Review current surveillance and treatment recommendations for hereditary cardiomyopathies.

KEY TERMS

Brugada syndrome
Cardiomyopathy
Fabry disease

Left ventricular
  hypertrophy (LVH)
Myocardium

Sarcomere
Wolff-Parkinson-White
  syndrome

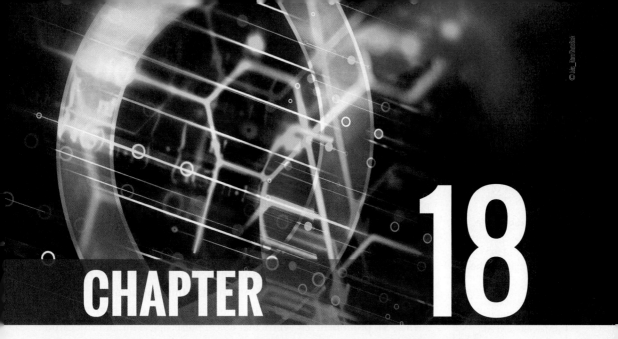

CHAPTER 18

Hereditary Cardiomyopathies

Cardiomyopathy is any condition in which the heart muscle (**myocardium**) is dysfunctional. Affected individuals are at increased risk for arrhythmias and sudden cardiac death. Cardiomyopathies are categorized based on the pathological features of the heart tissue itself. They may occur secondary to other diseases or may be hereditary in nature. This chapter discusses the two most common types of *hereditary* cardiomyopathies: familial hypertrophic cardiomyopathy (HCM) and arrhythmogenic right ventricular dysplasia or cardiomyopathy (ARVD/C).

Familial HCM (formerly known as idiopathic hypertrophic subaortic stenosis) is characterized by unexplained **left ventricular hypertrophy (LVH)** that develops in the absence of other known causes. Mutations in various genes encoding for the contractile unit (**sarcomere**) of the heart muscle cells cause the muscle to be weakened, which impairs contractility. The clinical presentation of individuals affected by HCM may include dyspnea on exertion, palpitations, chest pain, and syncope, but some patients are asymptomatic. Unexplained LVH occurs in 1 in 500 persons. Known mutations in various sarcomere-associated genes are identifiable in approximately 70% of HCM cases.

ARVD/C is characterized by the replacement of normal heart muscle in the right ventricle by fibrous and fatty tissue. Similar to what happens with HCM, this abnormal tissue structure weakens the heart muscle and leads to impaired contractility. As in HCM, the clinical presentation of ARVD/C includes arrhythmias, palpitations, chest pain, and syncope. Incidence of ARVD/C has been reported to be 1 per 1,000 persons in the overall population, with incidence reaching as high as 4.4 cases per 1,000 population in the southern United States and in certain Mediterranean populations.

Both HCM and ARVD/C are associated with an increased risk for sudden cardiac death. HCM has been reported to be the leading cause of sudden cardiac death in competitive athletes in the United States, while ARVD/C is the second most common cause of sudden cardiac death and is more common in those younger than the age of 35. Both HCM and ARVD/C are inherited in autosomal dominant patterns.

Diagnosis

Familial HCM and ARVD/C can be difficult to diagnose. This challenge makes obtaining a thorough personal history and family history critical in patients being evaluated for fatigue, arrhythmias, palpitations, presyncope, syncope, or chest pain. Any of these physical symptoms in a person younger than the age of 35 or a positive family history of sudden cardiac death or unexplained death in first-degree relatives should raise the index of suspicion for HCM or ARVD/C. A family history of heart failure, HCM, heart transplant, stroke, or blood clots is also important in this evaluation.

Physical examination findings in HCM may include extra heart sounds such as S4, prominent left ventricular apical pulse, apical lift, or brisk carotid upstroke. Abnormal electrocardiogram (ECG) findings are very common in both HCM and ARVD/C (**Figure 18-1**). The diagnosis of HCM is made based on a positive family history and/or molecular genetic testing in patients who have LVH in a nondilated ventricle as determined by echocardiography. The LVH must be present in the absence of predisposing factors such as hypertension or aortic stenosis. Although a myocardial biopsy can also establish the presence of LVH on the cellular level, this technique is usually reserved for autopsy.

The age of onset varies widely for HCM. Notably, LVH may become evident during the second decade of life (adolescence), with its development thought to be related to the onset of puberty. Development of LVH may occur as early as infancy and childhood, however, or it may not become apparent until later in life. This variation in the age of onset can occur within families and is thought to be attributed to variations in the phenotypic expression of the gene mutation. It also explains why some people who inherit the mutation do not develop the disease—a phenomenon known as *reduced penetrance*.

Four clinically observable phases of ARVD/C are distinguished. In the first, the concealed phase, the patient shows no clinical manifestations but possesses a hidden risk of sudden cardiac death. This phase is followed by the second phase, in which there is the development of symptomatic arrhythmias. In the third phase, right ventricular failure occurs. The fourth phase is marked by pump failure. It should be noted that left ventricular involvement can occur in any of the phases.

Although the physical examination is normal in at least 50% of patients with ARVD/C, one striking diagnostic clue is the presence of an extra heart sound, such as a wide-split S2, S3, or S4. When the right ventricle is significantly dilated, asymmetry of the chest wall may be noticeable.

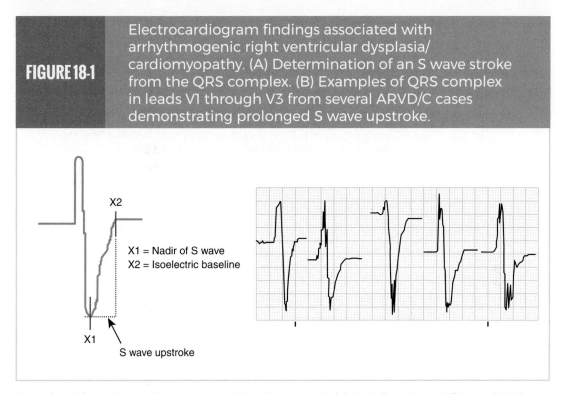

FIGURE 18-1 Electrocardiogram findings associated with arrhythmogenic right ventricular dysplasia/cardiomyopathy. (A) Determination of an S wave stroke from the QRS complex. (B) Examples of QRS complex in leads V1 through V3 from several ARVD/C cases demonstrating prolonged S wave upstroke.

X2

X1 = Nadir of S wave
X2 = Isoelectric baseline

X1

S wave upstroke

Reproduced from Nasir, K., Bomma, C., Tandri, H., Roguin, A., Dalal, D., Prakasa, K., . . . Calkins, H. (2004). Electrocardiographic features of arrhythmogenic right ventricular dysplasia/cardiomyopathy according to disease severity: A need to broaden diagnostic criteria. *Circulation, 110*, 1527–1534.

Characteristic ECG findings are evident in as many as 90% of affected individuals (**Figure 18-2**) and have been incorporated into the major and minor diagnostic criteria for ARVD/C (**Table 18-1**). Patients diagnosed with ARVD/C are typically between the ages of 19 and 45, and the majority are male.

Standard cardiac testing used in diagnosing cardiomyopathies such as HCM and ARVD/C includes a 12-lead ECG, signal-averaged ECG, exercise stress test, echocardiogram, cardiac MRI, and 24-hour Holter monitoring. Other tests, such as electrophysiological studies and myocardial biopsy, may be performed to complete the evaluation.

Genetic Testing and Counseling

As mentioned previously, ARVD/C and HCM are most commonly inherited in an autosomal dominant manner (McNally, MacLeod, & Dellafave, 2009). New mutations in an individual (de novo mutations) are also transmissible to

FIGURE 18-2 Electrocardiograms from arrhythmogenic right ventricular dysplasia/cardiomyopathy (ARVD/C) patients. (A) Diffuse ARVD/C. (B) Localized ARVD/C.

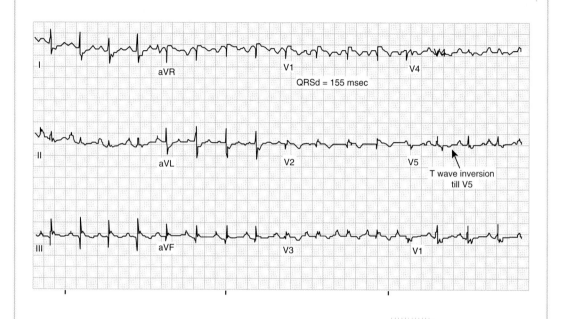

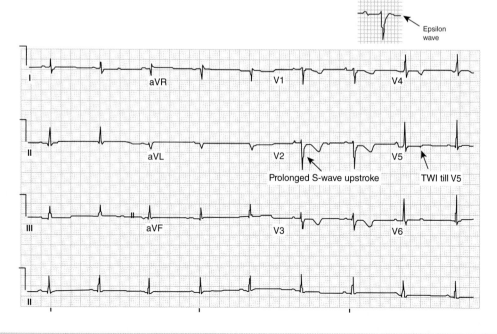

FIGURE 18-2 (C) ARVD/C with right bundle branch block pattern.

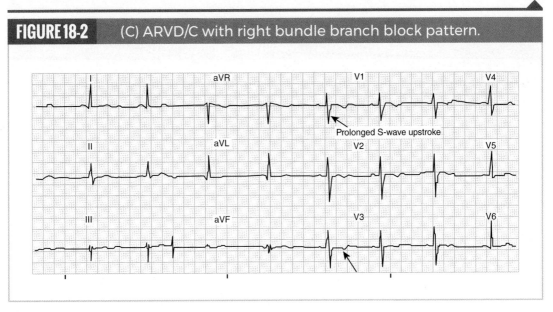

TWI: T wave inversion.
Reproduced from Nasir, K., Bomma, C., Tandri, H., Roguin, A., Dalal, D., Prakasa, K., . . . Calkins, H. (2004). Electrocardiographic features of arrhythmogenic right ventricular dysplasia/cardiomyopathy according to disease severity: A need to broaden diagnostic criteria. *Circulation, 110*, 1527–1534.

TABLE 18-1 Major and Minor Diagnostic Criteria for Arrhythmogenic Right Ventricular Dysplasia/Cardiomyopathy

Diagnosis requires either two major criteria, one major and two minor criteria, or four minor criteria from the following categories.

Category	Major Criteria	Minor Criteria
Global and/or regional dysfunction and structural alterations	Severe right ventricular dilation and reduction of right ventricular function with no (or only mild) left ventricular impairment Localized right ventricular aneurysms (akinetic or dyskinetic areas with diastolic bulging) Severe segmental dilation of the right ventricle	Mild global right ventricular dilation and/or ejection fraction reduction with normal left ventricle Mild segmental dilation of right ventricle Regional right ventricular hypokinesis

TABLE 18-1	Major and Minor Diagnostic Criteria for Arrhythmogenic Right Ventricular Dysplasia/Cardiomyopathy *(Continued)*

Category	Major Criteria	Minor Criteria
Tissue characterization of walls	Fibrofatty replacement of myocardium observed on endomyocardial biopsy	
Major repolarization abnormalities		Inverted T waves in right precordial leads (V2 and V3) (age >12 years, in absence of right bundle branch block)
Minor depolarization/ conduction abnormalities	Epsilon waves or localized prolongation (>110 ms) of the QRS complex in right precordial leads (V1–V3) Late potential (signal-averaged ECG)	Left bundle branch block-type ventricular tachycardia (sustained and nonsustained) on ECG, Holter monitor, or exercise testing Frequent ventricular extrasystoles (>1,000/24 h on Holter monitoring)
Family history	Familial disease confirmed at necropsy or surgery	Familial history of premature sudden death (<35 years) suspected to be caused by right ventricular dysplasia Familial history (clinical diagnosis based on present criteria)

Data from McKenna, W. J., Thiene, G., Nava, A., Fontaliran, F., Blomstrom-Lundqvist, C., Fontaine, G., & Camerini, F. (1994). Diagnosis of arrhythmogenic right ventricular dysplasia/cardiomyopathy. *British Heart Journal, 71*, 215–218.

the offspring of that individual. Although its occurrence is rare, ARVD/C may also be inherited in an autosomal recessive pattern, especially in families from Greece. Some individuals have inherited multiple mutations. In these cases, evaluation should include an effort to determine the mode of inheritance through construction of a pedigree.

Eight genes are known to be associated with ARVD/C, whereas 12 genes are linked to HCM. Testing of at-risk adult relatives for both disorders is

TABLE 18-2	Screening Guidelines for Healthy Relatives of Probands with Familial Hypertrophic Cardiomyopathy

Age	Screening Guidelines
<12 years	Optional but recommended, particularly if any of the following are present: family history of early HCM-related death, early development of LVH, or other adverse complications. Competitive athlete in intense training program. Symptoms: other clinical findings that suggest early LVH.
12–18 years	Repeat evaluation every 12–18 months.
>18–21 years	Repeat evaluation approximately every 3–5 years or in response to any change in symptoms. Tailor the evaluation if the family has late-onset LVH or HCM-related complications.

HCM: hypertrophic cardiomyopathy; LVH: left ventricular hypertrophy.
© American Heart Association, Inc. Reprinted with permission. *Circulation, 11*(124), 2761–2796.

routinely performed once the specific mutation has been identified in the proband. Unfortunately, mutation testing cannot predict the age of onset, constellation, or severity of symptoms. It can, however, identify those persons who require close surveillance. Screening guidelines have been proposed for asymptomatic relatives of the probands with HCM (**Table 18-2**). In particular, all first-degree family members of a proband with ARVD/C should undergo initial screening with the onset of puberty and have follow-up testing every 2–3 years.

Management and Treatment

No treatment exists to prevent or delay disease expression for either HCM or ARVD/C. The primary goal of medical management is to prevent arrhythmias, syncopal episodes, and sudden cardiac death. Arrhythmias such as atrial fibrillation may initially be managed with pharmacological therapies. Implantable cardioverter-defibrillators are indicated for persons who have survived a cardiac arrest, are at high risk of cardiac arrest, or have arrhythmias that cannot be managed pharmacologically (e.g., sustained ventricular tachycardia). Persons who develop atrial fibrillation should receive anticoagulation therapy to prevent thromboembolism. Obstructive cardiac physiology in any person should be managed with prophylactic antibiotics to prevent endocarditis.

KEY TERMS

Wolff-Parkinson-White syndrome: an electrocardiographic pattern sometimes associated with paroxysmal tachycardia; it consists of a short P-R interval (usually 0.1 second or less, occasionally normal) together with a prolonged QRS complex with a slurred initial component (delta wave).

Fabry disease: an inherited lipid storage disease that results from a deficiency in the enzyme alpha-galactosidase found on the X chromosome. This defect leads to the accumulation of glycosphingolipids in the plasma and lysosomes of vascular endothelial and smooth muscle cells.

Pregnancy, even in stable patients, necessitates care by an obstetrician who specializes in high-risk pregnancies. Circumstances that patients should be advised to avoid include endurance training, burst activities, and isometric exercise. Patients with outflow obstruction should be encouraged to keep hydrated and cautioned about the use of diuretics, angiotensin-converting enzyme (ACE) inhibitors, angiotensin-receptor blockers, and medications used for erectile dysfunction.

Dyspnea in HCM is common because of diastolic dysfunction; beta blockers and calcium-channel blockers can be used to slow heart rate and improve this diastolic function by extending the filling period. Unfortunately, even with proper management, patients with cardiomyopathy often progress to heart failure. Heart transplantation remains a consideration when failure cannot be managed medically.

Associated Syndromes

LVH occurs in 1 in 500 persons, with almost 70% of all such cases being attributable to HCM. The remainder are due to either the associated syndromes discussed in this section or other, idiopathic causes.

Acquired LVH is found in competitive athletes who have undergone vigorous training. It may be distinguished from hereditary cardiomyopathies by observing whether a restriction imposed on physical training results in a decreased wall thickness of the myocardium.

Metabolic cardiomyopathy should be considered when LVH is found in conjunction with a pre-excitation syndrome such as **Wolff-Parkinson-White syndrome**.

As much as 10% of unexplained LVH in young adult males has been attributed to **Fabry disease**, an inherited lipid storage disease. Fabry disease results from a deficiency in the enzyme alpha-galactosidase found on the X chromosome. This defect leads to the accumulation of glycosphingolipids in the plasma and lysosomes of vascular endothelial and smooth muscle cells. As a consequence, a fatty component of the cell wall cannot be broken down and builds up inside the cells, especially the cells lining the arteries and blood vessels. This accumulation of lipid clogs the blood vessels, which in turn damages the heart (heart attack) and kidneys (kidney failure). Lipid deposits are also found in cells of the cornea, kidney tubules, muscle fibers of the heart, and cells of the nervous system.

Cardiac amyloidosis is caused by deposition of an amyloid protein in the myocardium that displaces functional tissue. Normal cardiac movement is restricted by this accumulation; thus, this disorder is categorized as a "restrictive cardiomyopathy." Amyloidosis may be either inherited or occur as a de novo mutation.

Brugada syndrome is characterized by ST segment abnormalities in leads V1–V3 on the ECG. This condition, which is associated with ventricular fibrillation and sudden cardiac death, most commonly occurs in young males of Asian descent.

Childhood cardiomyopathies have been associated with three major causes: inborn errors of metabolism, malformation syndromes, and neuro-muscular disorders. The most common associated disorders in these categor-ies are glycogen storage disease type II, Noonan syndrome, and Friedreich ataxia, respectively.

> **KEY TERM**
>
> **Brugada syndrome:** a condition that causes ventricular arrhythmias and can lead to fainting (syncope), seizures, difficulty breathing, or sudden death.

Chapter Summary

» A cardiomyopathy is any condition in which the heart muscle (myocardium) is dysfunctional.

» Cardiomyopathies are categorized based on the pathological features of the heart tissue itself. They may either occur secondary to other diseases or be hereditary in nature.

» Familial hypertrophic cardiomyopathy is characterized by unexplained left ventricular hypertrophy that develops in the absence of other known causes.

» Arrhythmogenic right ventricular dysplasia/cardiomyopathy is characterized by the replacement of normal heart muscle in the right ventricle by fibrous and fatty tissue.

» Both familial hypertrophic cardiomyopathy and arrhythmogenic right ventricular dysplasia/cardiomyopathy are inherited in autosomal domin-ant patterns.

» No treatment exists to prevent or delay disease expression for these heredi-tary cardiomyopathies. Therefore, the primary goal of medical manage-ment is to prevent arrhythmias, syncopal episodes, and sudden cardiac death.

Chapter Review Questions

1. The majority of hereditary cardiomyopathies are attributed to
   _____ and _____.
2. The most life-threatening complications associated with cardiomyopa-thies are _____ and _____.

3. Both familial hypertrophic cardiomyopathy and arrhythmogenic right ventricular dysplasia/cardiomyopathy are inherited in a/an _____ pattern.

4. Signs and symptoms that raise clinical suspicion for familial hypertrophic cardiomyopathy include _____, _____, _____, and _____.

5. Electrocardiogram findings for arrhythmogenic right ventricular dysplasia/cardiomyopathy may include _____ and _____.

Bibliography

Fabry disease. (n.d.). In *Stedman's online medical dictionary*. Retrieved from http://www.stedmansonline.com

Hamid, M. S., Norman, M., Quraishi, A., Firoozi, S., Thaman, R., Gimeno, J. R., & Sachdev, B. (2002). Prospective evaluation of relatives for familial arrhythmogenic right ventricular cardiomyopathy/dysplasia reveals a need to broaden diagnostic criteria. *Journal of American College of Cardiology, 40*, 1445–1450.

McKenna, W. J., Thiene, G., Nava, A., Fontaliran, F., Blomstrom-Lundqvist, C., Fontaine, G., & Camerini, F. (1994). Diagnosis of arrhythmogenic right ventricular dysplasia/cardiomyopathy. *British Heart Journal, 71*, 215–218.

McNally, E., MacLeod, H., & Dellafave, L. (2009). Arrhythmogenic right ventricular dysplasia/cardiomyopathy, autosomal dominant. *GeneReviews*. Retrieved from http://www.ncbi.nlm.nih.gov/bookshelf/br.fcgi?book=gene&part=arvd

Nasir, K., Bomma, C., Tandri, H., Roguin, A., Dalal, D., Prakasa, K., . . . Calkins, H. (2004). Electrocardiographic features of arrhythmogenic right ventricular dysplasia/cardiomyopathy according to disease severity: A need to broaden diagnostic criteria. *Circulation, 110*, 1527–1534. Retrieved from http://circ.ahajournals.org/content/110/12/1527

Nava, A., Bauce, B., Basso, C., Muriago, M., Rampazzo, A., Villanova, C., . . . Thiene, G. (2000). Clinical profile and long-term follow-up of 37 families with arrhythmogenic right ventricular cardiomyopathy. *Journal of American College of Cardiology, 36*, 2226–2233.

Peters, S., Trummel, M., Koehler, B., & Westermann, K. U. (2007). The value of different electrocardiographic depolarization criteria in the diagnosis of arrhythmogenic right ventricular dysplasia/cardiomyopathy. *Journal of Electrocardiology, 40,* 34–37.

Sen-Chowdhry, S., Syrris, P., Ward, D., Asimaki, A., Sevdalis, E., & McKenna, W. J. (2007). Clinical and genetic characterization of families with arrhythmogenic right ventricular dysplasia/cardiomyopathy provides novel insights into patterns of disease expression. *Circulation, 115,* 1710–1720.

What is Fabry disease? (n.d.). Retrieved from http://www.fabrydisease.com/

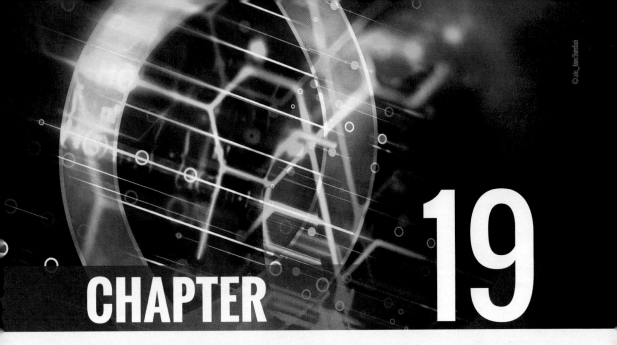

CHAPTER 19

Marfan Syndrome

Marfan syndrome is caused by a defect of the connective tissue that manifests itself as a series of disorders of multiple organs, including the eye, aorta, and skin, as well as overgrowth of the long bones. This syndrome results from either an inherited mutation or a new (de novo) mutation of the *fibrillin-1* gene (*FBN1*) on chromosome 15. Phenotypically, these mutations are indistinguishable from each other. The heritable form follows an autosomal dominant pattern of inheritance, meaning that only one copy of the mutated gene is required to produce disease. De novo mutations produce disease in people without a positive family history of the disorder. Although such cases are not as common as those involving inherited mutations, it is estimated that 25% of Marfan syndrome cases result from a new mutation in the *FBN1* gene. The incidence of Marfan syndrome ranges between 1 in 5,000 and 1 in 10,000 individuals; it shows no obvious predilection by race, ethnicity, or gender.

Phenotypic Features

Skeletal abnormalities that are commonly associated with Marfan syndrome include tall stature with long, thin arms and legs and arachnodactyly (spiderlike fingers and long, slender fingers and toes in comparison with the palms of the hands and soles of the feet). Another hallmark phenotypical feature is an arm span exceeding the body height of the individual (dolichostenomelia). In addition, common findings include an elongated, narrow face; a highly arched palate; overcrowded teeth; scoliosis; hyperflexible joints; and chest deformities (pectus excavatum or pectus carinatum).

Ocular disorders associated with Marfan syndrome include myopia, the most common disorder, and lens displacement from the center of the pupil (ectopia lentis), which is observed in approximately 60% of affected individuals. Individuals with Marfan syndrome are also at increased risk for retinal detachment, glaucoma, and early development of cataracts.

Abnormalities of the heart such as valve defects are often observed in people with Marfan syndrome and are the major cause of morbidity and mortality in affected individuals. The mitral valve and the aortic valve are the most commonly affected. Valvular insufficiency may manifest as palpitations, murmurs, shortness of breath, and fatigue. Weakening of the vessel wall of the aorta may result in aortic aneurysms or aortic dissections due to stretching.

Stretching of the dural sac in the lumbosacral spine (dural ectasia), the development of bullae in the lungs, spontaneous pneumothorax, hernias, and stretch marks of the skin are other findings associated with Marfan syndrome. Pregnancy presents a special cause for concern, and increased surveillance is imperative because the risk for aortic dissection is increased in both the peripartum and postpartum stages.

A recent study identified that the average age at diagnosis of Marfan syndrome is 19 years, but overall, there is a wide variation among affected individuals regarding age at presentation, organ system manifestation, and severity and progression of the disease. Because physical findings tend to remain consistent among affected family members, however, the predominant determinate of phenotype is presumed to be the *FBN1* genotype.

Genetics of Marfan Syndrome

The *FBN1* gene is the only known gene associated with Marfan syndrome. In healthy individuals, this gene carries instructions for making the protein fibrillin-1, which has two main functions: (1) it combines with other structural proteins to form microfibrils, and (2) it regulates the growth and repair of various body tissues. **Microfibrils** are integral fibers that lend strength and flexibility to all connective, load-bearing tissues. Thus, the characteristic features of Marfan syndrome created by the mutated *FBN1* gene are a product of dysfunction in each of these mechanisms. In addition, the mutated *FBN1* gene inhibits the production of the normal-functioning protein, blocking the formation of normal microfibrils (**dominant negative mutation**).

The specific *FBN1* mutations leading to Marfan syndrome vary widely among affected families and are often scattered across the gene (**genetic heterogeneity**). Because the penetrance of *FBN1* mutations is 100%, any offspring inheriting the mutated allele will develop Marfan syndrome, albeit with variable expressivity of the symptoms. **Variable expressivity** refers to the existence of variations in the symptoms associated with the disease. With Marfan syndrome, some affected individuals have multiple or severe symptoms, whereas others exhibit fewer or milder symptoms. It is important to note that the degree of severity in one affected individual will not dictate the degree of severity in that individual's offspring.

Marfan syndrome is inherited in an autosomal dominant pattern. Approximately 75% of affected individuals have an affected parent, while the remaining 25% cases involve random or de novo mutations. Therefore, the risk of inheriting the *FBN1* mutation and developing the syndrome when one parent is affected is 50%.

Diagnosis

The clinical diagnosis of Marfan syndrome is made based on both family history and the following physical examination findings: (1) aortic dilatation or dissection at the level of the sinuses of Valsalva, (2) ectopia lentis, (3) dural ectasia, and (4) four (of eight) specified skeletal features (see **Table 19-1**). In patients for whom no family history is available, the criteria are adjusted to require major involvement of two organ systems and minor involvement of one other system.

TABLE 19-1   Diagnostic Criteria for Marfan Syndrome

System	Major Criteria	Minor Criteria
Skeletal system	Presence of at least four of the following manifestations: ‹ Pectus carinatum ‹ Pectus excavatum requiring surgery ‹ Reduced upper-to-lower-segment ratio (torso lengths much shorter than legs) or arm-span-to-height ratio is greater than 1.05 ‹ Wrist and thumb signs (hypermobility of wrists and hand) ‹ Scoliosis >20 degrees or spondylolisthesis ‹ Reduced extension at the elbow (<170 degrees) ‹ Medial displacement of the medial malleolus causing pes planus ‹ Protrusio acetabulae of any degree (ascertained on radiographs)	‹ Pectus excavatum of moderate severity ‹ Joint hypermobility ‹ Highly arched palate with crowding of teeth ‹ Facial appearance (dolichocephaly, malar hypoplasia, enophthalmos, retrognathia, down-slanting palpebral fissures)
Ocular system	‹ Ectopia lentis (dislocated lens)	‹ Abnormally flat cornea (as measured by keratometry) ‹ Increased axial length of globe (as measured by ultrasound)

TABLE 19-1	Diagnostic Criteria for Marfan Syndrome *(Continued)*	
System	**Major Criteria**	**Minor Criteria**
Cardiovascular system	‹ Dilatation of the ascending aorta with or without aortic regurgitation and involving at least the sinuses of Valsalva **or** ‹ Dissection of the ascending aorta	‹ Mitral valve prolapse with or without mitral valve regurgitation ‹ Dilatation of the main pulmonary artery, in the absence of valvular or peripheral pulmonic stenosis or any other obvious cause, before the age of 40 ‹ Calcification of the mitral annulus before the age of 40 ‹ Dilatation or dissection of the descending thoracic or abdominal aorta before the age of 50
Pulmonary system	None	‹ Spontaneous pneumothorax ‹ Apical blebs (ascertained by chest radiography)
Skin and integument	None	‹ Stretch marks not associated with marked weight changes, pregnancy, or repetitive stress ‹ Recurrent incisional hernias
Dura	‹ Lumbosacral dural ectasia diagnosed by CT or MRI ‹ Having a parent, child, or sibling who meets these diagnostic criteria independently	None
Family/genetic history	‹ Presence of a mutation in the *FBN1* gene known to cause Marfan syndrome ‹ Presence of a haplotype around *FBN1*, inherited by descent, known to be associated with unequivocally diagnosed Marfan syndrome in the family	None

Data from National Marfan Foundation. Diagnosis. Retrieved from www.marfan.org/marfan /2319/Diagnosis#Criteria.

Genetic Testing and Counseling

Molecular genetic testing for *FBN1* mutations may be clinically useful to confirm a diagnosis, for prenatal diagnosis, and as predictive testing in families with known mutations. Clinical evaluation should include a medical history, thorough family history, and echocardiogram when there is high clinical suspicion for Marfan syndrome. Linkage analysis is available for those families in which an *FBN1* mutation has been previously identified.

Management and Treatment

Today, the life expectancy of individuals with Marfan syndrome approaches the life expectancy of the general population when cardiovascular risks are minimized. Cardiovascular surveillance should include annual echocardiograms. More frequent echocardiograms are recommended when the aortic root diameter is known to be enlarged above a defined threshold—that is, when it exceeds the expected rate of enlargement found in animal models— or when aortic regurgitation develops. Similar surveillance of the affected individual's relatives may be indicated if clinical suspicion is raised by the individual's phenotypic features or reported symptoms.

Affected individuals should be counseled to avoid contact sports, isometric exercise, caffeine, and decongestants because of increased stress that these factors place on the cardiovascular system. If individuals are found to be at increased risk for pneumothorax, they should be warned about the risks of breathing against resistance (such as playing brass instruments) and negative-pressure ventilation (e.g., scuba diving).

Annual eye examinations by an ophthalmologist are highly recommended to preserve vision. In addition to routine examination procedures, patients should also be assessed for glaucoma and cataracts. Any abnormalities should be managed by a specialist with experience in treating the ocular manifestations associated with Marfan syndrome. Severe scoliosis or other skeletal manifestations require the expertise of an orthopedist. Orthodontic evaluation is recommended particularly if the affected individual has a highly arched palate and/or overcrowded teeth.

Management and surveillance of Marfan syndrome are primarily aimed at early detection of symptoms and intervention to prevent disease progression. Recent studies suggest that losartan—an angiotensin receptor blocker used to treat hypertension—might be used to prevent the clinical manifestations of Marfan syndrome because it appears to inhibit aortic enlargement, reverse existing aortic root growth, and ameliorate lung and muscle tissue problems by blocking excess transforming growth factor-beta in mice models of Marfan syndrome.

Associated Syndromes

Numerous other phenotypes are associated with mutations of *FBN1* but do not meet the full diagnostic criteria for Marfan syndrome. Additionally, many of the characteristic skeletal features of Marfan syndrome are observed among the general population and may represent another underlying connective tissue disorder. Mitral valve prolapse syndrome may be present with variable expression of skeletal features. One specific phenotype associated with an *FBN1* mutation is known as MASS and involves myopia with mitral valve prolapse, aortic enlargement, and nonspecific skin and skeletal features. Aortic aneurysm, Marfanoid skeletal features, and familial ectopia lentis are all findings that the clinician must carefully differentiate from emerging Marfan syndrome.

Some genotypes, other than the *FBN1* mutation, can cause phenotypic features similar to those found in Marfan syndrome—referred to as **genocopy**. Examples include familial thoracic aortic aneurysms and aortic dissections (TAAD), Ehlers-Danlos syndrome, homocystinuria, and fragile X syndrome.

Chapter Summary

» Marfan syndrome involves connective tissue defects that result in a multiorgan system disorder involving skeletal, cardiovascular, pulmonary, skin, ocular, and dural abnormalities.

» Marfan syndrome may present in early childhood but is diagnosed, on average, at age 19.

» Marfan syndrome is a clinical diagnosis made based on family history and established findings across multiple organ systems.

» In this syndrome, mortality is related to cardiovascular disorders associated with this disease, such as aortic dissection.

» Surveillance guidelines include annual imaging of the aorta beginning in young adulthood.

» Pregnancy presents a special surveillance consideration because women are at increased risk for aortic dissection and rupture.

Chapter Review Questions

1. Marfan syndrome is the result of a mutation in the _____ gene.

2. _____(the presence of spiderlike fingers) and an arm span exceeding the _____ are hallmark phenotypic features of Marfan syndrome.

3. The most life-threatening complication associated with Marfan syndrome is _____.

4. The chance of an affected individual having offspring with Marfan syndrome is _____, which is described as _____ pattern of _____ inheritance.

5. Physical examination findings that raise clinical suspicion for Marfan syndrome include abnormalities of the _____, _____, _____, _____, and _____.

Bibliography

De Paepe, A., Devereaux, R. B., Dietz, H. C., Hennekam, R. C., & Pyeritz, R. C. (1996). Revised diagnostic criteria for the Marfan syndrome. *American Journal of Medical Genetics, 62*(4), 417–426.

Dietz, H. (2017, October). Marfan syndrome. Retrieved from https://www.ncbi.nlm.nih.gov/books/NBK1335/

Dietz, H. C., Loeys, B., Carta, L. A., & Ramirez, F. (2005). Recent progress towards a molecular understanding of Marfan syndrome. *American Journal of Medical Genetics Counselors Seminars in Medical Genetics, 139*(1), 4–9.

Gleb, B. (2006). Marfan syndrome and related disorders: More tightly connected than we thought. *New England Journal of Medicine, 355*(8), 841–844.

Groth, K. A., Hove, H., Kyhl, K., Folkestad L., Gaustadnes, M., Vejlstrup, N., . . . Gravhold, C. H. (2015). Prevalence, incidence and age at diagnosis in Marfan syndrome. *Orphanet Journal of Rare Diseases, 10*, 153.

Habashi, J. P., Judge, D. P., Holm, T. M., Cohn, R. D., Loeys, B. L., Cooper, T. K., . . . Dietz, H. C. (2006). Losartan, an AT1 antagonist, prevents aortic aneurysm in a mouse model of Marfan syndrome. *Science, 312*, 117–121.

Hiratzka, L. F., Bakris, G. L., Beckman, J. A., Bersin, R. M., Carr, V. F., Casey, D. E., . . . Society for Vascular Medicine. (2010). ACCF/AHA/AATS/ACR/ASA/SCA/SCAI/SIR/STS/SVM guidelines for diagnosis and management of patients with thoracic aortic disease: Executive summary. *Circulation, 121*, 1544–1579.

Milewicz, D. M., Dietz, H. C., & Miller, D. C. (2005). Treatment of aortic disease in patients with Marfan syndrome. *Circulation, 111*, e150–e157.

National Human Genome Research Institute. (2017). *Learning about Marfan syndrome*. Retrieved from https://www.genome.gov/19519224/learning-about-marfan-syndrome/

National Library of Medicine, National Institutes of Health, U.S. Department of Health and Human Services. (n.d.). *Genetics home reference*. Retrieved from http://ghr.nlm.nih.gov/

National Marfan Foundation. (n.d.). Retrieved from http://www.marfan.org

Sponseller, P. D., Erkula, G., Skolasky, R. L., Venuti, K. D., & Dietz, H. C. (2010). Improving clinical recognition of Marfan syndrome. *Journal of Bone Joint Surgery, 92*(9), 1868–1875.

‹ Describe the etiology and forms of polycystic kidney disease.
‹ Detail symptoms associated with polycystic kidney disease.
‹ Discuss triplet repeat expansion and anticipation.
‹ Review current surveillance and treatment recommendations for polycystic kidney disease.

KEY TERMS

Anticipation
Diverticula
Diverticulitis

End-stage renal disease (ESRD)
Genetic heterogeneity
Genetic modifiers

Hepatotoxic
Nephrotoxic
Renal cell carcinoma
Triplet repeat expansion

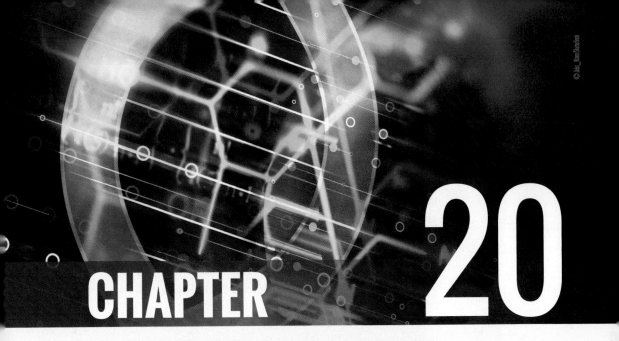

CHAPTER 20

Polycystic Kidney Disease

Polycystic kidney disease (PCKD) is a multisystem and progressive disorder that is one of the most common genetic diseases in humans. It is most often characterized by bilateral renal cysts, with the comorbidities of hypertension and worsening kidney function, often resulting in the need for dialysis and kidney transplantation. Although the most common cause of morbidity associated with PCKD is renal disease, other comorbidities exist, including intracranial aneurysms, aortic dissection with and without rupture, and cysts in other visceral organs (particularly in the liver). PCKD is caused by defects in the *PKD1* and *PKD2* genes, which encode for the membrane proteins polycystin-1 and polycystin-2, respectively. The majority of PCKD patients, 80–90%, have the *PKD1* defect, making the *PKD2* defect relatively uncommon. However, *PKD2* mutation has a slower progression and longer life expectancy than *PKD1*.

Fifty percent of adults will acquire renal cysts over the age of 50, however, these cysts are benign and have little clinical significance. They are unilateral, epithelium-lined cavities filled with fluid or semisolid material primarily from renal tubular elements. Renal cysts in those with PCKD are cysts throughout medulla and cortex of *both* kidneys and can progress to end-stage renal disease (ESRD).

Inheritance of PCKD most commonly follows an autosomal dominant pattern, in which it is known as autosomal dominant polycystic kidney disease (ADPKD). This variant is the most common potentially lethal single-gene mutation in the United States, with a prevalence of 1 case in every 500 people. It affects approximately 600,000 persons in the United States and 4–7 million people worldwide. PCKD may also follow an autosomal recessive pattern, in which case it is known as autosomal recessive polycystic kidney disease (ARPKD), which is relatively rare compared with ADPKD.

Phenotypic Features

PCKD may be diagnosed in adulthood or childhood, depending on the severity of disease and its manifestations. Hypertension, flank pain, and renal insufficiency are the most common renal sequelae. All affected persons eventually develop cysts within the kidneys, but the number of cysts, the size of individual cysts, and the rate of progression are highly variable among individuals and within PCKD-affected families. The mutated gene products also vary, as noted in phenotypical differences between persons with *PKD1* versus *PKD2* mutations. Typically, at diagnosis, persons with *PKD1* mutations have larger kidneys with more cysts than those with *PKD2* mutations. This is due to earlier development of cysts in individuals with the *PKD1* mutation.

As multiple cysts and associated scarring replace the normal anatomic structures of the kidney, the usual renal physiological exchange processes—including filtration, reabsorption, and concentration of urine—are disrupted. In the presence of increased solutes and other unfavorable conditions, kidney stones may form. Renal perfusion may also become disturbed because of the structural changes in the cystic kidney. Hypertension is the most common early manifestation of ADPKD, with 50–75% of patients presenting with hypertension even when renal function is still normal. Long-standing hypertension can result in glomerular damage and kidney failure, aneurysms, cardiac valve disease, and complications during pregnancy for both the mother and fetus. Therefore, early detection allows for earlier treatment and ideally will prevent the emergence of cardiovascular disease. Cardiovascular disease is the main cause of death in these patients.

Flank pain, hematuria, nocturia, proteinuria, kidney stones, abdominal bloating/fullness, constipation, headaches, and infections are common presenting features with this type of kidney disease. Factors that increase the risk of kidney stones in ADPKD are similar to the general risk factors for kidney stones—decreased flow, increased solutes, and favorable pH for precipitation of solutes. The occurrence of these individual factors in those with ADPKD and the structural changes of the kidneys caused by PCKD both contribute to increased prevalence of kidney stones in ADPKD patients. Most calculi in patients with ADPKD consist of uric acid with or without calcium oxalate, most likely due to decreased excretion of ammonia, acidic urinary pH, and decreased citrate concentration.

Females affected with ADPKD are more likely to develop urinary tract infections (UTIs) than their male counterparts. *Escherichia coli* and other enteric pathogens are the most common isolates of ascending infections. These UTIs may progress to pyelonephritis, emphysematous pyelonephritis (caused by gas-forming organisms), abscesslike infections of the renal cysts, or even sepsis if left untreated. These complications are especially common in diabetics or the immunocompromised.

Progression to **end-stage renal disease (ESRD)** occurs in approximately 50% of adults with PCKD by the time they are 60 years of age. This outcome results from several different mechanisms, starting with the initial loss of functional renal tissue that has been replaced or compressed by the cysts. Over time, the vessels become sclerosed, inflammation occurs, and fibrotic tissue replaces functional tissue, causing further obstruction. Death of renal tubular epithelial cells is the final contributing feature in this process. Overuse of **nephrotoxic** medications (nonsteroidal anti-inflammatory drugs [NSAIDs], aminoglycosides, vancomycin, diuretics, etc.) poor dietary habits (high protein/high salt intake, decreased water intake, etc.), and concomitant chronic illnesses (diabetes, hypertension, etc.) are also detrimental to renal function.

Other complications associated with renal cysts include the development of aggressive cancer with ensuing compression of surrounding structures. Although **renal cell carcinoma** occurs at the same frequency in patients with ADPKD as in the general population, it presents atypically and behaves more aggressively in ADPKD-affected individuals. As the kidneys become enlarged, nearby structures, such as the intestines and inferior vena cava, may become compromised, causing mass effect.

Extrarenal manifestations may arise related to the liver, pancreas, spleen, seminal vesicles, arachnoid membrane, colon, spinal meninges, cerebral vessels aorta, and cardiac valves. In fact, polycystic liver disease is the second most common finding associated with ADPKD. The incidence of liver (hepatic) cysts increases with patient age. This sequela develops at a younger age among women with ADPKD than among men with ADPKD. Generally, these cysts are asymptomatic and do not parallel the problems observed with renal cysts. Rarely, the mass effect of liver cysts may cause abdominal distention with or without pain, fullness, decreased appetite, or pain on inspiration. The liver cysts may also compress nearby structures, such as vessels or bile ducts, leading to complications that may include bleeding, infection, or rupture.

Pancreatic and splenic cysts occur less frequently than renal or hepatic cysts in ADPKD patients and are usually discovered incidentally. They tend to be small and do not usually interfere with pancreatic function or cause complications.

Cysts of the seminal vesicles are mostly asymptomatic and occur in almost 40% of affected males without diminishing fertility. However, women affected with PCKD have an increased risk for ectopic pregnancy.

Although arachnoid membrane cysts are usually asymptomatic, they may increase the risk of developing subdural hematomas.

KEY TERMS

End-stage renal disease (ESRD): the complete or almost complete failure of the kidneys to function. The dysfunctional kidneys can no longer remove wastes, concentrate urine, and regulate electrolytes.

Nephrotoxic: relating to an agent that damages renal cells.

Renal cell carcinoma: a type of kidney cancer in which the cancerous cells are found in the lining of very small tubes (tubules) in the kidney.

KEY TERMS

Diverticula: a pouch or sac opening from a tubular or saccular organ such as the intestines or the bladder.

Diverticulitis: inflammation of a diverticulum, especially of the small pockets in the wall of the colon, that fill with stagnant fecal material and become inflamed. Rarely, these sacs may cause obstruction, perforation, or bleeding.

Genetic heterogeneity: the character of a phenotype produced by mutation at more than one gene or by more than one genetic mechanism.

Genetic modifiers: genes that modify the expression of Mendelian traits.

While the incidence of **diverticula** of the colon and spinal meninges are slightly increased in persons with ADPKD, the most life-threatening manifestation is the development of aneurysms. Cerebral (intracranial/berry) aneurysms occur in 10–20% of persons affected with ADPKD, with the highest rates observed in individuals who have a positive family history of intracranial hemorrhage. Unlike in the general population, a history of renal dysfunction and hypertension does not usually precede the development of aneurysms in these families. In addition to diverticula of the spinal meninges, **diverticulitis** of the descending colon is more prevalent in persons affected with ADPKD, especially after patients develop ESRD. Diverticular disease outside the colon has also been reported.

Dilatation of the aortic root and cardiac valve abnormalities are associated with ADPKD as well. Aortic root dilatation may result in ascending aortic aneurysms that can propagate to involve the aortic arch and descending aorta. Recent evidence also suggests a link to thoracic aortic dissection. The most common valvular disorder is mitral valve prolapse, which is observed in 25% of affected individuals.

Genetics

ADPKD is inherited in an autosomal dominant pattern. Thus, persons with an affected parent have a 50% risk of inheriting the gene. Approximately 5% of all mutations involve de novo changes in the gene.

Polycystin-1 and polycystin-2 are proteins that are integral to specific membrane structures encoded by the *PKD1* and *PKD2* genes, respectively. When these genes are mutated, the protein complexes are rendered ineffective. These proteins are part of larger protein complexes located in the primary cilia of renal tubules, cardiac myocytes, and myofibroblasts of heart valves and vessels, which explains the multiple-organ system involvement that is characteristic of this disease.

Approximately 85% of disease expression is attributable to mutations of *PKD1*, with the remaining 15% due to mutations of *PKD2*. Furthermore, mutations of *PKD1* tend to yield more severe clinical symptoms than mutations of *PKD2*. Persons with *PKD1* mutations are typically younger at presentation and have increased severity of renal disease with faster progression to ESRD. The expression of other organ system manifestations is the same with both mutations (**genetic heterogeneity**).

Comorbid factors also influence disease expression. For example, hypertension before the age of 35, hematuria before the age of 30, hyperlipidemia at any age, and the coexistence of sickle cell trait all increase the likelihood and severity of PCKD.

Other factors that may contribute to disease expression include inherited genes that alter the expression of mutated genes (**genetic modifiers**). Some evidence also suggests that the position of the mutation leads to variability in disease expression. Homozygous expression is known to result in spontaneous abortion, usually in the second trimester of pregnancy. It can also increase the risk of ectopic pregnancy.

Because the penetrance of disease is very high for PCKD, virtually all adults with mutations develop some level of disease. Notably, the penetrance of *PKD1* mutations is greater than that of *PKD2* mutations. Offspring of affected individuals are likely to have the same or greater level of disease as the affected parent. When the number of repeating units of the defective gene increases, the gene is expressed to a higher degree. This increase is called **triplet repeat expansion**, and the prediction of worsening expression of disease associated with it is termed **anticipation**.

Diagnosis

Initial diagnosis of renal cysts is established by renal imaging, typically renal ultrasound first as a screening and then CT afterward to confirm. The etiology of PCKD is later confirmed by genetic testing. Imaging studies are indicated in the scenario of asymptomatic presentation with a positive family history or with the scenario of symptomatic presentation without a known family history. Different diagnostic criteria for ADPKD exist for each group, as outlined in **Table 20-1**.

When a parent is affected, his or her offspring should be clinically evaluated and undergo renal ultrasound to determine the presence and severity of cysts relative to patient age. In adult patients with ADPKD, the older the patient is at presentation, the more cysts he or she is likely to have compared with a younger patient (Table 20-1). The criteria given in Table 20-1 are 100% sensitive for patients with *PKD1* mutations who are older than the age of 30, but less sensitive for persons with *PKD2* mutations. In children, the PCKD-affected kidneys may appear enlarged and echogenic on ultrasound, but in most cases, no cysts can be visualized.

When there is a positive family history of disease, a physical exam finding of enlarged kidneys or liver should raise the level of clinical suspicion for disease. Mitral valve prolapse, abdominal hernias, and hypertension in these patients are also indicative of disease. In persons without a family history of ADPKD, renal cysts are considered less presumptive proof because renal cysts are a common incidental, insignificant finding in patients over the age of 50.

Imaging methods to identify and characterize cysts include abdominal ultrasound, computed tomography (CT), and magnetic resonance imaging (MRI). These techniques are also beneficial for examining extrarenal locations of disease, such as the liver. Although imaging is an invaluable tool, diagnosis of PCKD is confirmed by molecular genetic testing.

KEY TERMS

Triplet repeat expansion: a condition in which the number of repeating triplet units in a gene is so great that it interferes with gene expression and causes more severe disease.

Anticipation: the predictability of progressively earlier onset and increased severity of certain diseases in successive generations of affected persons.

TABLE 20-1	Diagnostic Criteria for Autosomal Dominant Polycystic Kidney Disease Based on Family History for Adults and Children

Type of Patient	No Family History*	Positive Family History
Adults	At least two unilateral or bilateral cysts in individuals younger than 30 years of age Two cysts in each kidney in individuals ages 30–59 years Four cysts in each kidney in individuals 60 years of age or older	Enlarged kidneys noted on physical examination Enlarged liver noted on physical examination Hypertension Mitral valve prolapse Abdominal wall hernia
Children	Large echogenic kidneys without distinct macroscopic cysts	

*Sensitivity of 100% in individuals with autosomal dominant polycystic kidney disease who are older than 30 years of age and in younger individuals with *PKD1* mutations. Sensitivity is 67% for *PKD2* mutations in persons younger than 30 years of age. Reproduced from Ravine, D., Gibson, R. N., Walker, R. G., Sheffield, L. J., Kincaid-Smith, P., & Danks, D. M. (1994). Evaluation of ultrasonographic diagnostic criteria for autosomal dominant polycystic kidney disease 1. *Lancet, 343*(8901), 824–827.

Genetic Testing and Counseling

Siblings of an affected proband have a 1 in 2 chance of being affected. Moreover, some affected individuals in the same family will become symptomatic before others. Testing for those at increased risk, including prenatal testing using amniotic fluid, is possible when the specific mutation has been identified in a family. Testing is also indicated for relatives of a proband in ESRD or when screening relatives as candidates for a living-donor kidney transplant. Genetic counseling is indicated for those who are known to be affected by, or are considered at risk of, PCKD because of a positive family history.

Management, Treatment, and Surveillance

Initial treatment of PCKD depends on the disease manifestations at diagnosis. In addition to the usual lifestyle modifications to treat hypertension, renal-protective drugs such as angiotensin-converting enzyme (ACE) inhibitors or angiotensin II receptor blockers (ARBs) are prescribed. These drugs increase blood flow in the kidney—an effect that is particularly important for ADPKD-affected patients, who lose renal function when blood flow to the kidney is obstructed by cysts and associated scar tissue. ACE inhibitors and angiotensin II receptor blockers also have a relatively benign side effect profile and have been shown to reduce development of arterial plaques (atherosclerosis), which may further complicate renal disease. However, if patients also have renal artery stenosis (RAS), ACEs and ARBs are contraindicated. Avoiding excessive dietary protein, salt, and potassium consumption is also recommended for patients with PCKD to minimize glomerular damage and preserve renal function.

Routine evaluation after initial diagnosis of PCKD includes monitoring blood pressure (keeping it under 130/80, unless positive for proteinuria, in which case the goal is under 125/75), evaluating renal function and structure (renal ultrasound and blood work), evaluating liver structure, evaluating blood lipids, and screening for valvular and aortic disease (**Box 20-1**). Pain management may be needed for chronic flank pain associated with cysts and renal cystic changes (avoid NSAIDs for pain management). In severe cases, cysts may be removed or decompressed to alleviate the pain. Infected cysts require special attention and treatment with intravenous antibiotics (typically fluoroquinolones). Screening for aneurysms is best accomplished by a brain MRI but is not recommended unless the patient has a positive family history of stroke or is undergoing elective surgery. Resources are available to patients who have PCKD through the American Association of Kidney Patients.

A list of nephrotoxic drugs, including over-the-counter medications, should be provided to patients. Patients should be advised to avoid caffeine because it may contribute to cyst growth. When there is liver involvement, patients should be warned about **hepatotoxic** agents as well. Because smoking damages the kidneys and independently increases the risk of renal cell carcinoma, efforts should be made to encourage smoking cessation and reduction of alcohol intake. It is also recommended that patients avoid contact sports because of the risk for cyst rupture, kidney/spleen trauma, or aneurysm rupture.

Recent clinical studies have focused on drugs that may help prevent cyst development and growth in PCKD. Several clinical trials have been

BOX 20-1	Surveillance Recommendations for Persons Affected by Autosomal Dominant Polycystic Kidney Disease

Renal ultrasound examination

Computed tomography (CT) imaging of the abdomen with and without contrast enhancement

Standardized blood pressure screening per recommendations of the American Heart Association

Measurement of blood lipids

Urine studies to detect the presence of microalbuminuria or proteinuria

Echocardiography or cardiac MRI to screen persons at high risk because of a family history of thoracic aortic dissections

Head MRI angiography or CT angiography to screen persons at high risk because of a family history of intracranial aneurysms

Reproduced from NCBI Bookshelf. *Gene Reviews*. Polycystic Kidney Disease, Autosomal Dominant. Retrieved from https://www.ncbi.nlm.nih.gov/books/NBK1246

completed that involved reviewing drugs that may address the prevention or reduction of cysts; however, the FDA has not approved any medications for this indication. Studied medications include vasopressin 2 receptor antagonists (tolvaptan) and somatostatin analogs (octreotide). In one study, octreotide did show some slowing in the growth of kidney and liver cysts, but the FDA does not currently indicate it for ADPKD. Although this drug's exact mechanism of action is not fully understood, it has been observed to reduce formation and growth of cysts. If a patient reaches ESRD with PCKD, then dialysis and/or kidney transplant will be considered.

Associated Syndromes

Besides PCKD, there are no known disorders associated with *PKD1* and *PKD2* mutations. However, numerous syndromes may present with renal cystic disease.

ARPKD is associated with bilateral renal cysts that have a different gross configuration and a distinct microscopic pathology from those observed in the autosomal dominant variant. Those persons affected with ARPKD do not have affected parents. Collectively, these features make ARPKD distinguishable from ADPKD.

Benign cystic kidney disease should be considered in the absence of a family history of ADPKD and when cystic disease is the only symptom. The prevalence of simple renal cysts increases with age, with such cysts being relatively rare in persons younger than age 50. Renal cysts are also associated with other disorders, such as tuberous sclerosis complex, von Hippel-Lindau syndrome, oral-facial-digital syndrome type 1, glomerulocystic kidney disease, and Hajdu-Cheney syndrome. Differentiating these disorders from ADPKD depends on the constellation of symptoms and other organ systems that are involved.

Chapter Summary

» Autosomal dominant polycystic kidney disease is a multisystem disorder that is most often characterized by bilateral renal cysts, intracranial aneurysms, aortic dissection and rupture, and cysts in other visceral organs, most often the liver.

» Autosomal dominant polycystic kidney disease is caused by defects in the *PKD1* and *PKD2* genes; it follows an autosomal dominant pattern of inheritance.

» Autosomal dominant polycystic kidney disease commonly manifests as hypertension, flank pain, and renal insufficiency in both children and adults.

» Diagnosis of autosomal dominant polycystic kidney disease requires renal imaging and confirmatory genetic testing.

» Although there is no cure for autosomal dominant polycystic kidney disease, treatment is targeted at preserving renal function through lifestyle modifications, avoiding nephrotoxic agents, and controlling hypertension.

Chapter Review Questions

1. Autosomal dominant polycystic kidney disease is the result of a mutation in the _____ and _____ genes.
2. The main cause of morbidity in polycystic kidney disease is

   _____.
3. The most life-threatening complication associated with autosomal dominant polycystic kidney disease is _____.
4. The chance of an affected person having offspring with autosomal dominant polycystic kidney disease is _____, which describes a/an _____ pattern of inheritance.
5. Physical exam findings associated with autosomal dominant polycystic kidney disease include _____ and _____.

Bibliography

Adeva, M., El-Youssef, M., Rossetti, S., Kamath, P. S., Kubly, V., Consugar, M. B., . . . Harris, P. C. (2006). Clinical and molecular characterization defines a broadened spectrum of autosomal recessive polycystic kidney disease (ARPKD). *Medicine (Baltimore), 85*, 1–21.

Belz, M. M., Fick-Brosnahan, G. M., Hughes, R. L., Rubinstein, D., Chapman, A. B., Johnson, A. M., . . . Gabow, P. A. (2003). Recurrence of intracranial aneurysms in autosomal-dominant polycystic kidney disease. *Kidney International, 63*, 1824–1830.

Ecder, T., & Schrier, R. W. (2001). Hypertension in autosomal-dominant polycystic kidney disease: Early occurrence and unique aspects. *Journal of the American Society of Nephrology, 12*, 194–200.

Fain, P. R., McFann, K. K., Taylor, M. R., Tison, M., Johnson, A. M., Reed, B., & Schrier, R. W. (2005). Modifier genes play a significant role in the phenotypic expression of PKD1. *Kidney International, 67*, 1256–1267.

Harris, P. C., & Torres, V. E. (2015, June 11). Polycystic kidney disease, autosomal dominant. *GeneReviews.* Retrieved from https://www.ncbi.nlm.nih.gov/books /NBK1246/

Hogan, M. C., Masyuk, T. V., Page, L. J., Kubly, V. J., Bergstralh, E. J., Li, X., . . . Torres, V. E. (2010). Randomized clinical trial of long-acting somatostatin for autosomal dominant polycystic kidney and liver disease. *Journal of the American Society of Nephrology, 21*(6), 1052–1061. doi:10.1681/ASN.2009121291

Ignatavicius, D. D., & Workman, M. L. (2010). *Medical-surgical nursing: Patient centered collaborative care* (6th ed.). St. Louis, MO: Saunders Elsevier.

Klahr, S., Breyer, J. A., Beck, G. J., Dennis, V. W., Hartman, J. A., Roth, D., . . . Yamamoto, M. E. (1995). Dietary protein restriction, blood pressure control, and the progression of polycystic kidney disease: Modification of diet in renal disease study group. *Journal of the American Society of Nephrology, 5*(12), 2037–2047.

National Kidney Foundation. (n.d.). Retrieved from http://www.kidney.org

Qian, Q., Harris, P. C., & Torres, V. E. (2001). Treatment prospects for autosomal-dominant polycystic kidney disease. *Kidney International, 59*, 2005–2022.

Ravine, D., Gibson, R. N., Walker, R. G., Sheffield, L. J., Kincaid-Smith, P., & Danks, D. M. (1994). Evaluation of ultrasonographic diagnostic criteria for autosomal dominant polycystic kidney disease 1. *Lancet, 343*(8901), 824–827.

Rossetti, S., & Harris, P. C. (2007). Genotype–phenotype correlations in autosomal dominant and autosomal recessive polycystic kidney disease. *Journal of the American Society of Nephrology, 18*, 1374–1380.

Torre, R. (2016, February). Polycystic kidney disease medication. *Medscape.* Retrieved from http://emedicine.medscape.com/article/244907-medication

Torres, V. E., & Harris, P. C. (2006). Mechanisms of disease: Autosomal dominant and recessive polycystic kidney disease. *Nature Clinical Practice Nephrology, 2,* 40–55.

Torres, V. E., Harris, P. C., & Pirson, Y. (2007). Autosomal dominant polycystic kidney disease. *Lancet, 369,* 1287–1301.

U.S. Renal Data System. (2002). *USRDS 2002 annual data report: Atlas of end-stage renal disease in the United States.* Bethesda, MD: National Institutes of Health, National Institute of Diabetes and Digestive and Kidney Diseases.

Wang, X., Wu, Y., Ward, C. J., Harris, P. C., & Torres, V. E. (2008). Vasopressin directly regulates cyst growth in polycystic kidney disease. *Journal of the American Society of Nephrology, 19,* 102–108.

CHAPTER OBJECTIVES

‹ Distinguish between unifactorial and multifactorial causes in rheumatic diseases.
‹ Identify the most common skeletal dysplasias.
‹ Identify cell lines that cause bone loss such as osteoporosis.
‹ Discuss gene penetrance and variable expressivity in osteoarthritis versus rheumatoid arthritis.
‹ Review the current surveillance, diagnosis, and treatment recommendations for systemic lupus erythematosus.

KEY TERMS

Achondrodysplasia
Apoptosis
Acetylsalicylic acid (ASA)
Concordance
Cytokines
DMARDs
Dysplasias

Eburnation
Enthesitis
Epitopes
Interleukins
MTX
Multifactorial
NSAIDs

Oligoarthritis
Osteopenia
Osteoporosis
Pannus
Rhizomelia
Senescence
Unifactorial

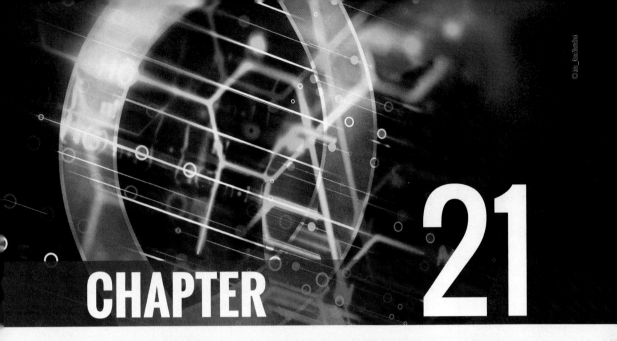

CHAPTER 21

Rheumatologic Disorders

Introduction

Rheumatic diseases encompass several medical conditions that directly affect the musculoskeletal system or have a broader involvement of the connective tissues. These diseases are inherited or familial, usually in clusters, with variable penetrance or expression of clinical signs and symptoms. Whether rheumatic diseases are **unifactorial** (one mutated gene locus), as in Marfan syndrome, or **multifactorial** (multiple genes and/or environmental triggers), as in rheumatoid arthritis, the vertical transmission to offspring is almost inevitable. It should be noted that most rheumatic diseases tend to be multifactorial in origin.

Environmental factors can turn on or activate a particular gene, triggering an autoinflammatory or autoimmune response. The utilization of identical versus fraternal twins in research studies has been helpful in identifying these **epitopes** (antigenic determinants on alleles) and their triggers by assessing the **concordance** rate. In general, the higher the concordance rate among twins, the stronger the genetic component. Conversely, lower concordance rates suggest more environmental factors as causes of the disease. This chapter provides an overview of some of the common rheumatologic diseases seen in clinical practice.

Skeletal Dysplasias

Skeletal **dysplasias** have more than 400 types of deformities, all of which are characterized by abnormalities of cartilage and bone growth, usually involving the long bones, spine, and head.

The pathophysiology is usually due to alteration of the genes and/or protein defects responsible for healthy cartilage and bone development. Look for a family medical history in first-degree relatives (autosomal dominant); consanguineous marriages, which have a higher expression of autosomal recessive diseases; or male preponderance, suggesting a sex-linked recessive inheritance. Most skeletal dysplasias have heterogeneous genetic and/or protein aberrations that appear early in newborns and children.

Achondroplasia

The lay term most people use to refer to a form of **achondrodysplasia** is dwarfism. Achondroplasia, the most common skeletal dysplasia, occurs in 1/20,000 live births. It is an autosomal dominant condition, but many de novo mutations also occur at the *fibroblast growth factor receptor 3 (FGFR3)* gene. Most children with achondroplasia present with a short stature, a condition known as **rhizomelia** (short lengths of the most proximal or "root" segment of the upper arms and legs compared with the distal segments), macroencephaly, lordosis or scoliosis, craniofacial abnormalities or a flat nasal bridge, prominent forehead (frontal bossing), and midfacial hypoplasia. The hands have a trident appearance, with short, broad digits splayed more distally than proximally. These children are on the growth curve at birth, but by 5 months of age, their length has fallen to <5th percentile. Note that children with achondroplasia have normal intellect and cognition.

Unfortunately, many medical complications are associated with achondrodysplasia. These children are at increased risk for serous otitis media, motor milestone delay, bowing of the legs, dental problems, obesity, spinal stenosis, and craniocervical junction abnormalities with compression of the upper cord, resulting in apnea, quadriparesis, growth delay, and hydrocephalus. The American Academy of Pediatrics recommends measuring the size and shape of the fontanelle and monitoring the occipitofrontal circumference (with growth curves standardized for achondroplasia) at every pediatric visit. If there are any concerns, further neurological examination, neuroimaging, and polysomnography are recommended.

Osteogenesis Imperfecta

Osteogenesis imperfecta (OI) refers to a disorder characterized primarily by osseous fragility leading to fractures. Most forms of OI are caused by the abnormal structure of type I collagen, which is responsible for skin, tendon, ligament, bone, and sclera formation. About 4–5 out of 100,000 patients are afflicted with some form of OI.

OI is most commonly caused by autosomal dominant mutations in genes encoding the alpha 1 and alpha 2 chains of type I collagen (*COL1A1* and *COL1A2*). The autosomal recessive forms are caused by mutations in genes encoding proteins involved in posttranslational modification of type I collagen (*FK506-binding protein 10* [*FKBP10*]; *cartilage-associated protein* [*CRTAP*]; *leprecan-like 1* [*LEPRE1*]; *peptidyl-prolyl isomerase B* [*PPIB*]) or other mechanisms of bone formation and homeostasis (*serpin peptidase inhibitor, clade, H, member 1 [SERPINH1]; serpin peptidase inhibitor, clade F, member 1 [SERPINF1]; specificity protein 7 [SP7]/osterix [OSX]; interferon-induced transmembrane protein 5 [IFITM5]).* Note that, regardless of the genetic aberration, OI has a wide range of phenotypes and variable expression. OI is discussed further in another chapter of this text.

Metabolic Bone Disorders

The most common metabolic bone disorder is osteoporosis, a microarchitectural loss of bone resulting in decrease in bone strength and quality and an increased risk for fracture.

Approximately, 44 million Americans have low bone mass (**osteopenia**) and porous bones (**osteoporosis**). There are many forms of osteoporosis: postmenopausal and senile in adults (most prevalent) and a rarer genetic form known as juvenile osteoporosis.

Juvenile Osteoporosis

Juvenile primary osteoporosis starts in early childhood as a skeletal disorder characterized by thinning of the bones, with multiple fractures in the long bones of the arms and legs, especially in the regions where new bone forms (metaphysis). In addition, there is a loss of trabecular or spongy bone (ribs, spine, distal forearm), which is more porous than cortical bone (sternum, femur) in these children. Hence, fractures at the spinal vertebra, known as vertebral compression fractures, are not unusual in children with juvenile osteoporosis.

The prevalence of juvenile osteoporosis is unknown. The inheritance pattern is an autosomal dominance pattern with a mutation in the gene *LDL receptor related protein 5* (*LRP5*). *LRP5* protein participates in the *Wnt* signaling pathway, which is important for the proliferation, adhesion, and migration of cells. During early childhood development, *LRP5* assists in the specialization of the retina, blood supply for the inner ear, and facilitating the use of calcium and other minerals into mineralized bone, causing an increase in bone density.

The diagnosis is made by the early loss of bone density without other signs and symptoms (unlike in OI). A whole bone density in children can identify the degree of bone loss. Bone turnover markers, genetic testing registry sites, and services for genetic counseling are recommended for patients with early bone loss. Treatment is aimed at augmenting calcium and vitamin D supplementation, along with weight-bearing exercises.

Paget's Disease of Bone

Paget's disease of bone (PBD) is an abnormal bone remodeling process, with osteoblast and osteoclast activity creating a haphazard organization of weak, woven bone. The disease is common in the elderly, is found more commonly

---

KEY TERMS

Osteopenia: a condition in which bone mineral density is lower than normal and a precursor to osteoporosis.

Osteoporosis: a medical condition in which the bones become brittle and fragile from loss of tissue, typically as a result of hormonal changes or deficiency of calcium or vitamin D.

in males than in females, and is usually asymptomatic until a lab abnormality (serum alkaline phosphatase) is discovered. However, there are familial forms of this disease, which is the focus here.

Genetic and environmental factors have been associated with PDB. Inheritance appears to be autosomal dominant with variable penetrance, and multiple genetic loci have been associated with PDB. The genes identified that affect bone remodeling and are associated with PDB are *SQSTM1*, *TNFRSF11A*, and *TNFRSF11B*. Mutations in the *SQSTM1* gene are the most common genetic cause of classic PDB, accounting for 10–50% of familial cases and 5–30% of sporadic cases. Variations in the *TNFRSF11B* gene also appear to increase the risk of the classic form of the disorder, particularly in women. *TNFRSF11A* mutations cause the early-onset form of PDB. There have been reports of infections with certain viruses (measles) and owning pets (dogs, cats) possibly being factors in triggering the disease. However, there are no consistent correlates in these circumstances. Patients with familial forms of PDB have abnormal bone patterns with earlier age of onset, hearing loss, and early loss of adult teeth.

The diagnosis of PDB is made by finding an elevated serum alkaline phosphatase and characteristic radiographic findings. The classic "salt and pepper" appearance on plain radiographs is consistent with the osteoblast (salt) and osteoclast (pepper) dysregulation of bone.

Baseline bone scans are also helpful in determining the extent of the disease. There is an increased risk of osteogenic sarcoma in patients with PDB. Effective first-line treatments for PDB are aminobisphosphonates or calcitonin.

Arthritides

Osteoarthritis

Osteoarthritis (OA) is the most common form of arthritis, affecting about 20 million people. Females are affected more commonly than males, and OA generally appears in older patients (over 65 years). Historically, OA was considered a noninflammatory, degenerative arthritis with a breakdown of the hyaline cartilage as a result of **senescence**. Instead, OA has been shown to be a complex arthritis with inflammatory components (**cytokines** and **interleukins**) affecting additional joint structures such as the synovium (typically seen in rheumatoid arthritis). OA tends to affect the proximal and distal phalanges of the hands, spine, and larger weight-bearing joints, such as the hips and knees, typically in an asymmetric pattern.

Evidence of a genetic influence of OA comes from epidemiological studies of family history, family clusters, and twin studies. Classic twin studies have shown that the influence of genetic factors is between 39% and 65% in radiographic OA of the hand and knee in women, about 60% in OA of the hip, and about 70% in OA of the spine. Studies have implicated linkages to OA on chromosomes 2q, 9q, 11q, and 16p, among others. Genes implicated in association studies include *VDR, AGC1, IGF-1, ER alpha, TGF beta, CRTM* (cartilage matrix protein), *CRTL* (cartilage link protein), and *collagen II, IX, and XI.* As with most diseases, the complexity of penetrance and expression of genes may vary in the two sexes and at different joint sites. For instance, the frizzled related gene protein, *FRZB* gene, has shown a strong correlation in younger females with hand OA.

Diagnosis of OA is made on clinical and radiographic assessment. Plain radiographs are cost-effective because of the classic findings of **eburnation**, subchondral cysts, and sclerosis with osteophytes. No labs are usually needed. Treatment modalities consist of NSAIDs, intra-articular steroids for weight control, hyaluronic injections, and physical therapy. For patients with intractable pain and limited function, arthroplasty and joint replacements are recommended. For OA, there is no specific genetic counseling available.

Rheumatoid Arthritis

Rheumatoid arthritis (RA) affects about 0.5–1% of people in the United States, with greater incidence in women than men. It affects the most productive years of one's life, with the typical age of onset between 30 and 40 years. RA usually presents as a chronic (longer than 6 weeks), symmetric (same hand joints affected bilaterally), polyarticular inflammatory arthritis with involvement of small joints more often than large joints.

The etiology of RA is unknown. RA does have some genetic basis; approximately 10% of patients have a first-degree relative with RA, and there is a higher concordance rate in identical twins than fraternal twins. RA is a heterogeneous disease with various genetic polymorphisms resulting in anything from mild joint involvement to severely erosive joint deformity. Genetic haplotypes such as *HLA-DR* and *HLA-DQ* have been associated with a more aggressive disease. Two genes known to be involved with the development of RA are the *HLA-DRB1* gene and the *protein tyrosine phosphatase 22* gene (*PTPN22*). It is not yet clear exactly how these genes predispose one to autoimmune disease, but it is known to be associated with a stronger likelihood of developing RA. As far as environmental factors, triggers such as viral infections (B19 virus), smoking, and hormones have correlated with the risk for RA.

The diagnosis of RA is made by achieving a good history and assessing physical signs and symptoms, followed by the appropriate labs and imaging studies. Signs and symptoms of RA include more than 1 hour of morning stiffness/pain that improves with activity. RA patients are prone to fatigue, low-grade fever, anorexia, and weight loss. The lab test specific for RA is the anticyclic citrullinated peptide antibodies. Aggressive RA disease and extra-articular manifestations are more common in the presence of RF and anti-CCP antibodies (seropositive RA) and, if not treated early, will result in

> **KEY TERM**
>
> **Eburnation:** hard, ivory.

pannus (scar) formation of the joints. These extra-articular manifestations of RA include various organs: eyes, skin, spleen, lungs, heart, and the central nervous system.

Treatment modalities consist of **NSAIDs**, disease-modifying anti-rheumatic drugs (**DMARDs**) such as methotrexate (**MTX**), corticosteroids, biologics, and other immunosuppressants.

Juvenile Idiopathic Arthritis

Juvenile idiopathic arthritis (JIA) is defined as persistent synovitis in one or more joints for at least 6 weeks in children younger than 16 years of age. JIA is not as common as adult RA, but it is still important to recognize its occurrence. Most cases of JIA are sporadic, which means they occur in people with no history of the disorder in their family. A small percentage of cases of JIA have been reported to run in families, although the inheritance pattern of the condition is unclear. The estimated risk of a sibling of a person with JIA developing the condition is about 12 times higher than for the general population.

Several subsets of JIA have been classified: systemic-onset arthritis, polyarthritis, **oligoarthritis**, **enthesitis**-related arthritis, and psoriatic arthritis. Many of these subsets are probably related to underlying genetic variations, not all of which have been identified. JIA appears to be influenced by genetic factors, both within and outside the HLA region. Although many of the HLA associations (*HLA-A*, *HLA-DR*, *HLA-DQ*, and *HLA-DP*) have been replicated in independent cohorts, only a few of the non-HLA associations (*PTPPN22*) have been replicated. The major reason for limited studies is the small number of JIA patients and enrollment at registry. Advances such as genomewide association studies and collaborative registry efforts are likely to result in the discovery of new genetic associations. There are current RA registries now available for this purpose.

Treatment goals for both adult RA and JIA are to preserve joint function and prevent disability and include use of NSAIDs, **ASA**, steroids in low doses, DMARDs (single or combination), and biologic modifiers (paired with MTX). In addition, physical/occupational therapy, nutrition, and weight control are also important.

Systemic Lupus Erythematosus

Systemic lupus erythematosus (SLE) is a prototypical autoimmune disease with a prevalence of 20–150 cases per 100,000. Peak incidences occur during one's most productive years of life (15–45 years of age), although children are also affected. Females are affected more than males partly because of hormonal estrogen effects. Hispanics and African Americans are afflicted more often than Caucasians and with more severe disease. SLE has a myriad of presentations, ranging from mild localized disease to severe multiorgan involvement abruptly or sequentially over the course of months to even years. Although there are many subtypes of lupus, SLE is the most recognized and is the type addressed here.

The pathogenesis of this disease has been recognized as being multifactorial, with a genetic predisposition triggered by hormonal and environmental factors. The *MHC HLA-DR2*, *HLA-DR3*, and *HLA-B8* alleles serve as antigenic determinants, known as epitopes, which contribute to the formation of pathogenic auto-antibodies due to dysregulation of self-tolerance, **apoptosis**, and cellular inflammation. There is no single gene polymorphism that creates high risk for SLE, except for the rare *TREX1* mutation or deficiencies of early components of complement (C1q, C2, C4).

In addition, some of the single-nucleotide polymorphisms (SNPs) in SLE risk genes predispose one to particular clinical subsets of SLE with or without nephritis. Note that the actual genetic polymorphism that actually imparts the increased risk of disease has not been identified. What is known is that SNPs are in linkage disequilibrium with the causal variant.

Be aware of the environmental triggers that generally predate and/or accompany the disease presentation by performing a thorough review of systems. Antecedent infections, stress, hormonal therapies, sunlight, and certain medications (hydralazine, infliximab) have been recognized as inciting triggers of lupus.

The diagnosis of SLE is made by a thorough history, physical examination, and lab test such as the antinuclear antibody (ANA). The ANA has a high sensitivity for diagnosing this disease but is nonspecific. Fractionation of the ANA antibody into its subtypes is helpful and can predict the course of disease for some patients. For example, the presence of anti-dsDNA antibodies correlates with a risk of nephritis.

Overall treatment for SLE will depend on disease severity and organ involvement, weighing the risks and benefits of each treatment modality. Mild cases of lupus without organ involvement can be controlled with NSAIDs and low-dose steroids. DMARDs are used for maintenance and long-term therapy for lupus patients. The profiles of these drugs range from slow-acting anti-rheumatic drugs (SAARDs) such as the antimalarials (hydroxychloroquine), to antimetabolites (methotrexate), to more immunosuppressive drugs (cyclophosphamide, mofetil mycophenolate).

Genetic screening and counseling for lupus are primarily done at the local level, with healthcare providers being the primary source of contact. Prenatal patients, familial history of SLE, and other comorbid diseases are generally the reason patients seek genetic counseling. The Centers for Disease Control and Prevention has sponsored longitudinal registries throughout the United States (MILES, the California Lupus Surveillance Project, and the Manhattan Lupus Surveillance Program), with the hope of obtaining more information on this disease.

KEY TERM

Apoptosis: programmed or gene-directed cell death.

Chapter Summary

» Rheumatic diseases are inherited or familial, usually in clusters, with variable penetrance or expression of clinical signs and symptoms.

» Skeletal dysplasias have more than 400 types of deformities, all of which are characterized by abnormalities of cartilage and bone growth, usually involving the long bones, spine, and head.

» OA tends to affect the proximal and distal phalanges of the hands, spine, and larger weight-bearing joints, such as the hips and knees, typically in an asymmetric pattern.

» RA usually presents as a chronic (longer than 6 weeks), symmetric (same hand joints affected bilaterally), polyarticular inflammatory arthritis with involvement of small joints more often than large joints.

» Juvenile idiopathic arthritis (JIA) is defined as persistent synovitis in one or more joints for at least 6 weeks in children younger than 16 years of age.

» SLE has variable presentations and the diagnosis is made by a thorough history, physical examination, and lab tests such as the antinuclear antibody (ANA). A fractionation of the ANA antibody into its subtypes is also helpful and can predict the clinical course of disease.

Chapter Review Questions

1. _____ is the definition of epitopes.
2. _____ is a common clinical manifestation of achondrodysplasia.
3. The cell that is predominantly the cause of bone loss in osteoporosis is _____.
4. The gene mutation that is the most common cause of classic Paget's disease of the bone is _____.
5. OA has been shown to be a complex arthritis with inflammatory components (cytokines and interleukins) affecting additional joint structures such as the _____ and _____.

Bibliography

Beary, J. F., & Chines, A. A. (2018). Osteogenesis imperfecta: Clinical features and diagnosis. *UpToDate.* Retrieved from https://www.uptodate.com/contents /osteogenesis-imperfecta-clinical-features-and-diagnosis

Bonafe, L., Cormier-Daire, V., Hall, C., Lachman, R., Mortier, G., Mundlos, S., . . . Unger, S. (2015). Nosology and classification of genetic skeletal disorders: 2015 revision. *American Journal of Medical Genetics A, 167A*(12), 2869–2892. doi:10.1002 /ajmg.a.37365

Centers for Disease Control and Prevention. (2017). *Lupus registries and longitudinal studies.* Retrieved from https://www.cdc.gov/lupus/funded/lupus-studies.htm

Cicuttini, F. M., & Spector, T. D. (1996). Genetics of osteoarthritis. *Annals of the Rheumatic Diseases, 55*(9), 665–667.

National Library of Medicine, National Institutes of Health, U.S. Department of Health and Human Services. (n.d.). *Genetics home reference.* Retrieved from http://ghr.nlm.nih.gov/

National Rheumatoid Arthritis Society. (2013). *The genetics of rheumatoid arthritis.* Retrieved from http://www.nras.org.uk/the-genetics-of-rheumatoid-arthritis

Scofield, H. (2015). Genetics of systemic lupus erythematosus. *Medscape.* Retrieved from http://emedicine.medscape.com/article/1884084-overview#a2

Todorov, A. B., Scott, C. I., Jr., Warren, A. E., & Leeper, J. D. (1981). Developmental screening tests in achondroplastic children. *American Journal of Medical Genetics, 9*(1), 19–23.

< Describe the etiology and various forms of neurofibromatosis.
< Review the genetics associated with neurofibromatosis types 1 and 2.
< Provide diagnostic criteria for neurofibromatosis to assist the primary care provider.
< Detail current medical management options and recommendations for neurofibromatosis.

KEY TERMS

Café-au-lait spot	Hypertrichosis	Neurofibromin
Crowe's sign	Lisch nodule	Schwannoma
Glioma	Merlin	Tumor suppressor gene
Hamartoma	Neurofibroma	

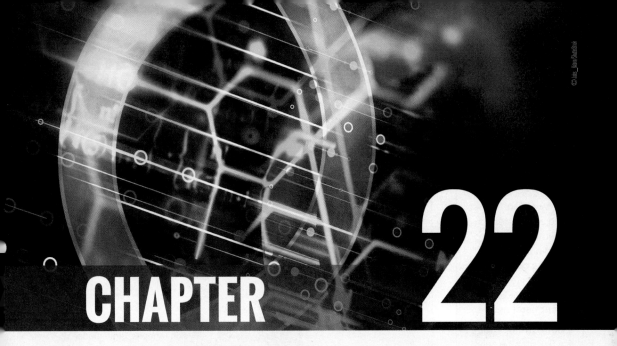

CHAPTER 22

Neurofibromatosis

A **neurofibroma** is defined as a benign, encapsulated tumor resulting from proliferation of Schwann cells that are of ectodermal (neural crest) origin and that form a continuous envelope around each nerve fiber of peripheral nerves. The autosomal dominant genetic disorder known as neurofibromatosis (NF) causes such tumors to grow on the sheaths of the nerves anywhere in the body at any time. This disorder affects 1 in 3,000–4,000 males and females of all races and ethnic groups worldwide and is one of the most common genetic disorders in the United States.

NF occurs in two distinctive forms: type 1 (NF-1) and type 2 (NF-2). The most common form is type 1 NF, which manifests as tumors of the subcutaneous tissues and hyperpigmented skin lesions known as **café-au-lait spots**.

In NF, multiple neurofibromas may develop anywhere along the peripheral nerve fibers, starting at the roots and extending distally. The resulting neurofibromas can become quite large, resulting in major disfigurement, bone erosion, and compression of various peripheral nerve structures. A small hamartoma (Lisch nodule) can be found in the iris of almost all patients. The effects of NF are unpredictable and have varying manifestations and degrees of severity (**Figure 22-1**).

NF type 2 has an incidence of 1 in 38,000 and occurs equally in males and females. This variant is characterized by the development of noncancerous tumors called **schwannomas** on the auditory and vestibular nerves that control hearing and balance. Although the tumors usually develop in late adolescence, some people do not develop problems until they are in their 40s and 50s. In the majority of cases, the schwannomas develop bilaterally but not necessarily at the same time, so there may be hearing loss of different degrees in both ears. In some cases, schwannomas develop on only one side (unilateral), and other nerves may be affected by different types of tumors that control swallowing, speech, eye movements,

KEY TERMS

Neurofibroma: a benign, encapsulated tumor resulting from proliferation of Schwann cells that are of ectodermal (neural crest) origin and that form a continuous envelope around each nerve fiber of peripheral nerves.

Café-au-lait spot: a flat spot on the skin that is the color of coffee with milk (café au lait) in persons with light skin. These spots are harmless by themselves, but in some cases they may be a sign of neurofibromatosis. The presence of six or more café-au-lait spots, each of which is 1.5 centimeters or more in diameter, is diagnostic for neurofibromatosis.

FIGURE 22-1 Body systems affected by neurofibromatosis type 1.

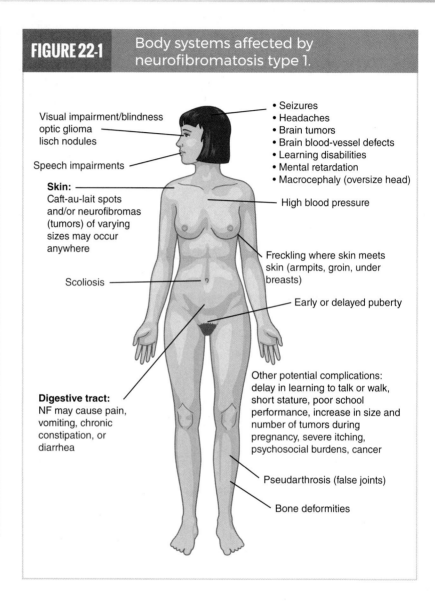

- Visual impairment/blindness optic glioma lisch nodules
- Speech impairments
- **Skin:** Caft-au-lait spots and/or neurofibromas (tumors) of varying sizes may occur anywhere
- Scoliosis
- **Digestive tract:** NF may cause pain, vomiting, chronic constipation, or diarrhea

- • Seizures
- • Headaches
- • Brain tumors
- • Brain blood-vessel defects
- • Learning disabilities
- • Mental retardation
- • Macrocephaly (oversize head)
- High blood pressure
- Freckling where skin meets skin (armpits, groin, under breasts)
- Early or delayed puberty
- Other potential complications: delay in learning to talk or walk, short stature, poor school performance, increase in size and number of tumors during pregnancy, severe itching, psychosocial burdens, cancer
- Pseudarthrosis (false joints)
- Bone deformities

and facial sensations. Tumors may also occur in the central nervous system (i.e., brain and spinal cord), but NF-2 has few cutaneous manifestations (**Figure 22-2**).

Genetics of Neurofibromatosis

As mentioned, NF is an autosomal dominant genetic condition. Approximately 50% of those affected by this disease have a family history of NF; the

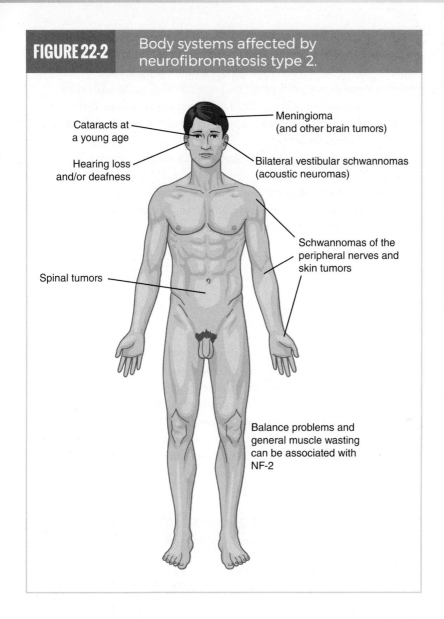

FIGURE 22-2 Body systems affected by neurofibromatosis type 2.

Cataracts at a young age

Hearing loss and/or deafness

Spinal tumors

Meningioma (and other brain tumors)

Bilateral vestibular schwannomas (acoustic neuromas)

Schwannomas of the peripheral nerves and skin tumors

Balance problems and general muscle wasting can be associated with NF-2

other 50% appear to be the first members of their family to have the disorder. Two explanations for the latter scenario are possible: (1) one of the parents actually does have NF-1, but its manifestations are so mild that he or she is unaware of it; or (2) neither parent has the disorder. However, if neither parent is affected, the mutation occurred in the sperm or egg. In that case, the parents do not have NF and cannot pass it on to other children.

KEY TERMS

Neurofibromin: a tumor suppressor gene encoded on chromosome 17 (*NF-1* gene). Loss of tumor suppression due to a mutation in this gene leads to the formation of neurofibromas associated with type 1 neurofibromatosis.

Tumor suppressor gene: a gene that encodes a protein involved in controlling cellular growth; inactivation of this type of gene leads to deregulated cellular proliferation, as in cancer.

NF type 1, also known as von Recklinghausen disease, is caused by a mutation in the *NF-1* gene located on chromosome 17 that encodes for **neurofibromin.** The normal *NF-1* gene is a **tumor suppressor gene** that probably suppresses activity of the ras protein following stimulation by nerve growth factor or other agents. Loss of tumor suppression due to *NF-1* mutation presumably permits uncontrolled ras activation, which leads to the formation of neurofibromas.

Although there appear to be similarities between NF-1 and NF-2, evidence of distinct origins exists for each. Type 2 NF is also characterized by autosomal dominant inheritance and is caused by mutation in the *NF-2* gene on chromosome 22 that encodes for **merlin.** Because merlin is also a tumor suppressor gene, the NF-related mutation disrupts this activity and leads to the formation of schwannomas.

Even though the genes for both NF-1 and NF-2 have been identified, there is no known cure for either form of NF.

Diagnosis

Although mutation analysis is 60–70% accurate in detecting the mutations associated with NF-1 and NF-2, this type of genetic testing is not widely available. As a consequence, a family history (even though 50% of patients diagnosed with NF are the first in their family to have this disorder) and a thorough physical examination are needed to diagnose NF. Generally, most individuals who develop NF are not born with café-au-lait macules; rather, these skin lesions develop during the first 3 years of life and prompt parents to seek medical attention for their child. Neurofibromas start to form in late adolescence. **Box 22-1** lists the diagnostic criteria for NF-1.

BOX 22-1   Diagnostic Criteria for Neurofibromatosis Type 1

Two or more of the following must be present:

1. Six or more café-au-lait spots 0.5 cm or larger in prepubertal individuals, 1.5 cm or larger in postpubertal individuals
2. Two or more neurofibromas of any type or one or more plexiform neurofibromas
3. Freckling in the axillary or inguinal region
4. Optic glioma (tumor of the optic pathway)
5. Two or more Lisch nodules (benign iris hamartomas)
6. A distinctive bony lesion: dysplasia of the sphenoid bone or dysplasia or thinning of long bone cortex
7. A first-degree relative with neurofibromatosis type 1

Data from Neurofibromatosis: National Institutes of Health Consensus Development Conference Statement (1987, July 13–15). Retrieved from https://consensus.nih.gov/1987/1987Neurofibromatosis064html.htm

The presence of multiple café-au-lait spots strongly suggests—but does not prove—the diagnosis of NF-1. In rare cases, individuals may have as many as six café-au-lait spots, and yet they do not exhibit other features of NF-1. In children between the ages of 5 and 12 years, the presence of café-au-lait macules greater than 0.5 cm in diameter is highly suggestive of NF; it is recommended that further testing be pursued in these children. Although healthy individuals may have one or two macules of this kind, children with three or more macules warrant further workup. Because many features associated with NF-1 may not appear until late childhood or adolescence, it is often impossible to make a definitive diagnosis of NF-1 in a young child whose only manifestations are multiple café-au-lait spots. Even if the child is affected, it could take years before another feature of the disorder appears and confirms the diagnosis. Consequently, healthcare providers should reexamine these children for the appearance of new features on an annual basis. If any additional features are found, the diagnosis can be made; if not, the question remains unanswered.

Lisch nodules are dome-shaped **hamartomas** of the iris that are found superficially on slit lamp examination. Although they are asymptomatic, their presence helps in confirming the diagnosis of NF. Axillary freckling (as well as freckling on the perineum), known as the **Crowe's sign**, is another helpful diagnostic feature in NF. Both axillary freckling and inguinal freckling often develop during puberty. Areas of freckling and regions of **hypertrichosis** (abnormal amount of hair growth) occasionally overlay plexiform neurofibromas, which are often large, infiltrative tumors that cause severe disfigurement of the face or an extremity. Bone involvement can include pseudoarthrosis of the tibia, bowing of the long bones, and orbital defects. Mild scoliosis may be encountered, and localized hypertrophy of bone, especially on the face, may be identified. Whether these bone changes are caused by diffuse neurofibromas or other kinds of mesodermal defects is not entirely clear. **Gliomas** of the optic nerve may also occur.

Neurofibromas are classified into one of three categories according to their gross pathology: (1) cutaneous, (2) subcutaneous, or (3) plexiform. They vary from brown to pink or flesh in color and may be either soft or firm to palpation. Various central nervous system tumors (e.g., astrocytomas, meningiomas, intramedullary gliomas, and ependymomas) occur with greater frequency in these patients. Any of these tumors may manifest as seizures, increased intracranial pressure, ataxia, or cranial nerve pathologies. In NF-2, schwannomas are the most common tumor and involve cranial and peripheral nerves (**Box 22-2**).

The incidence of learning disabilities and mental retardation among persons with NF-1 is as high as 40% and 10%, respectively. Common learning disabilities include neuromotor dysfunction, attention-deficit/hyperactivity

---

KEY TERMS

Merlin: a tumor suppressor gene encoded on chromosome 22 (*NF-2* gene). Mutation of this gene disrupts tumor suppressor activity and leads to the formation of schwannomas associated with type 2 neurofibromatosis.

Crowe's sign: axillary and inguinal freckling, often associated with type 1 neurofibromatosis.

Hypertrichosis: growth of hair in excess of the normal.

Glioma: any neoplasm derived from one of the various types of cells that form the interstitial tissue of the brain, spinal cord, pineal gland, posterior pituitary gland, and retina.

Lisch nodules: iris hamartomas, typically seen in type 1 neurobromatosis.

Hamartoma: a focal malformation that resembles a neoplasm, grossly and even microscopically, but results from faulty development in an organ.

BOX 22-2	Diagnostic Criteria for Neurofibromatosis Type 2

Confirmed (Definite) Neurofibromatosis Type 2

1. Bilateral vestibular schwannomas (VS; also known as acoustic neuroma)

Presumptive (Probable) Neurofibromatosis Type 2

1. Family history of neurofibromatosis type 2 (first-degree family member or relative) plus:
2. Unilateral VS or any two of the following:
   » Meningioma
   » Posterior subcapsular lenticular opacity
   » Glioma
   » Cortical cataract
   » Schwannoma

Individuals with the following clinical features should be evaluated for neurofibromatosis type 2:

» Unilateral VS plus at least two of any of the following: meningioma, glioma, schwannoma, juvenile posterior subcapsular lenticular opacities/juvenile cortical cataract
» Multiple meningiomas (two or more) plus unilateral VS or any two of the following: glioma, schwannoma, juvenile posterior subcapsular lenticular opacities/juvenile cortical cataract

Data from Neurofibromatosis: National Institutes of Health Consensus Development Conference Statement (1987, July 13–15). Retrieved from https://consensus.nih.gov/1987/1987Neurofibromatosis064html.htm

disorder, and visuospatial processing disorders. In addition, endocrine disorders, short stature, and growth hormone deficiency are noted to coexist in a higher than normal prevalence in this population.

Medical Management

Because there is no cure for NF-1 or any medical or surgical treatment that can reverse or prevent most related complications, medical management of NF-1 is limited to early detection of treatable complications. Examples of such care include assessment and management of learning disabilities or surgery referral to remove or reduce the size of neurofibromas. Anticipation of such problems and prompt intervention can greatly improve the outcome of treatment.

A person with NF-1 should have a complete medical evaluation at least once a year, to be conducted by a healthcare provider who is familiar with this disorder. During this evaluation, the provider should update the medical history and perform physical, neurological, and ophthalmologic examinations. Careful attention should be paid to any new signs or symptoms of NF-1, especially changes in skin manifestations, such as growth of or pain in a neurofibroma. If specific problems are found, a referral should be made to appropriate medical consultants or specialists for assistance. In the pediatric patient, cognitive development and school progress should be discussed because early identification of potential learning disabilities related to NF-1 is essential for proper intervention.

In general, any signs or symptoms of neurological problems should be fully investigated, including ordering a CT or MRI scan of the brain. In patients suspected of having NF-2, an MRI of the head is recommended in early adolescence. The value of such a scan in the absence of signs or symptoms of neurological impairment is not as clear, however, and different medical providers may make different recommendations. Some providers see these additional tests as a way to obtain as complete a picture as possible of a person's NF-1, whereas others believe that they are unnecessary in the absence of symptoms given the likelihood that nothing treatable would be found. It has been suggested that healthcare providers have an open discussion with patients and their families regarding the risks, benefits, and costs associated with these screening tests.

Regular slit lamp eye examinations are also an important part of managing NF-1. The presence of Lisch nodules can help in establishing a diagnosis of NF-1, so the primary care provider should consider referral to an ophthalmologist in patients with the suspected diagnosis. Lisch nodules are not medically significant and do not interfere with vision, but complications relating to optic glioma or problems with the bones of the orbit may occur in people with NF-1. Other recommendations for specialist referral are shown in **Table 22-1**.

TABLE 22-1	Recommendations for Specialist Referral for Neurofibromatosis Patients	
Disorder	**Specialist**	
Tibial bowing	Orthopedic surgeon	
Skin (especially facial) deformities	Plastic surgeon	
Self-esteem issues, language disorders, learning disabilities	Psychiatrist/psychologist	
Hearing deficit	Ears, nose, and throat specialist	

Chapter Summary

» The autosomal dominant genetic disorder known as neurofibromatosis causes tumors to grow on the nerve sheaths anywhere in the body at any time.

» Type 1 neurofibromatosis is the most common variant of this disease; it is characterized clinically by the combination of patches of hyperpigmentation and cutaneous and subcutaneous tumors.

» Type 1 neurofibromatosis, also called von Recklinghausen disease, is caused by a mutation in the *NF-1* gene located on chromosome 17, which encodes for neurofibromin.

» There is no cure for type 1 neurofibromatosis, so medical management is limited to the early detection of treatable complications.

» Type 2 neurofibromatosis is characterized by the development of noncancerous tumors called schwannomas on the nerves that control hearing and balance.

» Type 2 neurofibromatosis is caused by a mutation in the *NF-2* gene located on chromosome 22, which encodes for merlin.

Chapter Review Questions

1. _____ neurofibromatosis is the most common variant and is characterized clinically by the combination of patches of hyperpigmentation and cutaneous and subcutaneous tumors.
2. Type 2 neurofibromatosis is characterized by the development of noncancerous tumors called _____ on the nerves that control hearing and balance.
3. Loss of tumor suppression due to *NF-1* mutation presumably permits uncontrolled _____, which leads to the formation of neurofibromas.
4. True or False: The presence of multiple café-au-lait spots proves that a patient has type 1 neurofibromatosis.
5. Neurofibromatosis is a/an _____ genetic condition, and approximately 50% of those affected have a family history of this disorder.

Bibliography

Hersh, J. H. (2008). Health supervision for children with neurofibromatosis. *Pediatrics, 121*(3), 633. Retrieved from https://pediatrics.aappublications.org/content/121/3/633

Interactive dermatology atlas. (n.d.). Retrieved from http://www.dermatlas.net

Kam, J. R., & Helm, T. H. (2008). Neurofibromatosis. *Medscape.* Retrieved from http://emedicine.medscape.com/article/1112001-overview

Neurofibromatosis: National Institutes of Health Consensus Development Conference Statement (1987, July 13–15). Retrieved from https://consensus.nih.gov/1987 /1987Neurofibromatosis064html.htm

Neurofibromatosis type 2. (2007, June). Centre for Genetics Education, Fact Sheet 52. Retrieved from http://www.genetics.com.au/factsheet/fs52.html

Understanding NF1. (n.d.). University of Alabama and WGBH Educational Foundation. Retrieved from http://www.understandingnf1.org/id/int_id_win.html

< Distinguish between sporadic cutaneous malignant melanoma and familial malignant melanoma.
< Describe the etiology and various forms of familial malignant melanoma.
< Identify the risk factors associated with a predisposition to malignant melanoma.
< Discuss gene penetrance, variable expressivity, and skin phenotype.
< Use clinical assessment tools at the bedside.
< Review the current surveillance, diagnosis, and treatment recommendations for familial malignant melanoma.

KEY TERMS

Computed tomography (CT) scan
Covariates
Head and neck squamous cell carcinoma
Lymph node mapping

Magnetic resonance imaging (MRI)
Melanomagenesis
Penetrance
Phototype
Positron emission tomography (PET) scan

Recurrent melanoma
Satellite moles
Sentinel node
Variable expressivity
Wide local excision

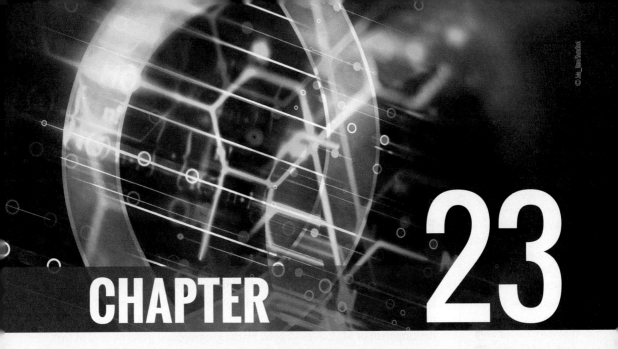

CHAPTER 23

Familial Malignant Melanoma

Malignant melanoma (MM) is one of the most aggressive and lethal skin cancers. It originates from melanocytes, the pigment-producing cells commonly found in the basal layer of the epidermis. In 2014, there were approximately 76,100 new cases of MM and 9,710 deaths from MM in the United States. The lifetime risk of melanoma has increased even more, with 1 in 1,500 of all people born in the early 1900s, 1 in 50 (2%) Caucasians, 1 in 200 Hispanics, and 1 in 1,000 African Americans. MM can affect all ages, and the incidence has been rising over the past several decades. It is the most common cancer among young women between the ages of 25 and 29. Note that these statistics apply to all MM cases, with sporadic cutaneous malignant melanoma being far more common (80%) than familial forms of malignant melanoma (20%). Because MM exhibits early metastasis and shows poor response to treatment once it has progressed, its emergence qualifies as a health crisis, and surveillance is necessary for high-risk individuals. Environmental and/or genetic factors are involved in the development of all malignant melanomas (**melanomagenesis**). This chapter focuses on the inheritance patterns of malignant melanoma.

MM that occurs in the familial pattern known as familial atypical multiple mole and melanoma (FAMMM) syndrome—also known as dysplastic nevus syndrome (DNS) and atypical mole syndrome (AMS)—is characterized by the appearance of a large number of dysplastic nevi or atypical moles at an *early* age, in combination with MM. The term "atypical" describes the gross appearance of the mole on visual examination, while "dysplastic" refers to the microscopic appearance of the tissue from biopsy. When MM does occur in these patients, it occurs at a younger age (usually younger than 30 years) and exhibits a more aggressive disease progression than is observed with sporadic melanoma; this is most likely due to higher gene **penetrance**.

Risk Factors for Malignant Melanoma

Several risk factors have been identified as indicators for increased development of MM for both sporadic and familial cases (see **Table 23-1**). Each of these risk factors is discussed independently.

Environmental Factors

Although the reason for the increased incidence of MM is unclear, exposure to ultraviolet (UV) radiation is the most recognized risk factor. In particular, sunburns, tanning beds, and early childhood exposure to UV rays are known to increase one's risk for developing MM. Certain aspects of UV light may affect overall survival from MM. Intensity of UV light is also a factor in development of MM, as evidenced by the geographical patterns of MM that occur relative to equatorial latitude. Furthermore, UV exposure may play an additive role in MM families because it tends to be a common environmental factor among kindreds.

Phenotypic Features

Physical characteristics have been reported in numerous studies to infer a higher risk of MM, regardless of genotype or family history. These associated risk factors include light skin color, **phototype** (ability to tan), hair color, number of freckles, number of atypical nevi, and anatomical distribution pattern of atypical nevi. Red hair and freckles are associated with the *MC1R* gene, which has also been shown to predispose individuals to MM. This gene association with MM is present even in the absence of red hair, making both freckles and red hair independent phenotypic risk factors for MM.

TABLE 23-1   Risk Factors for Malignant Melanoma

Environmental	UV radiation
Phenotypes	Light complexion, inability to tan, red hair, atypical nevi >10, location of atypical nevi (especially back), freckles
Genes with High-Risk Loci	*CDKN2A, 9p21* (MM or pancreatic cancer), *p14ARF* (brain tumors), *BRCA2* (breast or ovarian), *MC1R* (red hair, freckles), *OCA2* (albinism), *CDK4* (very rare)
Familial MM Aggregates	First- or second-degree relatives, three or more occurrences among any family members, multiple primaries in one parent or in any one individual, multiple cases on the same side of the family, any family member at young age

Atypical nevi are well-documented precursors to MM. Studies have suggested that AMS and DNS are associated with FAMMM syndrome and are seen in approximately 15% of the general population. Multiple moles and positive family history are also well-known risk factors for developing MM because dysplastic nevi occur as precursors in familial patterns of MM. These "atypical moles" have been found to be related to an autosomal dominant trait encoded on chromosome *9p16*.

An increased number of atypical nevi and the anatomical distribution of nevi are independent risk factors for MM. A finding of more than 100 nevi, or six or more dysplastic nevi, is significantly associated with a family history of MM. In addition, some melanoma-affected families show aggregation of phenotypes for factors such as number of nevi and skin phototypes. These phenotypes may be associated with MM independent of shared genes and common environmental exposures among family members.

Genetics

In studies of families in which multiple cases of melanoma have developed among kindreds, the chromosomal region *9p21* has been implicated as a causative factor. In addition to this locus, other gene sets appear to be involved in the process of nevi differentiation into melanoma (see Table 23-1). Although there are numerous gene variations identified in MM patients, mutations in four specific genes—*CDKN2A*, *CDK4*, *p14ARF*, and *MC1R*—have been identified in only some of known familial MM cases. However, many familial MM cases have no identified genetic association, and the etiologies of these remaining cases are currently unknown. Even though **variable expressivity** and gene penetrance are thought to play a partial role in disease expression among mutation carriers, interaction between **covariates** and melanoma genes is also suspected.

The FAMMM or AMS phenotypes have been associated with specific genetic mutations, but it is important to note that these phenotypes alone are not indicators of mutation status. Because the absence of these genetic mutations does not confer a decreased risk in MM families, it is probable that familial MM involves the interplay of environmental factors with genetic predisposition. Phenotypic expression has also been shown to vary among MM-affected families depending on ancestry (i.e., British, Swedish, Italian, Brazilian, or Scottish families).

Familial History

When accurately reported, risk assessment by family history is the most reliable indicator of risk for MM, regardless of mutation status (**Box 23-1**). Barriers to obtaining an accurate family history may include an unknown biological family history, inability of patients to differentiate between melanoma and non-melanoma skin cancers, and a fear of having an unfavorable medical history

KEY TERMS

Variable expressivity: variation in disease symptoms among persons with the same mutation.

Covariates: the interplay of environmental factors with genetic predisposition.

BOX 23-1	Associated Diseases Predictive of an Increased Risk for Malignant Melanoma

Cancers: pancreatic, *BRCA*+ breast and ovarian, and CNS tumors
Xeroderma pigmentosa
Li-Fraumeni syndrome
Werner's syndrome
Retinoblastoma

appear in the medical record. Not only have patients with more than two family members with MM been found to be more likely to develop MM themselves, but the disease also has an earlier age of onset in these individuals and tends to produce multiple primary lesions. While all first- and second-degree relative occurrences of MM are considered significant risk factors, the greatest familial risk indicator is a parent affected by multiple primary melanomas. The need to collect a detailed extensive family history at the initial visit, followed by annual review and updates, cannot be overstated.

Associated Diseases

Increased incidence of various other cancers associated with MM and FAMMM syndromes has been described (Box 23-1). For example, MM has been reported to account for approximately 7% of all second primary cancers that occur among retinoblastoma patients and their kindreds. Atypical nevi are also associated with this group. Pancreatic carcinoma has been positively linked to familial MM, especially in the presence of *CDKN2A* mutations. More specifically, it has been shown that MM, multiple nevi, and pancreatic carcinoma are inherited as autosomal dominant traits in some MM-affected families. Ocular MM has also been shown to have a correlation with atypical nevi and cutaneous MM within high-risk families. Breast cancer has been reported in association with MM, especially among *BRCA1* and *BRCA2* mutation carriers. Other nonmelanoma skin cancers, particularly squamous cell carcinoma and cancers of the nervous system such as neuroblastoma, show an association with MM-affected families who exhibit *CDKN2A* mutations.

Diagnosis

As with any medical condition, a thorough history and physical exam are essential in all patients. A detailed medical history that involves looking for the risk factors previously mentioned is the first step. A full head-to-toe physical skin (scalp and nails included) examination is also important. Melanoma can occur anywhere on the body. In males, it is more frequently found on the trunk, head, and neck, whereas females tend to develop melanoma predominantly on the arms and legs. Bedside clinical tools used by most primary care providers that have shown validity include the ABCDE checklist, the Glasgow 7-point criteria, and the "ugly duckling" sign—all of which involve looking for changes in the appearance of a mole or pigmented lesion suggestive of an MM (see **Box 23-2**). Any mole that exhibits changes in size, shape, or color; that has irregular borders; that demonstrates asymmetry; that itches; that has discharge; or that bleeds is cause for concern. A patient with any lesion that forms **satellite moles**— moles that grow in a pattern around existing moles—or a mole that is different from other moles should be referred to a qualified healthcare provider such as a dermatologist. Suspicious lesions can then be biopsied to remove as much of the lesion as possible. The tissue is then examined microscopically by a histopathologist to detect cancer cells and provide the level of staging. Such lesions should never be shaved, frozen, cauterized, or removed with a laser.

Management and Treatment

Staging takes into consideration the characteristics of the original melanoma such as tumor size (T), the presence or absence of nodes (N), and/or metastasis (M)—the TNM classification. Staging is required to develop the appropriate treatment plan. Approaches used in staging include **wide local excision, lymph node mapping**, various imaging studies, and laboratory assays. Wide local excision involves removal of some normal tissue surrounding the area of the primary melanoma. This tissue is then examined microscopically to determine whether melanoma cells are present. If any cancer cells remain, the excision is widened to ensure that no melanoma remains at the primary site.

BOX 23-2	Clinical Assessment Tools for Suspicious Moles

ABCDE Rule

» Asymmetry
» Border irregularities
» Color variegation (brown, red, black or blue/gray, and white)
» Diameter ≥6 mm
» Evolving: changes in size, shape, or color, or a new lesion forms

Glasgow 7-Point Criteria

3 major criteria: change in size/new lesion, shape, or color
4 minor criteria: diameter ≥7 mm, presence of inflammation, crusting or bleeding, or sensory change

The "Ugly Duckling" Sign

Any pigmented lesion that looks different from other surrounding lesions must be considered suspicious because most benign moles tend to have a morphologically similar appearance.

KEY TERMS

Satellite moles: new moles that grow in a pattern around existing moles.

Wide local excision: a surgical procedure to remove some of the normal tissue surrounding the area where melanoma was found to check for cancer cells not visible on gross examination.

Lymph node mapping: a procedure in which a radioactive substance or blue dye is injected near the tumor, then flows through lymph ducts to the first lymph node or nodes where cancer cells are likely to have spread. Lymph nodes that are marked with the dye are then surgically removed and examined microscopically by a pathologist for evidence of cancer cells.

KEY TERMS

Sentinel node: the first lymph node to receive lymphatic drainage from a tumor.

Computed tomography (CT) scan: an imaging procedure in which a computer linked to an x-ray machine is used to produce a series of detailed pictures of areas inside the body taken from different angles.

Magnetic resonance imaging (MRI): a procedure that uses a magnet, radio waves, and a computer to make a series of detailed images of areas inside the body.

Positron emission tomography (PET) scan: an imaging procedure used to locate malignant tumor cells in the body by identifying areas of tissue with greatest glucose utilization.

Clark's levels are used to classify thin tumors in terms of how deeply the cancer has spread into the skin. Tumors may be confined to the epidermis (Clark's level I), spread into different depths of the dermis (Clark's levels II, III, and IV), or spread into subcutaneous tissue (Clark's level V).

Lymph node mapping with sentinel lymph node biopsy is a procedure in which a radioactive substance or a dye is injected near the tumor. The substance flows through the lymph system and into the first major lymph node (**sentinel node**), which is the most likely location for cancer cells to spread. The nodes that are "mapped" are then removed and examined microscopically for evidence of cancer cells. If no cells are detected in the sentinel node, it is not necessary to remove the remaining lymph nodes in this area. Other diagnostic tests include a chest x-ray to screen for lung and bone metastases. **Computed tomography (CT) scans** of the chest, abdomen, and pelvis are also usually performed, whereas **magnetic resonance imaging (MRI)** is the preferred scanning modality for gross observation of brain metastases. The detection of smaller metastases requires a full-body **positron emission tomography (PET) scan**. This imaging procedure detects glucose uptake by cancer cells—such cells have a faster metabolic rate than noncancerous cells. It should be noted that PET scans are able to detect smaller tumors (micrometastases) that are not identifiable through other imaging studies.

The laboratory assay most commonly used in staging is serum lactate dehydrogenase (LDH). This enzyme is found in the cells of many tissues, such as the lungs, liver, kidneys, skeletal muscles, and brain. When injury (such as invasion by a tumor) occurs in these tissues, LDH is released in greater quantity into the serum. Because this enzyme is found in many tissues, however, an increase in total LDH is not very specific. Nevertheless, LDH is relatively sensitive for solid-tumor malignancies, and its level may be significantly elevated when cancer cells are present. These characteristics make LDH a good screening tool for detecting occult metastases.

More recently introduced staging systems take into account other factors that are independent variables for prognosis. The overall thickness of the primary tumor (both above and below the epidermis) is considered more important than the Clark's level, for example. The presence of ulceration in the primary tumor and the number of lymph nodes involved is also more valuable information than the size of positive lymph nodes. Elevated serum LDH in stage IV disease is a negative prognostic indicator.

Treatment of stage I melanoma involves surgical removal of both the lesion and a margin of unaffected skin. The amount of unaffected skin removed depends on the thickness of the melanoma. No more than 2 cm of normal skin needs to be removed from all sides of stage I melanoma; wider margins have not been found to improve overall survival. Standard treatment of stage II melanoma comprises wide excision of skin around the tumor site. Sentinel lymph node biopsy is optional at this stage because deeper tumors have an increased risk of spreading to a lymph node. Stage III melanoma requires the same surgical treatment of the primary lesion as accorded to stage II melanoma, along with lymph node dissection. Adjuvant therapy with a-interferon has been shown to increase disease-free survival in some patients but has little effect on overall survival. Clinical trials are also an option at this stage. Stage IV melanoma has a very poor prognosis, given that melanoma cells have spread to distant areas of the body at this stage. Surgery may be performed to debulk the tumors and relieve symptoms depending on the location. Metastases that cannot be removed may be treated with regional radiation or adjuvant chemotherapy. Chemotherapy drugs such as dacarbazine and temozolomide can be used, either by themselves or in combination with other drugs, to shrink tumors and slow disease progression. In general, their use does not improve overall survival. Recurrence of melanoma (**recurrent melanoma**) after initial diagnosis is not uncommon regardless of staging. Other modalities of treatment, such as immunotherapy with interferon and ipilimumab, have also played a role for more aggressive cases of MM.

> **KEY TERM**
>
> **Recurrent melanoma:** cancer that has returned, either to the original site or in other areas of the body, after it has been treated.

Genetic Testing, Counseling, and Surveillance

In general, dermatologists and other clinicians agree that genetic testing should not be routinely performed for MM patients. Because risk heterogeneity occurs even among carriers of known familial MM genes, such as *CDKN2A*, other unknown genetic variants are thought to also be involved in the development of MM. According to the Melanoma Genetics Consortium, testing for mutations in genes known to be associated with MM should be almost exclusively restricted to research laboratories because of the unknown penetrance of these mutations, the probable existence of unidentified mutations, and limited data related to prevention and surveillance. It is recommended that clinical testing for specific genetic mutations be reserved for patients with a personal or family history of MM, but only when patients can participate in a genetic counseling program. Some families require special attention and consideration for further counseling based on risk alone.

Moderation—if not outright avoidance—of sun exposure and skin self-examinations (SSE) of nevi are recommended for relatives of affected patients at high risk for developing MM. Melanoma risk is also more highly associated with UV radiation that is intermittent and intense. These factors emphasize the point that patient education is the key to developing a prevention strategy among those deemed at risk for developing this disease.

There are no American Academy of Dermatology consensus guidelines regarding surveillance and screening recommendations for relatives of MM patients in high-risk categories. Although some investigators recommend that family members of MM patients have any pigmented lesions evaluated, others recommend annual screening of first- and second-degree relatives beginning between 10 and 12 years of age. Specifically, these annual evaluations should include full-body photography, close-up photographs of any atypical nevi, and patient education for SSE; they should be continued at 6-month intervals until nevi are deemed to be stable and the patient is judged to be competent in SSE. Remaining follow-up visits should occur annually thereafter, at which time the pedigree should be revised.

Patients who report a personal or family history of ocular melanoma, especially in conjunction with atypical nevi, should be screened for ocular and cutaneous MM. The correlation between *CDKN2A* mutations in MM-affected patients and the development of pancreatic cancer is strong enough to warrant routine surveillance. In members of high-risk families, it is recommended that endoscopic ultrasonography be performed annually beginning at age 50 or 10 years earlier than the age of the youngest relative diagnosed with pancreatic cancer. For individuals who develop **head and neck squamous cell carcinoma** at a young age, annual screening for pancreatic carcinoma and melanoma is recommended.

In summary, high-risk patients for MM based on the presence of multiple atypical nevi, strong history of familial MM, and red hair or freckle phenotypes should be educated regarding the need for regular full-skin examinations by clinicians with skin expertise, skin self-examination, and sun protection. Because most autosomal dominantly inherited mutations in MM susceptibility genes are only a small proportion of cutaneous melanomas, genetic screening should be limited to these patients willing and able to participate in a research program.

Chapter Summary

» Risk factors for sporadic cutaneous melanoma and familial malignant melanoma are both interchangeable and independent of each other.

» Malignant melanoma is complex in etiology; multiple pathways are involved in melanomagenesis.

» An accurate family history is the most reliable indicator of risk for development of malignant melanoma, regardless of mutation status.

» Familial atypical multiple mole and melanoma syndrome involves the coexistence of familial malignant melanoma and atypical nevi within families.

» Diagnosis of malignant melanoma requires a thorough risk assessment and a full head-to-toe skin examination, including scalp and nails.

» High-risk patients and their families should be counseled on the importance of prevention and surveillance measures such as avoidance of sun exposure, skin self-examinations, and referral to a dermatologist.

Chapter Review Questions

1. The single greatest indicator of risk for malignant melanoma is
   _____.
2. Patients who exhibit familial malignant melanoma are often clinically distinguished from those patients with sporadic cutaneous malignant melanoma because they are at a _____ age at the time of diagnosis.
3. Which risk factor confers the highest risk among patients who have melanoma? _____
4. Three important preventive measures for patients at high risk for malignant melanoma are _____, _____, and _____.
5. Other cancers associated with familial malignant melanoma include
   _____, _____, _____, and _____.
6. The three clinical risk assessment aids for malignant melanoma used at the bedside are _____, _____, and _____.

Bibliography

Bishop, J. N., Harland, M., Randerson-Moor, J., & Bishop, D. T. (2007). Management of familial melanoma. *Lancet Oncology, 8*(1), 46–54.

Debniak, T. (2004). Familial Malignant Melanoma–Overview. *Hereditary Cancer in Clinical Practice, 2*(3), 123–129. Advance online publication. doi:10.1186/1897-4287-2-3-123

GeneReviews. (n.d.). Retrieved from http://www.genetests.org

Gershenwald, J. E., Scolyer, R. A., Hess, K. R., Sondak, V. K., Long, G. V., Ross, M. I., Lazar, A. J., . . . Wong, S. L. (2017). Melanoma of the skin. In M. B. Amin (Ed.), *AJCC cancer staging manual* (8th ed., p. 563). Chicago, IL: American Joint Committee on Cancer.

Gunder, L. M. (2008). Update on familial melanoma: Understanding risk, surveillance and the role of genetic testing. *Journal of Dermatology for Physician Assistants, 2*(2), 16–21.

Kaufman, H. L., Kirkwood, J. M., Hodi, F. S., Argawala, S., Amatruda, T., Bines, S. D., Clark, J. I., . . . Atkins, M. B. (2013). The Society for Immunotherapy of Cancer consensus statement on tumour immunotherapy for the treatment of cutaneous melanoma. *Nature Reviews Clinical Oncology, 10,* 588.

National Cancer Institute, U.S. National Institutes of Health. (2018). *Breast cancer treatment (PDQ®) – Patient Version.* Retrieved from http://www.cancer.gov /cancertopics/pdq/treatment/breast/Patient/page5#Keypoint25

National Cancer Institute, U.S. National Institutes of Health. (2018). *Melanoma treatment (PDQ®).* Retrieved from https://www.ncbi.nlm.nih.gov/books/NBK65950/

National Library of Medicine, National Institutes of Health, U.S. Department of Health and Human Services. (n.d.). *Genetics home reference.* Retrieved from http://ghr.nlm.nih.gov/

Pho, L., Grossman, D., & Leachman, S. A. (2006). Melanoma genetics: A review of genetic factors and clinical phenotypes in familial melanoma. *Current Opinions in Oncology, 8*(2), 173–179.

CHAPTER OBJECTIVES

< Describe and differentiate between the mood disorders described in this chapter.
< Describe the criteria for substance abuse and understand how to stratify.
< Understand the genetic relationships between mood disorders and substance abuse.
< Differentiate between the different mood disorders and substance predilection.
< Identify the different pathways involved in mood disorders and substance abuse disorders.

KEY TERMS

Anhedonia
Bipolar disorder
Generalized anxiety disorder (GAD)

Hypomania
Major depressive disorder (MDD)

Major mood disorder (MMD)
Tolerance

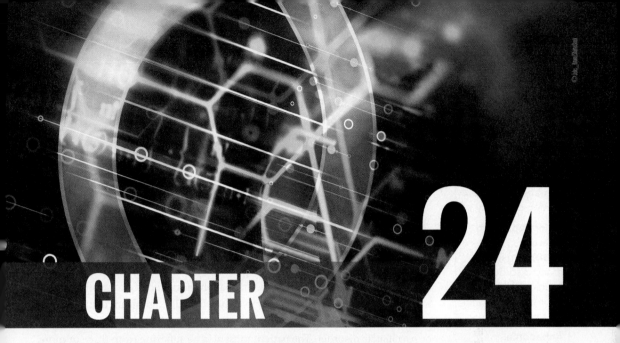

CHAPTER 24

Behavioral Medicine

It is estimated that between 30% and 60% of Americans suffer from a psychiatric disorder, particularly those termed "major mood disorders," or substance abuse disorders. The term **major mood disorder (MMD)** is a blanket term that encompasses the most common psychiatric disorders, including major depressive disorder, generalized anxiety disorder, and bipolar disorder. Of these patients, approximately 15% have a coexisting substance abuse disorder. The genetic association between these two disorders has been poorly assessed. It has been assumed that major mood disorders predispose people to substance abuse disorders because of compulsivity and poor self-control, so a genetic link has not been thoroughly explored. This chapter discusses the heritability of MMDs, substance abuse disorders, and the potential coheritability of these two illnesses.

Diagnosis

Major depressive disorder (MDD) is defined by the *Diagnostic and Statistical Manual of Mental Disorders (DSM-5)* as having five or more depressive symptoms during a 2-week period that represent a change in previous functioning. The symptoms must cause clinically significant distress or impairment in functioning and must not be attributable to a substance or other medical condition. A depressive episode must include either depressed mood *or* **anhedonia** (loss of interest of pleasure). Additionally, a depressive episode must include at least four of the following symptoms:

» Significant weight loss when not dieting, or weight gain (>5% total body weight in 1 month), or significant changes in appetite
» Insomnia or hypersomnia every night
» Psychomotor agitation or retardation (observable by others)

Major mood disorder (MMD): a family of behavioral health disorders that affect a large portion of society.

Major depressive disorder (MDD): a major mood disorder characterized by depressed mood for at least 2 weeks.

Anhedonia: not able to feel pleasure.

Generalized anxiety disorder (GAD): a major mood disorder characterized by at least 6 months of anxious symptoms.

Bipolar disorder: a major mood disorder characterized by the presence of mania and depression.

» Fatigue/loss of energy
» Feelings of worthlessness or inappropriate/excessive guilt
» Diminished ability to think/concentrate or indecisiveness
» Recurrent thoughts of death or suicide, suicidal ideation, or suicide attempt/planning

Additionally, the episode must not be attributed to schizoaffective disorder, schizophrenia, or delusional/psychotic disorders. The patient must not have ever suffered a manic or hypomanic episode.

Generalized anxiety disorder (GAD) is defined by the *DSM-5* as having excessive anxiety/worry on more days than not for at least 6 months, often about multiple events or activities. The patient has difficulty controlling this worry, and it is significant enough to cause clinically significant distress or impairment. The anxiety cannot be attributed to a substance or other medical or psychiatric disorder. The patient must also be suffering from three or more of the following symptoms, with some symptoms present more often than not for at least 6 months:

1. Restlessness/feeling on edge
2. Being easily fatigued
3. Difficulty concentrating or mind going blank
4. Irritability
5. Muscle tension
6. Sleep disturbance

Bipolar disorder is now categorized as either bipolar I disorder or bipolar II disorder under the *DSM-5*. This disorder is characterized by the presence of both elevated moods (mania) and deeply depressed moods, simultaneously. Bipolar I disorder is distinguished from bipolar II disorder by the presence of manic episodes that affect the patient's ability to function. The *DSM-5* diagnostic criteria for a manic episode are as follows:.

1. Persistent elevated/expansive/irritable mood for at least 1 week (unless hospitalization is required)
2. At least three of the following symptoms also present (four if the primary mood is irritability)
   a. Inflated self-esteem/grandiosity
   b. Decreased need for sleep
   c. Increased talkativeness
   d. Flight of ideas/racing thoughts
   e. Distractibility
   f. Increase in goal-directed activity and/or psychomotor agitation
   g. Increase in risky behavior
3. Symptoms cannot meet the criteria for a mixed episode

4. Symptoms cause significant social or occupational impairment and/or hospitalization, or involve psychotic features
5. Symptoms cannot be attributed to a substance or other medical condition

A mixed episode must meet the criteria for both a manic and a major depressive episode for at least 1 week.

Bipolar I disorder is defined by the presence of at least one manic or mixed episode at least once, at any time, in a person's life. Bipolar II disorder has episodes of **hypomania**, in which some features of mania are present, but they are not severe enough to significantly impair a person's social or occupational life.

The *DSM-5* criteria for a substance abuse disorder is stratified into mild (two to three criteria), moderate (four to five criteria), and severe (six or seven criteria). The drug of choice does not impact the ability to use these criteria for diagnosis.

1. Taking the substance in a larger amount and for a longer period than intended
2. Wanting to cut down/quit but being unable to do so
3. Spending a great deal of time acquiring the substance
4. Craving/strong desire for the substance
5. Repeatedly unable to carry out major obligations (work or social) because of use
6. Continued use despite recurring interpersonal issues due to the use of the substance
7. Stopping/reducing important social/occupational activities because of use
8. Recurrent use in physically hazardous situations
9. Consistent use despite acknowledgment of physical or psychological difficulties from use
10. **Tolerance** for the substance
11. Withdrawal displayed as the traditional characteristic syndrome, or using the substance to avoid withdrawal

It should be noted that the final two criteria do not apply if the substance is being used under medical supervision.

> **KEY TERMS**
>
> **Hypomania:** a state of elevated or irritable mood that is abnormal but does not impair one's ability to function.
>
> **Tolerance:** no longer responding to the substance in the same way as when initially used, and a larger dose is required to achieve the initial effect.

Genetic Testing and Counseling

At this time, there is no definitive genetic test for any mood disorder or substance abuse disorder. All research into the genetics of behavioral health is relatively new and not considered a standard of care. This chapter highlights some of the studies that have been conducted to investigate the genetics of behavioral health because it is important to understand the strong pattern of heritability of these extremely common disorders. The majority of genetic studies in behavioral health have been performed seeking single nucleotide polymorphisms in candidate genes that appear to be different from those in control groups.

Substance Abuse

Several genetic studies have been performed on patients who have been diagnosed with a substance abuse disorder, and several pathways have been implicated in this process. Many of these genes are involved in neurocognitive impulse control, specifically *DRD2, DRD4,* and *SLC6A2*. A list of genes believed to be involved in substance abuse heritability can be seen in **Table 24-1**. Many of these genes could be stratified into which substance was likely to be abused. The majority of these genes are associated with alcohol, opiate, and nicotine addictions (as seen in **Figure 24-1**), likely because of the high usage and easy access of these substances. Most genes implicated are involved in serotonin or dopamine signaling pathways, which are often associated with impulse control and mood disorders.

Major Mood Disorders

Several genetic studies have been conducted seeking a genetic culprit for all the major mood disorders. As seen with substance abuse, many of these genes are involved in dopamine and serotonin signaling pathways. These genes are outlined in **Table 24-2** and are organized by their associated mood disorder. The genetic overlap between the three most common major mood disorders is illustrated in **Figure 24-2**. It should be noted that bipolar disorder seems to have the most genetic variability but shares the most overlap with major depressive disorder, likely because it shares many of the same features. One unique gene is found to contribute to general anxiety disorder alone, *CHRNA4*, which is associated with acetylcholine transport in the brain.

Relationship Between Substance Abuse and Mood Disorders

A few genetic studies have ventured into the relationship between major mood disorders and substance abuse disorders. A list of 13 candidate genes that are involved in both types of disorders has been compiled and is shown in **Table 24-3**. Of these 13 genes, 9 were seen to be associated with bipolar disorder, 6 of which were also seen in alcohol abuse. There has always been a strong sense that bipolar disorder and substance abuse were seen together; however, now there is perhaps a genetic explanation for that relationship as well. Major depressive disorder was associated with seven genes, five of which overlap with

TABLE 24-1	Genes Associated with Substance Abuse, with Specific Substance Associations*								
Gene	**Name**	**Chromosome**	**Alcohol**	**Amphetamines**	**Cannabis**	**Cocaine**	**Opiates***	**Nicotine**	
ALDH2	Aldehyde dehydrogenase 2 family	12	X				X	X	
AVPR1A	Arginine vasopressin receptor 1A	12	X				X		
CHRNA4	Cholinergic receptor, nicotinic, α4	20					X	X	
COMT	Catechol-O methyl-transferase	22			X		X		
*DAT**	Dopamine transporter	5						X	
DDC	Dopa decarboxylase	7						X	
DRD2	Dopamine receptor D2	11	X		X				
DRD3	Dopamine D3 receptor	3	X			X	X		
DRD4	Dopamine receptor D4	11	X					X	
GABRG2	γ-aminobutyric acid A receptor, γ2	5	X				X	X	
MAOA	Monoamine oxidase A	X	X						

TABLE 24-1 Genes Associated with Substance Abuse, with Specific Substance Associations* (Continued)

Gene	Name	Chromosome	Alcohol	Amphetamines	Cannabis	Cocaine	Opiates*	Nicotine
MAOB	Monoamine oxidase B	X	X			X		
SLC6A2	Solute carrier family 6 member 2	16	X			X	X	
NRXN1	Neurexin 1	2						X
NTRK2	Neurotrophic tyrosine kinase receptor, type 2	9						X
OPRD1	Opioid receptor, δ1	1	X				X	
OPRK1	Opioid receptor, 1	8	X			X	X	
PENK	Proenkephalin	8			X			
SLC6A3	Solute carrier family 6 member 3	5	X	X		X	X	X
SLC6A4	Solute carrier family 6 member 4	17	X					
VMAT2	Solute carrier family 18 member 2	10				X		

*Includes heroin, morphine, and general opioids.
**No specified substance.

FIGURE 24-1	Venn diagram demonstrating the genetic relationship for susceptibility for opiate, cocaine, and alcohol addiction.

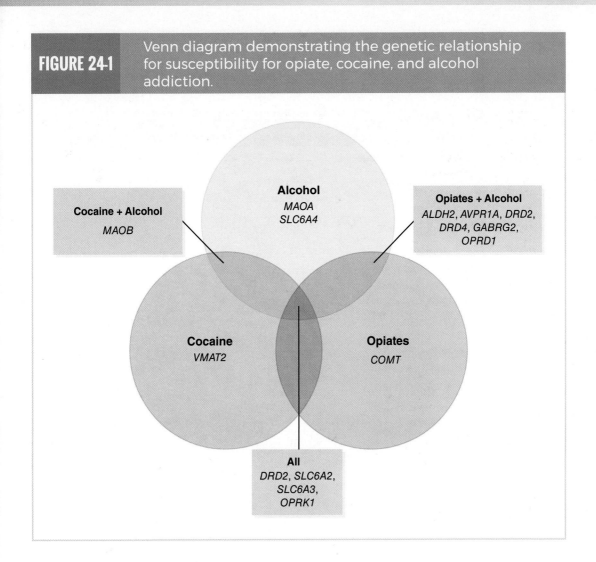

alcoholism. Generalized anxiety disorder has the smallest overlap with substance abuse, with only three of the six implicated genes involved in any substance abuse. However, all three of those genes are associated with opiate abuse, not alcohol abuse, perhaps due to the calming tendencies of opiates.

TABLE 24-2	Genes Associated with Major Mood Disorders Categorized by the Specific Disorders in Which They Are Implicated

Gene	Name	Chromosome	Anxiety	Major Depression	Bipolar
ALDH2	Aldehyde dehydrogenase 2 family	12			X
ANK3	Ankyrin 3, node of Ranvier	10		X	X
APOE	Apolipoprotein E	19		X	
BDNF	Brain-derived neurotrophic factor	11	X		X
CACNA1C	Calcium channel, voltage-dependent, α 1C	12		X	X
CHRNA4	Cholinergic receptor, nicotinic, α4	20	X		
COMT	Catechol-O-methyltransferase	22	X		X
DAT	Dopamine transporter	5			X
DRD4	Dopamine receptor D4	11			X
GABRG2	γ-aminobutyric acid A receptor, γ2	5			X
GNB3	Guanine nucleotide binding protein β polypeptide 3	12		X	X
GRIK1	Glutamate receptor, ionotropic, kainite 1	21		X	
GRIN2B	Glutamate receptor, ionotropic, N-methyl D-aspartate 2B	12			X

Gene	Name	Chromosome	Anxiety	Major Depression	Bipolar
HTR1A	5-hydroxytryptamine (serotonin) receptor 1A	5	X		X
HTR2B	5-hydroxytryptamine (serotonin) receptor 2B	2		X	
MAOA	Monoamine oxidase A	X	X	X	X
MAOB	Monoamine oxidase B	X	X	X	
MTHFR	Methylenetetrahy-drofolate reductase (NAD(P)H)	1		X	X
NCAN	Neurocan	19			X
SLC6A2	Solute carrier family 6 member 2	16	X	X	
NRXN1	Neurexin 1	2			X
NTRK2	Neurotrophic tyrosine kinase receptor, type 2	9		X	
OPRK1	Opioid receptor, 1	8			X
PENK	Proenkephalin	8			X
SLC6A3	Solute carrier family 6 member 3	5	X	X	
SLC6A4	Solute carrier family 6 member 4	17	X	X	X
VMAT2	Solute carrier family 18 member 2	10		X	X
ZNF804A	Zinc finger protein 804A	2			X

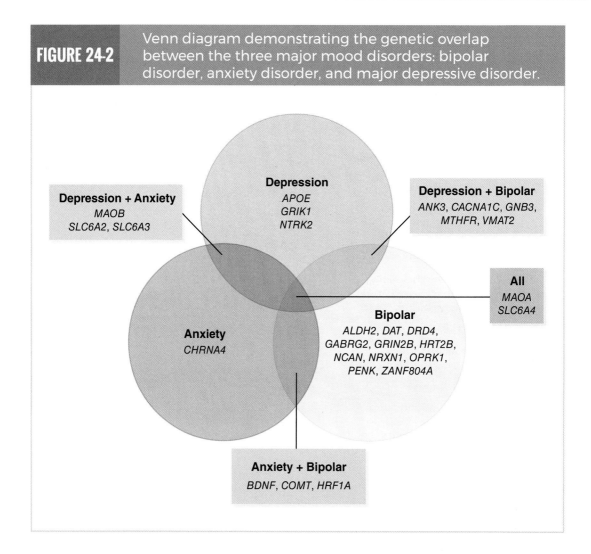

FIGURE 24-2 Venn diagram demonstrating the genetic overlap between the three major mood disorders: bipolar disorder, anxiety disorder, and major depressive disorder.

Depression
APOE
GRIK1
NTRK2

Depression + Anxiety
MAOB
SLC6A2, SLC6A3

Depression + Bipolar
ANK3, CACNA1C, GNB3,
MTHFR, VMAT2

All
MAOA
SLC6A4

Anxiety
CHRNA4

Bipolar
ALDH2, DAT, DRD4,
GABRG2, GRIN2B, HRT2B,
NCAN, NRXN1, OPRK1,
PENK, ZANF804A

Anxiety + Bipolar
BDNF, COMT, HRF1A

Management and Treatment

Behavioral health problems are often difficult to treat but do respond well to some types of medications. Substance abuse disorders specifically are extremely difficult to treat because it seems that one addiction is often easily replaced by another; thus, they often are best treated through the use of various forms of psychotherapy. However, the purpose of this chapter is not to expound on the different classes of medications and therapy available.

When treating patients with major mood disorders, it is important to keep in mind that these patients are at high risk of having or developing a concurred substance abuse disorder. These patients need to be properly screened

TABLE 24-3 Genes Associated with Major Mood Disorders and the Abuse of Alcohol, Cocaine, or Opioids

Gene	Name	Chromosome	Anxiety	Depression	Bipolar	Alcohol	Cocaine	Opioids*
ALDH2	Aldehyde dehydrogenase 2 family	12			X	X	X	X
COMT	Catechol-O methyltransferase	22	X		X	X		X
DRD4	Dopamine receptor D4	11			X	X		X
GABRG2	γ-aminobutyric acid A receptor, γ2	5			X	X		
GRIK1	Glutamate receptor, ionotropic, kainite 1	21		X		X		
GRIN2B	Glutamate receptor, ionotropic, N-methyl-D-aspartate 2B	12			X	X		
MAOA	Monoamine oxidase A	X	X	X	X	X		
MAOB	Monoamine oxidase B	X	X	X		X	X	
SLC6A2	Solute carrier family 6 member 2	16	X	X		X	X	X
OPRK1	Opioid receptor, 1	8			X	X	X	X
SLC6A3	Solute carrier family 6 member 3	5	X	X		X	X	X
SLC6A4	Solute carrier family 6 member 4	17	X	X	X	X	X	
VMAT2	Solute carrier family 18 member 2	10		X	X		X	

*Includes heroin, morphine, and other opiate medications.

for preexisting substance abuse conditions or history. It is also important to educate them on their risks for possibly developing these conditions. Be diligent when prescribing highly addictive substances, and follow these patients closely.

Chapter Summary

» Major mood disorders affect between 30% and 60% of Americans.

» The term *major mood disorder* encompasses three separate disorders: major depressive disorder, bipolar disorder, and generalized anxiety disorder.

» A statistically significant portion of patients with major mood disorders have a concurrent substance abuse problem.

» There is no definitive genetic test or pattern of heritability for any behavioral health condition.

» Some studies indicate a genetic link between the heritability of major mood disorders and substance abuse disorders.

» The pathways implicated in both substance abuse and major mood disorders predominantly involve the serotonin and dopamine pathways in the brain.

» Most of these pathways are also involved in impulse control.

Chapter Review Questions

1. Approximately _____ of Americans suffer from a psychiatric disorder.
2. A major depressive episode must include either _____ or _____ and last for at least _____.
3. According to the *DSM-5*, all psychiatric disorders must not be attributable to _____ or _____.
4. To be diagnosed with generalized anxiety disorder, the symptoms must last for _____.
5. Bipolar disorder is characterized by the presence of _____.
6. Bipolar I disorder differs from bipolar II disorder by the presence of _____ that _____.
7. If a person _____ a substance, he or she requires larger and larger doses to achieve the same effect as the initial dose.
8. Pathways involving the signaling of _____ and _____ are implicated in both substance abuse and major mood disorders.
9. Generalized anxiety disorder has the most genetic predisposition for _____.

Bibliography

Deo, A. J., Huang, Y. Y., Hodgkinson, C. A., Xin, Y., Oquendo, M. A., Dwork, A. J., . . . Haghighi, F. (2013). A large-scale candidate gene analysis of mood disorders: Evidence of neurotrophic tyrosine kinase receptor and opioid receptor signaling dysfunction. *Psychiatric Genetics, 23*(2), 47–55. doi:10.1097 /YPG.0b013e32835d7028

Doherty, J. L., & Owen, M. J. (2014). Genomic insights into the overlap between psychiatric disorders: Implications for research and clinical practice. *Genome Medicine, 6*(4), 29. doi:10.1186/gm546

Fineberg, N. A., Chamberlain, S. R., Goudriaan, A. E., Stein, D. J., Vanderschuren, L. J., Gillan, C. M., . . . Potenza, M. N. (2014). New developments in human neurocognition: Clinical, genetic, and brain imaging correlates of impulsivity and compulsivity. *CNS Spectrums, 19*(1), 69–89. doi:10.1017/s1092852913000801

Flint, J., & Kendler, K. S. (2014). The genetics of major depression. *Neuron, 81*(3), 484–503. doi: 10.1016/j.neuron.2014.01.027

Hall, F. S., Drgonova, J., Jain, S., & Uhl, G. R. (2013). Implications of genome wide association studies for addiction: Are our a priori assumptions all wrong? *Pharmacology & Therapeutics, 140*(3), 267–279. doi:10.1016/j.pharmthera .2013.07.006

Hopfer, C. (2014). Community, siblings, heritability and the risk for drug abuse. *American Journal of Psychiatry, 171*(2), 140–141. doi:10.1176/appi.ajp.2013.13111508

Kessler, R. C., Nelson, C. B., McGonagle, K. A., Edlund, M. J., Frank, R. G., & Leaf, P. J. (1996). The epidemiology of co-occurring addictive and mental disorders: Implications for prevention and service utilization. *American Journal of Orthopsychiatry, 66*(1), 17–31.

National Institute on Drug Abuse. (2017, March 1). Monitoring the future study: Trends in prevalence of various drugs. Retrieved from http://www.drugabuse.gov /trends-statistics/monitoring-future/monitoring-future-study-trends-in -prevalence-various-drugs

Oquendo, M. A., Ellis, S. P., Chesin, M. S., Birmaher, B., Zelazny, J., Tin, A., . . . Brent, D. A. (2013). Familial transmission of parental mood disorders: Unipolar and bipolar disorders in offspring. *Bipolar Disorders, 15*(7), 764–773. doi:10.1111/bdi.12107

Regier, D. A., Farmer, M. E., Rae, D. S., Locke, B. Z., Keith, S. J., Judd, L. L., & Goodwin, F. K. (1990). Comorbidity of mental disorders with alcohol and other drug abuse: Results from the Epidemiologic Catchment Area (ECA) study. *JAMA: The Journal of the American Medical Association, 264*(19), 2511–2518.

Reus, V. I. (2012). Mental disorders. In D. L. Longo, A. S. Fauci, D. L. Kasper, S. L. Hauser, J. L. Jameson, & J. Loscalzo (Eds.), *Harrison's principles of internal medicine* (18th ed., pp. 1059–1081). New York, NY: McGraw-Hill.

Safran, M., Dalah, I., Alexander, J., Rosen, N., Iny Stein, T., Shmoish, M., . . . Lancet, D. (2010). GeneCards Version 3: The human gene integrator. *Database, 2010.* doi:10.1093/database/baq020

< Define pharmacogenomics.
< Detail some of the challenges associated with drug therapy.
< Review example applications of pharmacogenomics.
< Identify limitations and pitfalls to this developing technology.

KEY TERMS

International Normalized
    Ratio (INR)
Pharmacogenetics

Pharmacogenomics
Polymorphisms

Prodrug
Prothrombin time

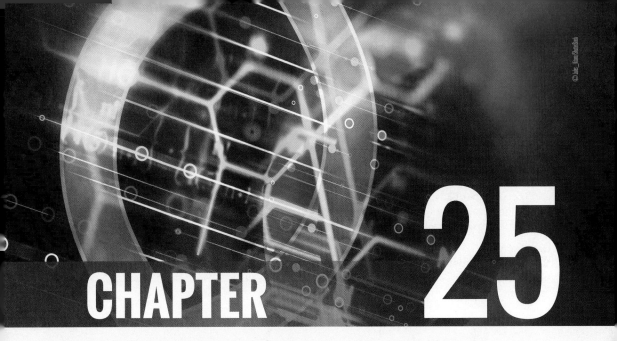

CHAPTER 25

Pharmacogenomics

Every practicing clinician has noticed differences among patients in terms of how they react to medicines. This includes not only prescription medications but also over-the-counter medications (i.e., those obtained without a prescription). Unfortunately, the only way to determine how a patient will react to a medication is via trial and error. Generally, a patient will try some new medicine and then report an adverse reaction soon after starting the treatment. The range of potential reactions varies, from a mild, itchy skin rash to a full-blown anaphylactic reaction that includes lip and tongue swelling and closing of the airway. Obviously, all healthcare providers want to avoid these types of adverse events in their patients.

Pharmacogenomics is the study of how genes affect a person's response to drugs. A relatively new field, it combines pharmacology and genomics to develop effective and safe medications so that doses can be tailored to a person's genetic makeup. Along the way, it attempts to explain variability of drug responses based on genetic differences between individuals. The goal is to understand the role that an individual's genetic makeup plays in how well a medicine works, as well as which side effects are likely to occur in the individual's body. This information can help tailor the development of drugs so that they are best suited for a particular individual or group. **Pharmacogenetics** refers to the role of inheritance in individual variation in drug metabolism. For most purposes, the terms *pharmacogenetics* and *pharmacogenomics* can be used interchangeably. Some potential benefits of pharmacogenomics are shown in **Box 25-1**.

Many drugs are altered by enzymes during their metabolism within the body. In some cases, an active drug may be made inactive or less active through metabolism. In other cases, an inactive or less active drug may be made more active through metabolism. The challenge in drug therapy is to make sure that the active form of a drug stays around long enough to do its job: Some people have enzymes that may

---

BOX 25-1 Potential Benefits of Pharmacogenomics

More accurate methods of determining drug dosages

Development of drugs that maximize therapeutic effects but decrease damage to nearby healthy cells

Drug prescribing based on a patient's genetic profile rather than by trial and error; decreased occurrence of adverse reactions

Vaccine development using genetic material, which could activate the immune system similar to current vaccines but with reduced risks of infections

Data from Barlow-Stewart, K., & Saleh, M. (2015). *Pharmacogenomics/pharmacogenetics.* The Center for Genetics Education. Retrieved from http://www.genetics.edu.au/Publications-and -Resources/Genetics-Fact-Sheets/FactSheetPHARMACOGENETICSPHARMACOGENOMICS.pdf.

KEY TERMS

Pharmacogenomics: the study of the combination of pharmacology and genomics; the aim is to develop effective and safe medications to compensate for genetic differences in patients that cause varied responses to a single therapeutic regimen.

Pharmacogenetics: the study of the interrelation of hereditary constitution and response to drugs.

metabolize a drug too quickly, too slowly, or not at all. Therefore, depending on the situation, the drug may be completely metabolized before it has its intended effect or metabolized very little, leading to unsafe concentrations within the body.

Many currently available drugs are marketed as "one size fits all" therapies even though they do not work the same way for everyone. It can be difficult to predict who will benefit from a medication, who will not respond at all, and who will experience negative side effects. Unfortunately, adverse drug reactions are a significant cause of hospitalizations and deaths in the United States. Knowledge gained from the Human Genome Project is being used to determine how inherited differences in genes affect the body's response to medications. In the future, these genetic differences may be used to predict whether a medication will be effective for a particular person and to help prevent adverse drug reactions.

The small differences in the genes between different population groups or some families within a population group that have built up over the course of many generations can mean that they react differently to medicines. For example, if one group of people break down a medicine very quickly or very slowly compared with others, then their genes may offer a clue as to why they respond that way. If so, then it may be predicted, based on his or her genes, how someone would react to a medicine before giving it.

It is clear that many nongenetic factors (e.g., age, organ function, drug interactions) influence the effects of medications. Nevertheless, genetic variation may account for as much as 95% of variability in some drugs' disposition and effects. There are numerous examples of interindividual differences in drug response caused by common genetic variations (called **polymorphisms**) in genes encoding drug-metabolizing enzymes, drug transporters, or drug targets.

The human genes involved in many pharmacogenetic traits have been identified, and polymorphisms within these genes are in various stages of being exploited as molecular diagnostics in medicine. At present, clinical applications are mostly limited to medications with narrow therapeutic indices (e.g., anticancer agents, some antidepressants, warfarin).

Drug Metabolism

Several different types of liver enzymes are involved in the metabolism of medications. Genetic variations in these enzymes that affect metabolic rate are relatively common, but the prevalence of the variations differs significantly by ethnic background. Among these enzymes are the cytochrome P450 family (CYP), N-acetyltransferase, thiopurine methyltransferase (TPMT), and UDP-glucuronosyltransferase. Although there are many clinically relevant polymorphisms that have been discovered with all these enzyme families, this chapter aims to focus on a few relevant examples to introduce the reader to the concept of pharmacogenetics and the role that it may play in his or her patients. Readers who would like to learn more about other clinically relevant polymorphisms are encouraged to review the resources listed in the bibliography section of this chapter.

The CYP enzymes include approximately 57 liver enzymes that metabolize more than 30 classes of drugs, including antidepressants, antiepileptics, and cardiovascular drugs. Based on variations in the associated CYP gene, patients can generally be separated into poor, normal, and ultrarapid drug metabolizers. Depending on the type of medication, a significant proportion of the population may fall into the poor or ultrarapid metabolizer category. When a patient who is a poor metabolizer of a particular drug is given a standard dose, he or she will process the drug more slowly than expected, resulting in increased levels of the drug in the person's bloodstream. Consequently, there is increased risk for side effects and toxicity. In the case of an ultrarapid metabolizer, the same dose may be ineffective because the drug is metabolized too rapidly to achieve its maximal effects. Therefore, dosages of these drugs must be modified to accommodate the rate of metabolism.

N-acetyltransferase is a liver enzyme that activates some drugs and deactivates others. Some patients can acetylate (a type of metabolic change) drugs slowly, whereas others acetylate drugs quickly. Those persons who are slow acetylators may experience toxicity when taking drugs such as procainamide, isoniazid, hydralazine, and sulfonamides, whereas those who are fast acetylators may not respond to isoniazid or hydralazine. Between 40% and 70% of Caucasians and African Americans are considered to be slow acetylators.

Azathioprine and other thiopurine medications (such as 6-mercaptopurine and 6-thioguanine) are used to treat children afflicted with acute lymphocytic

KEY TERM

Polymorphisms: natural variations in a gene, DNA sequence, or chromosome that have no adverse effects on the individual and occur with fairly high frequency in the general population.

International Normalized Ratio (INR): a system established by the World Health Organization and the International Committee on Thrombosis and Hemostasis for reporting the results of blood coagulation (clotting) tests. All results are standardized using the international sensitivity index for the particular thromboplastin reagent and instrument combination used to perform the test. Regardless of which laboratory checks the prothrombin time, the result should be the same even if different thromboplastins and instruments are used.

leukemia; they are also used to treat inflammatory bowel disease, rheumatoid arthritis, and transplant immune suppression. These immune suppressants are metabolized by TPMT. Because each copy of the *TPMT* gene will produce some TPMT enzyme, three different groups of enzyme activity levels are distinguished: deficient, intermediate, and normal. Although less than 1% of the general population have a TPMT deficiency, approximately 11% have moderately reduced levels of the enzyme. Therefore, if these patients are given a standard drug dose, they may suffer severe hematopoietic toxicity. Some of these individuals are able to achieve the desired therapeutic effect from a dose that is 1/10 of the recommended dose.

UDP-glucuronosyltransferase is involved in the metabolism of irinotecan, a chemotherapeutic drug that is used in the treatment of metastatic colorectal cancer. Variations in the gene that codes for this enzyme can influence the patient's ability to break down the major active metabolite in irinotecan. The inability to degrade the metabolite can lead to increased blood concentrations and increased risk of side effects, including reduced white blood cell count and severe diarrhea.

Warfarin

Warfarin is used to prevent dangerous blood clots from forming in the blood vessels of certain patients, but it can significantly increase the risk of bleeding into the brain or gastrointestinal tract. It is widely known that many clinical and demographic factors, such as age, sex, drug interactions, and diet, affect warfarin's metabolism. In addition, strong evidence indicates that genetic variation contributes to interindividual variability in warfarin's metabolism. Warfarin acts by inhibiting vitamin K epoxide reductase complex subunit 1 (VKORC1) and is a major substrate of cytochrome CYP2C9. Any genetic variation in the gene sequence coding for both of these enzymes can potentially vary the efficacy and toxicity of warfarin treatment.

The *CYP2C9* gene has been linked to toxicity and altered dosage requirements, despite clinicians' ability to titrate warfarin dosing to a clear, effective endpoint (i.e., **International Normalized Ratio [INR]**). For example, in the best-case scenario, a person taking warfarin might maintain an INR of 2 to 3. Patients with a variant *CYP2C9* genotype take a median of 95 days longer to achieve stable dosing compared with patients who have a wild-type genotype, however. They also have a higher risk of acute bleeding complications. Patients with the two most common variant alleles require 15–30% lower maintenance doses of warfarin to achieve the target INR. When added to other clinical factors that are known to affect warfarin dosing, the *CYP2C9* genotype has been shown to incrementally improve prediction of warfarin dose maintenance.

Clearly, understanding clinical as well as genetic factors has the potential to improve warfarin therapy. Clinical and demographic variables account for approximately 20% of interindividual variability in warfarin dosing, while the *CYP2C9* genotype accounts for 15–20% of this variability, and the *VKORC1* genotype accounts for an additional 14%. Collectively, 50% to 60% of the total variation in warfarin dosing is predictable before administration—which is very valuable information to the prescribing clinician.

Cytochrome P450 2D6

Probably the most extensively studied polymorphic drug-metabolizing liver enzyme in humans is cytochrome P450 2D6 (CYP2D6). More than 30 medications are metabolized by this enzyme, including analgesics, antidepressants, and antiemetics. Polymorphisms in the *CYP2D6* genotype can cause exaggerated or diminished drug effects, depending on whether the medication is inactivated (e.g., nortriptyline, fluoxetine, 5-hydroxytryptamine inhibitors) or activated (e.g., codeine).

For example, approximately 10% of patients will receive no pain relief from codeine because of the absence of a functional CYP2D6 enzyme, which is responsible for producing the active agent from the **prodrug**. Notably, people with Asian, Caucasian, or Middle Eastern heritage are less likely to convert codeine into its active morphine form. In contrast, some women are ultrarapid metabolizers of codeine and are warned against taking the drug during pregnancy or lactation because of increased risk of adverse effects from excessive conversion to morphine. Consequently, it has been suggested that poor or ultrarapid metabolizers should not be prescribed this particular agent.

Pharmacogenomic Tests

Because enzymes involved in drug metabolism arise from multiple genes, pharmacogenomic test results can be difficult to interpret. These test results constitute predictions based on information about the specific genetic variations and on information about the associated diseases, adverse drug reactions, and patient outcomes that have been gathered during studies and clinical trials. In many cases, the predictions will be very accurate, but physicians cannot use the information to state with absolute certainty what will happen with an individual patient. Furthermore, these test results do not incorporate or make allowances for other factors in a patient's life related to the disease condition or to the individual that may affect the response to treatment. Therefore, the results are intended to be used in conjunction with other relevant clinical findings.

KEY TERMS

Prothrombin time: a clotting test done to test the integrity of part of the clotting scheme, which is commonly used as a method of monitoring the accuracy of blood thinning treatment (anticoagulation) with warfarin. The test measures the time needed for clot formation after thromboplastin (plus calcium) has been added to plasma.

Prodrug: a class of drugs in which the pharmacologic action results from conversion by metabolic processes within the body.

TABLE 25-1 — Some Currently Available Pharmacogenomic Tests

Test	Purpose
DNA microarray that tests for 29 *CYP2D6* genetic variants and two *CYP2C19* genetic variants	Meant to be used as an aid in individualizing treatment selection and dosing for drugs metabolized through these genes. Helps predict poor, intermediate, extensive, or ultrarapid metabolizers.
A test that detects variations in the *UGT1A1* gene, which produces the enzyme UDP-glucuronosyltransferase	Used to identify patients who may be at increased risk of adverse reaction to irinotecan.
Tests that detect genetic variants of the CYP2C9 and VKORC1 (vitamin K epoxide reductase) enzymes	Used to identify patients who have genetic variations and need a reduced dose of warfarin to avoid bleeding episodes.

Data from *Pharmacogenetic tests*. American Association for Clinical Chemistry. Retrieved from https://labtestsonline.org/understanding/analytes/pharmacogenetic-tests/start/2

Some currently available pharmacogenomic tests are shown in **Table 25-1**. In 2005, a Food and Drug Administration advisory committee voted in favor of changing warfarin's label to indicate that pharmacogenomic information can be useful in deciding a patient's individual dose.

Limitations and Ethical Issues

Because many genes are likely to play at least some role in how someone reacts to a drug, the idea of targeting different drugs represents a very complex challenge (**Box 25-2**). Another consideration is that interactions with other drugs and environmental factors may influence a specific drug reaction. Consequently, the influence of these factors will need to be elucidated before conclusions are drawn about how a specific drug is working.

Although the idea of individually targeted drug therapy is very attractive, it is likely to be very expensive—a consideration that will affect the access to such drugs for many people. Of course, there is always the issue of whether health insurance plans will cover the cost. Given these factors, the future of pharmacogenomics will most likely focus on the development of drugs that work well with certain population groups. However, any program will need to be carefully implemented to avoid a perception of stigma based on ethnicity.

BOX 25-2	Limitations to Taking Full Advantage of Pharmacogenomics

Many genes are likely involved in how someone reacts to a drug, making targeted drugs very complex.

Identification of the small variations in everyone's genes that may influence drug metabolism or how the condition develops is very difficult and time consuming.

Interactions with other drugs and environmental factors will need to be determined before any conclusions are reached about genetic influence on how the drug is working.

Data from Barlow-Stewart, K., & Saleh, M. (2015). *Pharmacogenomics/pharmacogenetics*. The Center for Genetics Education. Retrieved from http://www.genetics.edu.au/Publications-and-Resources/Genetics-Fact-Sheets/FactSheetPHARMACOGENETICSPHARMACOGENOMICS.pdf/view.

Because not all people who belong to a particular ethnic group will have the same genetic variations, the assumption that an individual's race can indicate his or her genetic profile for drug response can be a potential problem. A possible consequence of such genetic profiling is denial of treatment based on race if a pharmacogenomic test is not available for a particular drug. Thus, people from different ethnic groups who are affected by the same condition may be given different access to treatment.

Chapter Summary

» Pharmacogenomics combines pharmacology and genomics to develop effective and safe medications so that doses can be tailored to a person's genetic makeup.

» Many currently available drugs are marketed as "one size fits all" options, even though they do not work the same way for everyone.

» Adverse drug reactions are a significant cause of hospitalizations and deaths in the United States.

» Pharmacogenomic test results are predictions based on information about the specific genetic variations and on information about the associated diseases, adverse drug reactions, and patient outcomes that have been gathered during studies and clinical trials.

» While the idea of individually targeted drug therapy is very attractive, it is likely to be very expensive, a factor that will affect the accessibility of such drugs for many people.

Chapter Review Questions

1. Pharmacogenomics attempts to explain variability of drug responses based on _____ between individuals.
2. Many drugs are altered by _____ during metabolism in the body.
3. Genetic variation can account for as much as _____ of variability in drug disposition and effects.
4. Approximately 50 liver cytochrome P450 enzymes metabolize more than 30 classes of drugs, including _____, _____, and _____.
5. Many clinical and demographic factors, such as _____, _____, _____, and _____ affect warfarin dosing.

Bibliography

American Association for Clinical Chemistry. (2018). *Pharmacogenomic tests.* Retrieved from https://labtestsonline.org/understanding/analytes/pharmacogenetic -tests/start/2

Centre for Genetics Education. (2015). *Pharmacogenomics/pharmacogenetics: Fact sheet 21.* Retrieved from http://www.genetics.edu.au/publications-and-resources /facts-sheets/fact-sheet-21-pharmacogenomics-pharmacogenetics/view

Higashi, M. K., Veenstra, D. L., & Kondo, L. M. (2002). Association between CYP2C9 genetic variants and anticoagulation-related outcomes during warfarin therapy. *Journal of the American Medical Association, 287*(13), 1690–1698.

Kalow, W., Meyer, U. A., & Tyndale, R. (2001). *Pharmacogenomics.* New York, NY: CRC Press.

Lanfear, D. E., & McLeod, H. L. (2007). Pharmacogenetics: Using DNA to optimize drug therapy. *American Family Physician, 76,* 1179–1182.

National Human Genome Research Institute. (2016). *Frequently asked questions about pharmacogenomics.* Retrieved from https://www.genome.gov/27530645/faq -about-pharmacogenomics/

National Institute of General Medical Sciences. (n.d.). *NIH Pharmacogenomics Research Network.* Retrieved from https://www.nigms.nih.gov/Research/Specific Areas/PGRN/Pages/default.aspx

Personalized Healthcare Report 2008: *Warfarin and genetic testing.* (n.d). Retrieved from https://crediblemeds.org/files/1713/7727/6113/warfarin_brochure.pdf

U.S. National Library of Medicine. (n.d.). Pharmacogenomics [Search results]. Retrieved from http://clinicaltrials.gov/ct2/results?term=pharmacogenomics

U.S. National Library of Medicine, National Center for Biotechnology Information. (n.d.). Retrieved from https://www.ncbi.nlm.nih.gov

U.S. National Library of Medicine, National Institutes of Health, U.S. Department of Health and Human Services. *Genetics home reference*. (2018). *What is pharmacogenomics?* Retrieved from http://ghr.nlm.nih.gov/handbook/genomic research/pharmacogenomics

‹ Describe the basic principles of gene therapy.
‹ Identify the various types of gene therapy.
‹ Detail how various viruses are used as delivery vehicles for new genetic information.
‹ Review the problems and pitfalls associated with gene therapy.

KEY TERMS

Adeno-associated virus
Adenovirus
CFTR gene
Fifth disease
Gain-of-function mutation
Herpes simplex virus
Lentivirus

Liposome
Loss-of-function mutation
Neoplastic
Oligonucleotide
Oncogene
Packaging cells
Proto-oncogene

Ribozymes
Severe combined immune
 deficiency
Thalassemia
Transduction
Vector

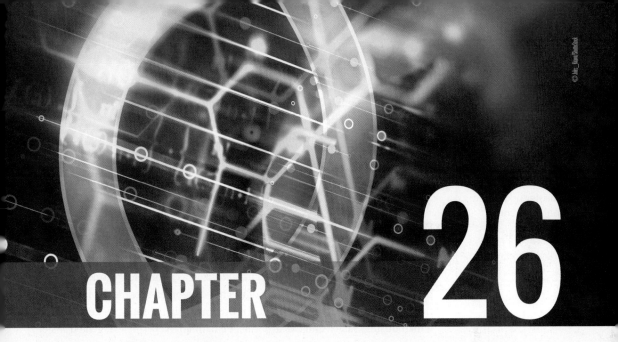

CHAPTER 26

Gene Therapy

Given the exciting genetic progress that has been made over the past 25 years, such as through the Human Genome Project, it is natural to speculate how this new information might be used to address various human genetic diseases. On an almost daily basis, an announcement is released to the media that another important gene involved in some disease has been identified. Thus, it might seem that the concept of taking out the "bad" gene and replacing it with a "good" gene would lend itself to rather straightforward application. In fact, the basic premise of gene therapy is to insert a "normal" gene into the genome to replace an "abnormal" disease-causing gene. Even though this sounds simple, in reality, it is very challenging.

Some approaches currently under investigation include using gene therapy for the following purposes:

» Exchange an abnormal gene for a normal gene through homologous recombination
» Repair an abnormal gene through selective reverse mutation, which returns the gene to its normal function
» Alter the regulation (the degree to which a gene is turned on or off) of a particular gene

Basic Process

Because adding naked DNA or RNA to a cell is an inefficient process, most gene therapy uses some type of gene delivery vehicle. A carrier molecule, called a **vector**, is frequently used to deliver the therapeutic gene to the patient's target cells. Currently, the most common vector is a virus that has been genetically altered to carry normal human DNA. Viruses have evolved a way of encapsulating and delivering their genes to human cells in a pathogenic manner. Researchers have tried to take advantage of this capability by manipulating the virus genome, removing disease-causing genes and inserting therapeutic genes.

Gene transfer strategies involve three essential elements: (1) a vector, (2) a gene to be delivered, and (3) a relevant target cell to which the DNA or RNA is delivered. Gene delivery can take place *in vivo*, in which the vector is directly injected into the patient, or, in the case of hematopoietic and some other target cells, *ex vivo*, in which the target cells are removed from the patient, followed by return of the modified autologous cells after gene transfer in the laboratory. When the donated DNA enters the target cell and begins expression, this process is referred to as **transduction**.

Gene therapy is far from being characterized as a routine treatment regimen at this point. In fact, it is one of the most complex therapeutic modalities yet attempted. Each new disease represents a therapeutic problem for which dosing, safety, and efficacy must be defined. Nevertheless, gene transfer remains one of the most powerful and promising concepts in modern molecular medicine. It has the potential to address a host of diseases for which there are currently no cures or, in some cases, available treatment. More than 2,400 gene therapy clinical trials have taken place worldwide, and serious adverse events have been rare. As outlined in **Table 26-1**, gene therapies are being developed for a wide variety of disease processes, although the majority of

TABLE 26-1	Breakdown of Clinical Gene Transfer Studies by Disease Classification
Disease	**Percentage**
Cancer	64.5%
Monogenic diseases	10.3%
Infectious diseases	7.5%
Cardiovascular diseases	7.4%
Neurological diseases	1.8%
Ocular diseases	1.4%
Inflammatory diseases	0.6%
Other diseases	2.3%
Gene marking	2.1%
Healthy volunteers	2.2%

Data from Gene therapy clinical trials worldwide. (2016). *Journal of Gene Medicine*. Retrieved from http://www.abedia.com/wiley/indications.php

trials so far have addressed cancer, with monogenic disorders and infectious diseases representing the next most researched indications.

Types of Gene Therapy

In theory, it is possible to transform either somatic cells (most cells of the body) or cells of the germline (such as sperm cells, ova, and their stem cell precursors). Historically, gene therapy in people has been directed at somatic cells, whereas germline modification in humans remains highly controversial. Not all somatic cells are good candidates for gene therapy. Specifically, good candidates should be easily accessible and have a long life span within the body. Proliferating cells are preferred for some gene delivery systems because the vector carrying the gene of interest can integrate itself into the replicating DNA of the cell. Although bone marrow stem cells meet all of these requirements, they are difficult to manipulate and isolate from bone marrow. Therefore, a variety of other cell types are being investigated as potential targets, including skin fibroblasts, muscle cells, vascular endothelial cells, hepatocytes, and lymphocytes.

Most current gene therapy approaches involve the replacement of a missing gene product by insertion of a normal gene into a somatic cell to correct **loss-of-function mutations**. These types of mutations result in a nonfunctional or missing gene product; insertion of the normal gene corrects this defect. Potentially, many recessive disorders may be corrected with the production of only a small amount of the gene product.

Viruses as Gene Therapy Vectors

Many techniques have been developed for introducing genes into different cell types, although not all are applicable or feasible in somatic cells. Because viruses have evolved ways to insert their genes into cells with high efficiency, they have received a lot of focus as potential gene therapy vectors. As described in this section, several types of viruses are being investigated, with varying degrees of success. Note that these viral vectors have been modified using molecular techniques to prevent replication and subsequent infection of the host.

Retroviruses

A retrovirus can create double-stranded DNA copies of its RNA genome, which can then be integrated into the chromosomes of host cells. Such viruses become integrated into the host DNA with a high degree of efficiency and seldom induce an immune response. Because these modified retroviruses are unable to replicate, they are propagated in **packaging cells**, which allows for production of multiple copies that contain the human gene but cannot replicate themselves (**Figure 26-1**). The modified retroviruses are then incubated with the somatic cells (e.g., bone marrow stem cells) obtained from a patient,

FIGURE 26-1

Use of a retroviral vector for gene therapy. Replication of the retrovirus is prevented by removing most of its genome; a normal human gene is then inserted into the retrovirus and propagated in a packaging cell. Virions from the packaging cell are incubated with human somatic cells, which allow the retrovirus to insert copies of the normal human gene into the cell. Once integrated into the cell's DNA, the inserted gene produces normal gene product.

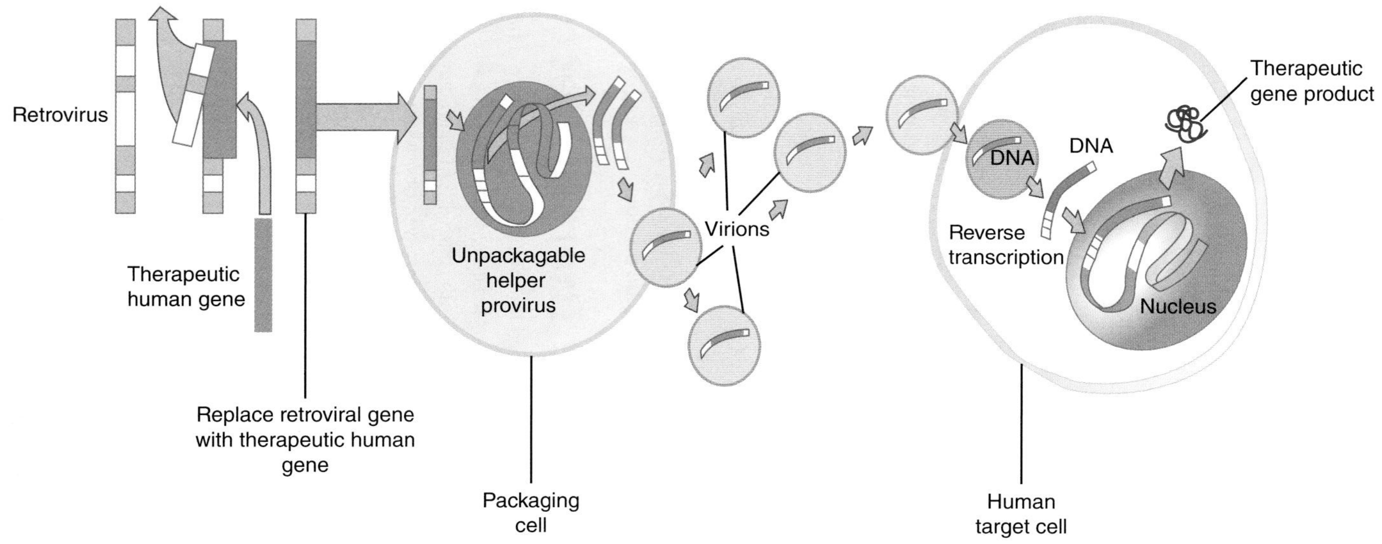

Reproduced with permission from Jorde, L. B., Carey, J. C., Bamshad, M. J., & White, R. L. (2006). *Medical genetics* (3rd ed.). St. Louis, MO: Mosby.

and the modified retrovirus inserts the normal human gene into the host cell. Once inserted, the normal gene will encode for a normal gene product in the patient's somatic cells. This approach has been used to treat many diseases, including **severe combined immune deficiency**.

Even though there are advantages to using retroviruses as vectors in gene therapy, this approach also has certain disadvantages. One important concern relates to their potential to induce tumor formation. Because a retrovirus becomes integrated into gene-rich regions of the host's DNA, it could activate a nearby **proto-oncogene**, resulting in tumor formation. Another disadvantage is that retroviruses infect only dividing cells; they are ineffective in nondividing or slowly dividing cells such as neurons. Of course, if the goal is to target only dividing cells, then this limitation may actually be beneficial. One example would be in the treatment of a brain tumor where the **neoplastic** cells are dividing but the nearby brain cells are not.

Adenoviruses

Adenoviruses contain double-stranded DNA. This class of viruses causes respiratory, intestinal, and eye infections in humans, including the common cold. Before their use as a gene therapy vector, adenoviruses must be modified so that they are unable to replicate. They are able to infect both dividing and nondividing cells but do not become integrated into the host cell's genome. Thus, gene expression following adenoviral gene transfer is short lived. However, because these viruses do not become integrated into the genome of the host, they will not activate a proto-oncogene, as might occur with a retrovirus. Based on their ability to infect nondividing cells, adenoviruses are being used in trials to deliver the normal **CFTR gene** to lung epithelial cells by an aerosol. Researchers hope that this novel approach will increase chloride-ion channel activity in patients with cystic fibrosis.

One disadvantage of their short life span is that eventually these adenoviruses will become inactivated and will then need to be readministered for therapeutic purposes. Another problem is that typically only part of the adenovirus genome is removed, which can lead to stimulation of the host's immune response. This problem increases with repeated adenovirus exposure as the foreign protein further stimulates the immune response. Researchers are attempting to remove more of the viral genome in an effort to reduce the immune response.

Adeno-Associated Viruses

Parvovirus is an example of an **adeno-associated virus**—one of a class of small, single-stranded DNA viruses that can insert their genetic material at a specific site on chromosome 19. **Fifth disease** is caused by infection with human parvovirus B19 and infects only humans. It manifests as a mild rash illness that occurs most commonly in children. Although adeno-associated viruses are smaller than either retroviruses or adenoviruses, they have the

KEY TERMS

Severe combined immune deficiency: any of a group of rare, sometimes fatal, congenital disorders characterized by little or no immune response.

Proto-oncogene: a gene whose protein product is involved in the regulation of cell growth. When altered, a proto-oncogene can become a cancer-causing oncogene.

Neoplastic: related to the pathologic process that results in the formation and growth of a neoplasm or abnormal tissue that may be either benign or malignant.

Adenovirus: any of a class of viruses that contain double-stranded DNA and cause respiratory, intestinal, and eye infections in humans.

CFTR gene: the cystic fibrosis transmembrane conductance regulator gene, which helps create sweat, digestive juices, and mucus. Cystic fibrosis develops because of mutations in this gene.

advantage that they stimulate little, if any, immune response from the host and can enter nondividing cells.

As discussed elsewhere in this text, hemophilia is caused by a deficiency of either factor VIII (hemophilia A) or factor IX (hemophilia B) and can require lifelong therapy. In early experiments with gene therapy to treat this condition, researchers injected an adeno-associated virus with the factor IX gene into the skeletal muscle of mice, which resulted in the production of sustained levels of this factor above the therapeutic range. More recently, similar experiments have been carried out in several human patients with hemophilia B. In one individual, the treatment resulted in sustained expression of factor IX at 1% of the normal level. Although this response is insufficient to cure this disease, this low level of expression significantly reduced the number of factor IX treatments needed to control bleeding.

Other Viral Sources

Herpes simplex viruses are a class of double-stranded DNA viruses that infect a particular cell type, specifically the neurons. These viruses are common human pathogens that can cause cold sores and genital lesions. This vector is being investigated in an attempt to take advantage of its ability to insert DNA into frequently inaccessible neurons.

In addition to simple retroviruses, complex retroviruses known as **lentiviruses** can enter nondividing cells through pores in the nuclear membrane. An example of a lentivirus is the human immunodeficiency virus (HIV). These viruses are stably integrated into the genome.

Challenges Associated with Viral Vectors

Although the carrier of choice in most gene therapy studies is some type of virus, use of this approach presents a variety of potential problems to the patient (**Box 26-1**). For example, because only some (not all) of the target cells may successfully incorporate the normal gene, the desired gene product may be expressed at subtherapeutic levels in the host. This result is not necessarily a negative outcome because transient expression may be adequate in some types of therapy.

As mentioned earlier, it may be difficult to target neurons associated with central nervous system disorders. By comparison, systemic disorders may prove relatively easy to target by modifying lymphocytes or bone marrow stem cells. Nevertheless, there is always the fear that the viral vector, once inside the patient, may recover its ability to cause disease.

Whenever a foreign object is introduced into human tissues, the immune system is induced to attack the foreign substance. Therefore, the possibility that the vector might stimulate the immune system in a way that reduces the

BOX 26-1	Potential Pitfalls Associated with Using Viral Gene Therapy

Transient and low-level expression
Toxicity
Immune and inflammatory response
Difficulty reaching target tissue
Need for precise regulation of gene activity
Potential for mutagenesis
Viral reactivation in host

Data from High, K. A. (2015). Gene therapy in clinical medicine. In D. Kasper, A. Fauci, S. Hauser, D. Longo, J. Jameson, & L. Loscalzo (Eds.), *Harrison's principles of internal medicine* (19th ed., pp. 1462–1470). New York, NY: McGraw-Hill; Jorde, L. B., Carey, J. C., Bamshad, M. J., & White, R. L. (2006). *Medical genetics* (3rd ed.). St. Louis, MO: Mosby.

KEY TERMS

Thalassemia: any of a group of inherited disorders of hemoglobin metabolism in which there is impaired synthesis of one or more of the polypeptide chains of globin.

Liposome: an artificial lipid sphere with an aqueous core.

gene therapy's effectiveness is always a risk. In addition, the immune system's enhanced response to intruders that it has seen before makes it difficult for gene therapy to be repeated in patients.

Another pitfall associated with current viral gene therapy is the inability to achieve precise regulation of gene activity. Although this factor may not be critical for some diseases, it is critical for diseases such as **thalassemia**, where the number of globin chains must be balanced in a narrow range.

Alternative Gene Delivery Systems

Besides virus-mediated gene delivery systems, several nonviral options are being explored as means to administer gene therapy. The simplest method involves the direct introduction of therapeutic DNA into target cells. Unfortunately, the main limitation to this approach is that it can be used only with certain tissues and requires large amounts of DNA.

Another nonviral alternative involves the creation of an artificial lipid sphere with an aqueous core, or **liposome**. Owing to the lipophilic nature associated with the liposome, the therapeutic DNA would be capable of passing through the target cell's membrane. One advantage of the liposome is that it does not stimulate an immune response because it does not contain any peptides. Conversely, the main disadvantage is that it does not have a transfer efficiency equivalent to that of viruses.

Therapeutic DNA can enter target cells by chemically linking the DNA to a molecule that will bind to special cell receptors. Once bound to these receptors, the therapeutic DNA molecules are engulfed by the cell membrane and passed into the interior of the target cell. This delivery system tends to be less effective than other options, however.

An interesting concept that has recently emerged focuses on the use of human artificial chromosomes. These synthetically constructed chromosomes contain functional centromeres and telomeres, so they should be able to integrate and replicate in human cell nuclei. **Table 26-2** summarizes some advantages and disadvantages of several proposed gene delivery vehicles.

Although gene replacement techniques are being investigated to correct loss-of-function mutations, these techniques are not adequate to correct gain-of-function or dominant negative mutations (e.g., those causing Marfan syndrome or Huntington's disease). Rather than trying to increase synthesis of a defective gene product, in neutralizing **gain-of-function mutations**, the defective gene product must be disabled or prevented from being synthesized. Several gene-blocking methods (antisense therapy, ribozyme therapy, and RNA interference) are being evaluated to see whether they might be effective in alleviating some of these diseases.

Antisense therapy involves the synthesis of an oligonucleotide containing DNA that is complementary to that of the messenger RNA sequence produced by a gain-of-function mutation. The binding of this **oligonucleotide**

TABLE 26-2 Advantages and Disadvantages of Gene Delivery Vehicles

Vector	Advantage	Disadvantage
Retroviral	Persistent gene transfer in dividing cells	Theoretical risk of insertional mutagenesis
Lentiviral	Persistent gene transfer in transduced tissues	Might induce oncogenesis in some cases
Adenoviral	Highly effective in transducing various tissues	Viral capsid elicits strong immune responses
Adeno-associated virus	Elicits few inflammatory responses, nonpathogenic	Limited packaging capacity
Herpes simplex virus 1	Large packaging capacity with persistent gene transfer	Residual cytotoxicity with neuron specificity
Liposomes	Transfects many cell types; large holding capacity to enable a high number of base pairs	Expensive to produce
Naked DNA	Efficient in gene transfer; limited immunogenicity	Transient and low-level expression

Data from High, K. A. (2015). Gene therapy in clinical medicine. In D. Kasper, A. Fauci, S. Hauser, D. Longo, J. Jameson, & L. Loscalzo (Eds.), *Harrison's principles of internal medicine* (19th ed., pp. 1309–1315). New York, NY: McGraw-Hill.

to the abnormal messenger RNA prevents translation of the harmful protein. This approach is being used to disrupt expression of **oncogenes** involved in pancreatic and colorectal cancers.

Ribozymes are RNA molecules with enzyme activity that can cleave messenger RNA. As a consequence, they might potentially be engineered to disrupt specific mutation-causing sequences within the messenger RNA molecule before translation occurs. This therapy is being explored as a way to prevent overexpression of certain receptors involved in many breast tumors.

The last type of gene blocking involves RNA interference, a strategy that cells have evolved to defend themselves against viral invasion. Many viruses contain double-stranded RNA. When cells of multicellular organisms detect this type of RNA, an enzyme is induced to digest the foreign RNA by breaking it into small pieces. These pieces are then used as a template to direct the destruction of any single-stranded viral RNA. By artificially synthesizing double-stranded RNA molecules that correspond to a disease-causing DNA sequence, RNA interference might potentially be induced to destroy the messenger RNA produced by a mutated sequence. This approach has shown some promise in reducing transcripts produced by some oncogenes as well as the *bcr/abl* fusion gene associated with chronic myelogenous leukemia.

In addition to the limitations detailed previously regarding viral gene therapy, several other factors may prevent gene therapy from becoming an effective treatment for genetic diseases. One goal is to ensure that the therapeutic DNA introduced into target cells remains functional and that the cells containing the therapeutic DNA are long lived and stable. Unfortunately, problems with integrating therapeutic DNA into the genome, as well as the rapidly dividing nature of many cells, prevent gene therapy from achieving any long-term benefits. Such a short-lived response means that patients will have to undergo multiple rounds of gene therapy.

Disorders that arise from single-gene mutations are currently the best candidates for gene therapy. However, some of the most commonly occurring disorders seen in everyday clinical practice—such as heart disease, high blood pressure, Alzheimer's disease, hyperlipidemia, arthritis, and diabetes—involve the combined effects of many gene variations. Therefore, multigene or multifactorial disorders present another limitation in that they are especially difficult to treat effectively using gene therapy.

Recent Progress

Table 26-3 summarizes a few recent developments in the use of gene therapy to address different disease processes in humans, although it is not meant to be an all-inclusive listing. Most gene therapy studies involve only a few patients, so their results usually do not reflect findings from large patient populations. Nevertheless, some of the results are very promising. To obtain more

> ## KEY TERMS
>
> **Oncogene:** a gene that can transform cells so that they enter into a highly proliferative state that causes cancer.
>
> **Ribozymes:** RNA molecules with enzyme activity that can cleave messenger RNA.

TABLE 26-3	Examples of Recent Progress in Gene Therapy Research	
Disease	**Gene Therapy**	**Result**
Leber's congenital amaurosis—a rare inherited eye disease due to mutation in the *RPE65* gene	Recombinant adeno-associated virus vector expressing *RPE65*	Significant improvement in visual function
Lung cancer tumors	Gene delivery using lipid-based nanoparticles	Tumor regression in mice has paved the way for human trials
Advanced metastatic melanoma	Normal lymphocytes infected with modified retrovirus	Tumor regression in human subjects

Data from U.S. National Library of Medicine. Retrieved from https://clinicaltrials.gov/ct2/home

up-to-date information regarding gene therapy clinical trials, the following websites are recommended:

» Clinicaltrials.gov: https://clinicaltrials.gov/ct2/results?term=gene+therapy&Search=Search
» Gene therapy clinical trials worldwide: http://www.abedia.com/wiley/

Chapter Summary

» The basic premise underlying gene therapy is the insertion of a "normal" gene into the genome to replace an "abnormal," disease-causing gene.

» A carrier molecule called a vector is frequently used to deliver the therapeutic gene to the patient's target cells.

» Because viruses have evolved ways to insert their genes into cells with high efficiency, they have received a great deal of attention as potential gene therapy vectors.

» Gene transfer strategies involve three essential elements: (1) a vector, (2) a gene to be delivered, and (3) a relevant target cell to which the DNA or RNA is delivered.

» Proliferating cells are preferred for some gene delivery systems because the vector carrying the gene of interest can become integrated into the replicating DNA of the cell.

» Gene therapy is far from being characterized as a routine treatment regimen because it is one of the most complex therapeutic modalities yet attempted. Each new disease represents a therapeutic problem for which dosing, safety, and efficacy must be defined.

Chapter Review Questions

1. A carrier molecule called a _____ is frequently used to deliver a therapeutic gene to target cells.

2. Gene transfer strategies involve three essential elements: _____, _____, and _____.

3. Most current gene therapy approaches involve the replacement of a missing gene product by inserting a normal gene into a somatic cell to correct _____.

4. The class of viruses whose members contain double-stranded DNA and cause respiratory, intestinal, and eye infections in humans is called _____.

5. In _____, the defective gene product must be disabled or prevented from being synthesized.

Bibliography

Fung, H., & Gerson, S. (2015). Gene therapy for hematologic diseases. In K. Kaushansky, M. A. Lichtman, J. T. Prchal, M. M. Levi, O. W. Press, L. J. Burns, & M. Caligiuri (Eds.), *Williams hematology* (9th ed., pp. 2200–2218). New York, NY: McGraw-Hill.

Gene Therapy Clinical Trials Worldwide. (2016, August). *Journal of Gene Medicine.* Retrieved from http://www.abedia.com/wiley/indications.php

High, K. A. (2015). Gene therapy in clinical medicine. In D. Kasper, A. Fauci, S. Hauser, D. Longo, J. Jameson, & L. Loscalzo (Eds.), *Harrison's principles of internal medicine* (19th ed., pp. 1462–1470). New York, NY: McGraw-Hill.

Jorde, L. B., Carey, J. C., Bamshad, M. J., & White, R. L. (2006). *Medical genetics* (3rd ed.). St. Louis, MO: Mosby.

Morgan, R. A., Dudley, M. E., Wunderlich, J. R., Hughes, M. S., Yang, J. C., Sherry, R. M., . . . Rosenberg, S. A. (2006). Cancer regression in patients mediated by transfer of genetically engineered lymphocytes. *Science Express, 314*(5796), 126–129.

National Human Genome Research Institute. (n.d.). Retrieved from http://www.genome.gov

Parvovirus B19 (Fifth Disease). (n.d.). National Center for Immunization and Respiratory Diseases, Division of Viral Diseases. Retrieved from https://www.cdc.gov/parvovirusB19/index.html

Robbins, P. F., Morgan, R. A., Feldman, S. A., Yang, J. C., Sherry, R. M., Dudley, M. E., . . . Rosenberg, S. A. (2011). Tumor regression in patients with metastatic synovial sarcoma and melanoma using engineered lymphocytes reactive with NY-ESO-1. *Journal of Clinical Oncology, 29*(7), 917–924. doi:10.1200/JCO.2010.32.2537

Severe combined immunodeficiency. (n.d.). *Genes and disease.* National Center for Biotechnology Information. Retrieved from https://www.ncbi.nlm.nih.gov/books/NBK22254/

Westman, J. A. (2006). *Medical genetics for the modern clinician.* Philadelphia, PA: Lippincott Williams & Wilkins.

< Discuss ethical, legal, and social issues related to genetic testing.
< Identify factors to discuss with a patient before and after genetic testing.
< Emphasize that complete confidentiality of genetic test results cannot be guaranteed.
< Review bioethics principles that all healthcare providers need to incorporate into their practice.

KEY TERMS

Genetic Information
    Nondiscrimination
    Act of 2008 (GINA)

Genetic test

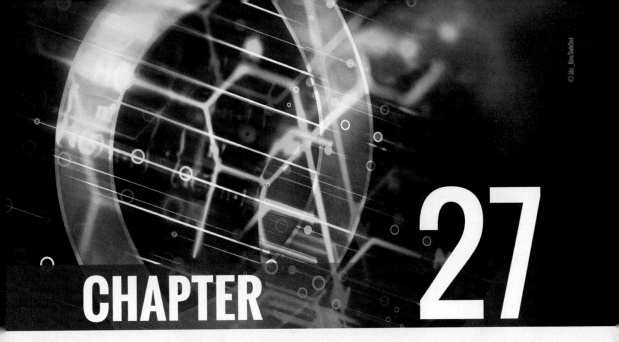

CHAPTER 27

Ethical, Legal, and Social Issues

It is anticipated that in the future, genetic information will play an increasingly larger role in the screening, diagnosis, and treatment of disease. Although these advances are intended to improve the health of the population, the potential for negative effects cannot be ignored. This chapter explores the question of how advances in medical genetics might adversely affect patients.

One important negative is the possibility that sensitive genetic information might be used by insurance companies and employers to discriminate against certain individuals. For example, if a person has a chronic long-term disease (e.g., sickle cell anemia, cystic fibrosis), a health insurance company may not want to deal with the economic consequences associated with the medical management of that disease and may refuse to provide coverage for a known genetic predilection. Similarly, if an insurance provider knows that an individual or family has a positive **genetic test** for hereditary breast and ovarian cancer or familial adenomatous polyposis, the economic consequences to the affected individuals and family members could be devastating if the insurance company denies coverage for that condition.

Genetic Testing

As genetic testing for disease susceptibility becomes incorporated into clinical practice to a greater extent, primary care providers will increasingly initiate genetic counseling and referrals for testing. However, genetic testing is associated with many ethical, social, and legal concerns that need to be addressed during the counseling process (**Box 27-1**). For example, informed consent requires discussion of the limitations of available genetic tests and interventions, implications of the test results for the patient and family members, and limits of confidentiality, as well as discrimination risks posed by such testing. Other issues include regulatory concerns associated with commercial testing and existing legal protections against genetic discrimination.

BOX 27-1	Guidelines for Pretest Education, Informed Consent, and Posttest Counseling

1. Obtain an accurate family history and confirm the diagnosis before testing.
2. Provide information about the natural history of the condition and the purpose of the test.
3. Discuss the predictive value of the test, the technical accuracy of the test, and the meaning of a positive versus negative result.
4. Explore options for approximation of risk without genetic testing.
5. Identify the patient's motives for undergoing the test, the potential impact of testing on relatives, and the risk of passing a mutation on to children.
6. Discuss the potential risk of psychosocial distress to the patient and family even if no mutation is found.
7. Explain the logistics of testing and the fees involved for testing and counseling.
8. Discuss issues involving confidentiality and risk of employment and insurance discrimination.
9. Describe medical options, efficacy of available surveillance and prevention methods, and recommendations for screening if test results are negative.
10. Provide a written summary of counseling session content.
11. Obtain informed consent for testing.
12. Provide test results in person and offer follow-up support.

Reproduced with permission from *The Journal of the American Medical Association, 278*(15), 1217–1220. (1997). Copyright © 1997 American Medical Association. All rights reserved.

KEY TERM

Genetic test: an analysis of human DNA, RNA, chromosomes, proteins, or metabolites that is intended to detect genotypes, mutations, or chromosomal changes.

Genetic testing for mutations that may influence disease susceptibility is appropriate for those relatively few patients who are known to be at high risk. Consequently, testing is not usually suggested until patients or their family members have received genetic counseling. Ideally, testing will begin with a living family member who has been diagnosed with a genetic disease. Such testing is performed to determine the presence or absence of a responsible mutation within the individual; this information can then be used to establish or confirm a diagnosis. Unfortunately, many genetic tests do not identify all possible mutations, so test results can be ambiguous in the absence of a known mutation.

Pretest counseling includes risk assessment, discussion of testing alternatives, and the predictive value and interpretive limitations of the test(s). Risk assessment involves taking a detailed family history, with the provider then estimating disease risks associated with specific mutations. Patients need to consider any medical benefits provided by this kind of testing, the psychological implications of the test result, and the significance of testing for family members. Potential benefits of testing typically include relief of anxiety, opportunities for behavior modification, and increased surveillance or interventions that may reduce risk (**Table 27-1**). Negatives include "survivor guilt,"

TABLE 27-1	Benefits and Risks Associated with Genetic Testing

Benefits	Risks
Provides emotional relief and/or reassurance	Psychological stress
Provides knowledge that may affect future decisions	Strained family relationships
Provides opportunities for increased surveillance or risk-reducing behaviors	Confidentiality/disclosure issues
	Insurance and/or employment discrimination

Reproduced from White, M. T., Callif-Daley, F., & Donnelly, J. (1999). Genetic testing for disease susceptibility: Social, ethical and legal issues for family physicians. *American Family Physician, 60*, 748, 750, 755, 757–758.

increased anxiety, depression, anger, and the potential for discrimination by insurers and employers. Whether a genetic test is positive or negative, its results have implications for major life decisions.

Posttest counseling ensures that the test results are interpreted correctly. It is important that patients fully understand that a positive test result represents only a probability; it does not necessarily guarantee that the patient will get that disease. Similarly, a negative test result does not guarantee that a disease will not develop. For example, a woman may receive a negative test result for known breast cancer mutations, but she needs to be educated that she is still at risk for developing breast cancer just like the other women in the general population without known breast cancer mutations.

Confidentiality

All patients need to be aware that their genetic information may be requested by third parties, including family members, insurers, employers, or other physicians. Before undergoing genetic testing, a patient needs to understand that complete confidentiality may be difficult to ensure and that disclosure of genetic information to insurers and employers may have discriminatory consequences. For example, patients could be denied access to health insurance, employment, education, and even loans based on their test results.

The Health Insurance Portability and Accountability Act of 1996 (HIPAA) was designed to provide some protection from discrimination. Unfortunately, HIPAA does not prohibit the use of genetic information as a basis for charging a group more for health insurance, limit the collection

KEY TERM

Genetic Information Nondiscrimination Act of 2008 (GINA): federal legislation that provides a baseline level of protection against genetic discrimination for all Americans.

of genetic information by insurers, prohibit insurers from requiring an individual to take a genetic test, limit the disclosure of genetic information by insurers, or apply to individual health insurers except if covered by the portability provision.

Many state legislatures have passed laws to govern health insurance and protect the rights to privacy of any individual. In general, these laws define what counts as "genetic information," prohibit insurers from engaging in discriminatory practices based on that information, and require written informed consent by a patient before disclosure of test results to third parties. Unfortunately, the main loophole in the state laws has related to the definition of genetic information, which is usually limited to results of DNA, RNA, or chromosomal analysis. In reality, genetic information may also be obtained from a patient's medical record, family history, and laboratory results to which these laws may not apply. Moreover, in some cases, employer-based group plans are exempt from state regulation.

To overcome the limitations associated with HIPAA and some state laws, a new federal law that prohibits discrimination in health coverage and employment based on genetic information was signed into law on May 21, 2008. The **Genetic Information Nondiscrimination Act of 2008 (GINA)** provides a baseline level of protection against genetic discrimination for all Americans. As mentioned, many states already have laws that protect against genetic discrimination in health insurance and employment situations, but the degree of protection they provide varies widely. Although most state provisions are less protective than GINA, some are more protective. All entities that are subject to GINA must, at a minimum, comply with all applicable GINA requirements, and they may also need to comply with more protective state laws.

In conjunction with HIPAA, GINA generally prohibits health insurers or health plan administrators from requesting or requiring genetic information of an individual or the individual's family members or using it for decisions regarding coverage, rates, or preexisting conditions. Employers are also prohibited from using genetic information for hiring, firing, or promotion decisions and for any decisions regarding terms of employment.

The federal statute has attempted to more clearly define "genetic information" and does not include information about the sex or age of any individual (**Box 27-2**). A genetic test is defined as an analysis of human DNA, RNA, chromosomes, proteins, or metabolites that detects genotypes, mutations, or chromosomal changes (Current Genetic Definitions in Minnesota Statutes and Federal Law, 2010). Routine laboratory tests that do not measure these genetic parameters (e.g., complete blood count, lipid tests, and liver function tests) are not protected under GINA. Specific information is also provided detailing what GINA will not do (**Box 27-3**).

BOX 27-2 Definition of Genetic Information According to the Genetic Information Nondiscrimination Act of 2008

An individual's genetic tests (including genetic tests done as part of a research study)

Genetic tests of the individual's family members (defined as dependents and up to and including fourth-degree relatives)

Genetic tests of any fetus of an individual or family member who is a pregnant woman, and genetic tests of any embryo legally held by an individual or family member using assisted reproductive technology

The manifestation of a disease or disorder in family members (family history)

Any request for, or receipt of, genetic services or participation in clinical research that includes genetic services (genetic testing, counseling, or education) by an individual or family member

Data from U.S. Department of Health and Human Services. (2009, April 6). *"Gina" The Genetic Information Nondiscrimination Act of 2008: Information for researchers and health care professionals.* Retrieved from http://www.genome.gov/Pages/PolicyEthics/GeneticDiscrimination /GINAInfoDoc.pdf

BOX 27-3 Areas That Are Not Protected by the Genetic Information Nondiscrimination Act of 2008

Health coverage nondiscrimination protections do not extend to life insurance, disability insurance, and long-term care insurance.

The act does not mandate coverage for any particular test or treatment.

Employment provisions generally do not apply to employers with fewer than 15 employees.

For health coverage provided by a health insurer to individuals, the act does not prohibit the health insurer from determining eligibility or premium rates for an individual based on the manifestation of a disease or disorder in that individual.

For employment-based coverage provided by group health plans, the act permits the overall premium rate for an employer to be increased because of the manifestation of a disease or disorder of an individual enrolled in the plan, but the manifested disease or disorder of one individual cannot be used as genetic information about other group members to further increase the premium.

The act does not prohibit health insurers or health plan administrators from obtaining and using genetic test results in making health insurance payment determinations.

The Equal Employment Opportunity Commission (EEOC) has reported up to 1,600 cases of infringement of the act since its inception. This has generally resulted in fines paid by the malefactor, in cumulative total exceeding $5,000,000.00. The EEOC filed the first lawsuit against an employer in Oklahoma in 2013. The facts of the action revolve around the employer discriminating against a temporary employee who was attempting to obtain permanent worker status. The employer requested that she fill out an extensive preemployment family history that led to further testing to rule out carpal tunnel syndrome. The employee complied and provided results, only to be denied employment by the employer. The Act specifically denies any discriminatory use of this type of information.

Another potentially discriminatory action was brought to the EEOC by two workers in Georgia. The plaintiffs worked in a warehouse that stored groceries for transport. Multiple cases of human defecation were noted to have occurred in the workplace, and through an internal investigation, the employer caused the plaintiffs to provide a DNA sample that was compared to the feces found in the warehouse. The plaintiffs sought relief through the EEOC, but the EEOC did not bring the case forward, stating the sample was used by the employer for identification only. Ultimately, a case was filed in civil court on behalf of the plaintiffs, and a jury found in their favor, awarding in excess of $2,000,000.00.

Both of these cases illustrate the need for continued training and monitoring on the part of the employer to protect the federally mandated rights of employees.

Data from U.S. Department of Health and Human Services. (2009, April 6). *"Gina" The Genetic Information Nondiscrimination Act of 2008: Information for researchers and health care professionals.* Retrieved from http://www.genome.gov/Pages/PolicyEthics/GeneticDiscrimination/ GINAInfoDoc.pdf; "Fabricut to pay $50,000 to settle disability and genetic information discrimination lawsuit." Retrieved from https://www.eeoc.gov/eeoc/newsroom/release/5-7-13b.cfm; *Lowe v. Atlas Logistics Retail Group Services (Atlanta) LLC* (N.D. Ga., May 5, 2015).

Conclusion

Almost all advances in scientific knowledge have brought with them ethical dilemmas. All healthcare providers need to be aware of the following principles of bioethics (adapted from Westman, 2006):

» Autonomy
  • Adults' right and ability to make their own decisions
  • Right to informed consent and confidentiality
  • Right not to know
» Beneficence
  • Act to improve the patient's welfare
» Nonmaleficence
  • Do no harm
» Justice
  • Fairness and equal access to care

Although genetic research offers much promise for improving health, we are currently engaged in a transitional period between new discoveries and an understanding of how that knowledge will be applied. The main question is, how will we apply our new knowledge without violating the basic rights and privileges of individuals? It is likely that the Human Genome Project will be recorded in history as one of the greatest accomplishments of this century. The knowledge and research present no real danger in and of themselves.

How their use is shaped and guided by policy, legislation, morals, and ethics, however, is critical.

It is imperative that genetic information be protected to prevent widespread discrimination against individuals and families by insurers, employers, and third-party payers. Because not all genetic tests have the same predictive value and most genetic diseases have been determined to be multifactorial in origin, using a genetic test to deny coverage and discriminate does not make sense scientifically. Moreover, as a matter of social justice, it is unfair to deny coverage based on a speculative system that we have just begun to understand.

As pointed out by Kahn (2000), health insurance is not only a precious commodity for those who have coverage, but a limited resource shared by the community. The entire insurance industry is based on the prediction of illness, injury, disability, or death. If those consumers who are likely to make claims can be eliminated, then the insurance companies will become nothing more than businesses operating on the principle of charging higher premiums to provide less coverage to more consumers.

Even though there has been much excitement regarding the potential applications of the information gleaned from the human genome, it is imperative that we as a society proceed with extreme caution. For members of the healthcare industry, a top priority has to be protecting the confidentiality of genetic information for our patients and their families. As healthcare providers, we need to be vigorous advocates for our patients and protect them as much as possible from unwarranted discrimination by outside entities such as insurance companies, employers, and government agencies. Therefore, in addition to expecting their caregivers to possess excellent clinical and diagnostic skills, our patients will rely on providers more and more in the future to guide them through the potentially complex maze of genetic diseases and genetic testing.

To obtain more up-to-date information regarding ethical, legal, and social issues, the following websites are recommended:

- » Genome.gov: http://www.genome.gov/10001618
- » Genetics Home Reference: http://ghr.nlm.nih.gov/handbook/hgp/elsi
- » Human Genome Project Information: http://www.ornl.gov/sci/techresources /Human_Genome/research/elsi.shtml

Chapter Summary

- » Genetic information and testing will play an increasingly larger role in the screening, diagnosing, and treatment of disease.

- » There is justifiable concern that sensitive genetic information might be used by insurance companies and employers to discriminate against certain individuals.

» As genetic testing for disease susceptibility becomes incorporated into clinical practice to a greater extent, primary care providers will increasingly initiate genetic counseling and referrals for testing.

» Genetic testing should not be performed until patients have received genetic counseling.

» The Genetic Information Nondiscrimination Act of 2008 provides a baseline level of protection against genetic discrimination for all Americans beyond those associated with the Health Insurance Portability and Accountability Act of 1996 and many state laws.

Chapter Review Questions

1. _____ is associated with many ethical, social, and legal concerns that need to be addressed during the counseling process.
2. Ideally, genetic testing begins with a _____ who has a diagnosis of the disease in question to determine if a responsible mutation can be found.
3. Potential benefits of genetic testing typically include _____ and _____ that may reduce risk.
4. Patients need to fully understand that a positive genetic test result represents only a _____ and does not necessarily guarantee that they will get that disease.
5. _____ generally prohibits health insurers or health plan administrators from requesting or requiring genetic information of an individual or the individual's family members or using it for decisions regarding coverage, rates, or preexisting conditions.

Bibliography

Clayton, E. W. (2003). Ethical, legal, and social implications of genomic medicine. *New England Journal of Medicine, 349,* 562–569.

Collins, F. S., Green, E., Guttmacher, A. E., & Guyer, M. S. (2003). A vision for the future of genomics research. *Nature, 422,* 835–847. Retrieved from http://www.genome.gov/11007524

Guidance on the Genetic Information Nondiscrimination Act: Implications for investigators and institutional review boards. Office for Human Research Protections, Department of Health and Human Services. Retrieved from https://www.hhs.gov/ohrp/regulations-and-policy/guidance/guidance-on-genetic-information-nondiscrimination-act/index.html

Gunder, L. M. (2006). *Ethical considerations in medical genetics* (Unpublished paper). Nova Southeastern University, Fort Lauderdale, FL.

Kahn, J. P. (2000). Genetic testing: The future is here. *CNN.com.* Retrieved from http://www.cnn.com/HEALTH/bioethics/9808/genetics.part1/index.html

U.S. Department of Health and Human Services. (2009, April 6). *"Gina" The Genetic Information Nondiscrimination Act of 2008: Information for researchers and health care professionals.* Retrieved from http://www.genome.gov/Pages/PolicyEthics /GeneticDiscrimination/GINAInfoDoc.pdf

Westman, J. A. (2006). *Medical genetics for the modern clinician.* Philadelphia, PA: Lippincott Williams & Wilkins.

White, M. T., Callif-Daley, F., & Donnelly, J. (1999). Genetic testing for disease susceptibility: Social, ethical and legal issues for family physicians. *American Family Physician, 60,* 748, 750, 755, 757–758.

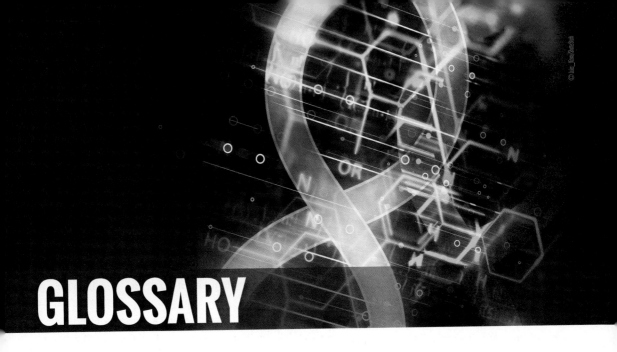

GLOSSARY

achondrodysplasia   the most common cause of dwarfism or significantly abnormal stature caused by an abnormal development of cartilage and bone.

acquired hemophilia   production of autoantibody that inactivates coagulation factors (VIII or IX) and results in the same clinical bleeding diathesis as occurs in inherited hemophilias.

acquired von Willebrand's disease   a form of von Willebrand's disease that is not inherited, but rather develops late in life. It is caused by the development of antibodies that attack and destroy a person's von Willebrand factor. This disease is commonly "acquired" in conjunction with another serious disease.

acute-phase reactant   any substance that can be elevated in inflammatory processes.

adeno-associated virus   any of a class of small, single-stranded DNA viruses that can insert their genetic material at a specific site on chromosome 19. Parvovirus is an example of this type of virus.

adenoma   a benign epithelial neoplasm in which the tumor cells form glands or glandlike structures.

adenomatous   relating to an adenoma and to some types of glandular hyperplasia.

adenomatous polyposis coli (APC)   a tumor suppressor gene on chromosome 5. Mutations in this gene result in familial adenomatous polyposis.

adenovirus   any of a class of viruses that contain double-stranded DNA and cause respiratory, intestinal, and eye infections in humans.

advanced maternal age   when a woman is 35 or older at the time of delivery.

allele   any one of a series of one, two, or more alternative forms of a gene that may occupy the same locus on a specific chromosome.

allelic variant   an alteration in the normal sequence of a gene.

amniocentesis   a prenatal test in which a small sample of the amniotic fluid surrounding the fetus is removed and examined.

amnion   a membrane that forms a fluid-filled sac around the embryo.

Amsterdam criteria   research criteria for defining Lynch syndrome established by the International Collaborative Group meeting in Amsterdam.

anemia   any condition in which the number of red blood cells per cubic millimeter (mm^3), the amount of hemoglobin in 100 mL of blood, and/or the volume of packed red blood cells per 100 mL of blood are less than normal.

aneuploidy   when a cell has an extra or missing chromosome.

angina   chest pain that is precipitated by exertion and relieved by rest; it is caused by inadequate oxygen delivery to the heart muscles.

anhedonia   not able to feel pleasure.

anticipation   the predictability of progressively earlier onset and increased severity of certain diseases in successive generations of affected persons.

aortic aneurysm   an abnormal dilation of the aorta at the level of the ascending aorta or the sinuses of Valsalva (descending aorta).

aortic dissection   a longitudinal tear between the layers of the aorta that may progress because of the high-pressure flow inside the aorta.

apoptosis   programmed or gene-directed cell death.

arcus corneus   a corneal disease caused by deposits of phospholipids and cholesterol in the corneal stroma and anterior sclera surrounding the iris of the eye.

ASA   Aspirin.

atherosclerosis   thickening and loss of elasticity of arterial walls caused by lipid deposition and thickening of the intimal cell layers within arteries.

atrophy   a decrease in size or wasting of a tissue or muscle.

autoantibody   a protein that attacks the body's own tissues.

autosomal dominant   a pattern of inheritance in which a child acquires a disease by receiving a normal gene from one parent and a defective gene from the other parent.

autosomal recessive   a pattern of inheritance in which both parents carry and pass on a defective gene to their child.

autosomes   all chromosomes other than the sex chromosomes.

azoospermia   the absence of spermatozoa in the semen.

biliary cirrhosis   cirrhosis to biliary obstruction, which may be a primary intrahepatic disease or occur secondary to obstruction of extrahepatic bile ducts.

biopsy   a procedure in which tissue or other material is removed from the body and studied for signs of disease.

bipolar disorder   a major mood disorder characterized by the presence of mania and depression.

blast cells   a very immature precursor cell (e.g., erythroblast, lymphoblast).

blast crisis   in a patient with chronic myelogenous leukemia, a disease stage characterized by high burden of blasts in the peripheral blood and/or bone marrow; it carries a clinically poor prognosis.

blastocyst   an early stage of embryo development that can be recognized through the presence of an inner cell mass.

bleeding diathesis   a group of distinct conditions in which a person's body cannot properly develop a clot, resulting in an increased tendency for bleeding.

BRCA1   a tumor suppressor gene on chromosome 17 that prevents cells with damaged DNA from dividing. Carriers of germline mutations in *BRCA1* are predisposed to develop both breast and ovarian cancer.

BRCA2   a tumor suppressor gene on chromosome 13. Carriers of germline mutations in *BRCA2* have an increased risk, similar to that of carriers of *BRCA1* mutations, of developing breast cancer and a moderately increased risk of ovarian cancer. *BRCA2* families also exhibit an increased incidence of male breast, pancreatic, prostate, stomach, skin, and uterine cancer.

brugada syndrome   a condition that causes ventricular arrhythmias and can lead to fainting (syncope), seizures, difficulty breathing, or sudden death.

café-au-lait spot   a flat spot on the skin that is the color of coffee with milk (café au lait) in persons with light skin. These spots are harmless by themselves, but in some cases they may be a sign of neurofibromatosis. The presence of six or more café-au-lait spots, each of which is 1.5 centimeters or more in diameter, is diagnostic for neurofibromatosis.

callus area of new bone that is laid down at the fracture site as part of the healing process.

cardiomyopathy a disease of the myocardium (heart muscle) that has variable etiologies and clinical presentations.

carrier a person (usually female) who can pass an altered gene to her children but generally does not express the disease herself.

cephalohematoma a collection of blood under the skull due to an effusion of blood, usually as a result of trauma.

CFTR gene a gene that codes for a protein involved in chloride and water transport across membranes. In patients with cystic fibrosis, a mutation in this gene disrupts chloride and water transport across membranes. The end result is production of thick and sticky mucus that obstructs the airways in the lungs and the ducts in the pancreas.

chelating agent a drug that binds to a substance in the body, rendering it unable to be used and/or less harmful to the body.

cholesterol the principal sterol found in all higher animals. It is distributed in body tissues, especially the brain and spinal cord, and in animal fats and oils.

chorionic villus sampling (CVS) a prenatal test that involves taking a tiny tissue sample from outside the sac where the fetus develops. It is performed between 10 and 12 weeks after a pregnant woman's last menstrual period.

chorea from the Greek word for "dance"; the incessant, quick, jerky, involuntary movements that are characteristic of Huntington's disease.

chromosomal aberration alteration in the number or physical structure of chromosomes.

chromosome a DNA molecule that contains genes in linear order to which numerous proteins are bound.

chromosome painting use of differentially labeled, chromosome-specific DNA strands for hybridization with chromosomes to label each chromosome with a different color.

chronic myelogenous leukemia (CML) a myeloproliferative disorder characterized by increased proliferation of the granulocytic cell line without the loss of their capacity to differentiate.

cirrhosis a degenerative disease of the liver characterized by formation of fibrous tissue and scarring, resulting in the inhibition of normal cellular function.

clinicians genetics counselors trained in the fundamentals of human disease and healthcare who use the most current genetic knowledge and testing to facilitate diagnoses and provide information regarding medical/developmental implications and management.

clotting factor any of several proteins that are involved in the blood coagulation process.

coagulation the chemical reaction mediated by coagulation factor proteins that results in a stable fibrin clot.

codon a sequence of three adjacent nucleotides in an mRNA molecule, specifying either an amino acid or a stop signal in protein synthesis.

colectomy surgical excision of part or all of the colon.

compound heterozygote an individual who carries two different mutant alleles for the same gene.

computed tomography (CT) scan an imaging procedure in which a computer linked to an x-ray machine is used to produce a series of detailed pictures of areas inside the body taken from different angles.

concordance the presence of the same trait in both members of a pair of twins.

confined placental mosaicism a condition in which there is a discrepancy in the genetic makeup between the cells of the placenta and the cells of the fetus.

consanguineous mating between related individuals.

consanguinity degree of relationship between persons who descend from a common ancestor.

contracture   chronic shortening of a muscle or tendon that limits movement of a bony joint, such as the elbow.

cor pulmonale   failure of the right ventricle of the heart secondary to enlargement and increased pressure caused by disease of the lungs or pulmonary blood vessels.

counselors   genetic counselors who are trained in psychological techniques and empathetic communication to help individuals and families adjust to and cope with the genetic condition or risk in question.

covariates   the interplay of environmental factors with genetic predisposition.

Cowden syndrome   caused by mutations in the *PTEN* gene (a tumor suppressor gene), this syndrome is associated with noncancerous growths known as hamartomas and malignancies such as breast, thyroid, colorectal, kidney, and endometrial cancer.

coxa vara   a deformed hip joint in which the neck of the femur is bent downward; the acute angle of the femur head is less than 120 degrees and subsequently affects the hip socket.

creatine kinase   a protein needed for the chemical reactions that produce energy for muscle contractions; high levels in the blood indicate muscle damage.

Crowe's sign   axillary and inguinal freckling, often associated with type 1 neurofibromatosis.

cystic fibrosis   a congenital metabolic disorder, inherited as an autosomal recessive trait, in which secretions of exocrine glands are abnormal. Excessively viscid mucus causes obstruction of passageways (including pancreatic and bile ducts, intestines, and bronchi), and the sodium and chloride content of sweat is increased throughout the patient's life.

cystic fibrosis-related diabetes mellitus   insulin deficiency and insulin resistance caused by complications from cystic fibrosis.

cytokines   cell signaling proteins.

degenerate   a feature of the genetic code in which an amino acid corresponds to more than one codon.

deletion   absence of a segment of DNA; it may be as small as a single base or large enough to encompass one or more entire genes.

de novo mutations   mutations that are not inherited, but rather appear first in the affected individual.

dentinogenesis imperfecta   characterized by discolored teeth, usually gray or brown, that easily degrade, break, or wear down.

deoxyribonucleic acid (DNA)   a macromolecule usually composed of two polynucleotide chains in a double helix that is the carrier of genetic information in all cells.

desmopressin acetate   a synthetic hormone that increases factor VIII levels.

disseminated intravascular coagulation   a condition of altered coagulation that results in consumption of clotting factors and platelets and yields a clinical presentation characterized by both excessive clotting and excessive bleeding.

diverticula   a pouch or sac opening from a tubular or saccular organ such as the intestines or the bladder.

diverticulitis   inflammation of a diverticulum, especially of the small pockets in the wall of the colon, which fill with stagnant fecal material and become inflamed. Rarely, these sacs may cause obstruction, perforation, or bleeding.

DMARDs   disease-modifying antirheumatic drugs.

dominant   refers to an allele whose presence in a heterozygous genotype results in a phenotype characteristic of the allele.

dominant negative mutation   a mutated allele that disrupts the function of a normal allele in the same cell.

Down syndrome   a chromosomal dysgenesis syndrome consisting of a variable constellation of abnormalities caused by triplication or translocation of chromosome 21. Affected individuals have some degree of mental retardation, characteristic facial features, and, often, heart defects and other health problems.

dyskinesia   difficulty in performing voluntary movements.

dysplasia the presence of cells of an abnormal type within a tissue, which may signify a stage preceding the development of cancer.

dystrophin muscle protein involved in maintaining the integrity of muscle.

eburnation describes a degenerative process of bone.

ectoderm the outer layer of cells in the embryo, after establishment of the three primary germ layers (ectoderm, mesoderm, endoderm); the germ layer that comes in contact with the amniotic cavity.

educators genetic counselors who transform complex genetic information and translate it to a form that is understandable and meaningful to patients and audiences of all levels of literacy.

embryo the developing human within the first two months after conception.

endoderm the innermost of the three primary germ layers of the embryo (ectoderm, mesoderm, endoderm). The epithelial lining of the primitive gut tract and the epithelial component of the glands and other structures (e.g., lower respiratory system) that develop as outgrowths from the gut tube are derived from the endoderm.

end-stage renal disease (ESRD) the complete or almost complete failure of the kidneys to function. The dysfunctional kidneys can no longer remove wastes, concentrate urine, and regulate electrolytes.

enthesitis inflammation of the entheses, the sites where tendons or ligaments insert into the bone.

epitopes antigenic determinants.

ethnic variation of allelic frequency a situation in which frequency of mutated alleles is higher among certain ethnic groups than others.

Fabry disease an inherited lipid storage disease that results from a deficiency in the enzyme alpha-galactosidase found on the X chromosome. This defect leads to the accumulation of glycosphingolipids in the plasma and lysosomes of vascular endothelial and smooth muscle cells.

factor assay a specialized lab test used to determine the level of circulating factor VIII or IX.

factor deficiency any of several rare disorders characterized by the complete absence or an abnormally low level of clotting factor in the blood.

factor inhibitors antibodies that develop in patients in response to factor replacement therapy.

factor replacement therapy replacement of a deficient clotting factor from another source (either human derived or recombinant) in an effort to stop or prevent abnormal bleeding.

familial adenomatous polyposis (FAP) an inherited colorectal cancer syndrome that leads to hundreds—sometimes even thousands—of polyps in the colon and rectum at a young age.

fetal alcohol effect the development of relatively mild degrees of mental deficiency and emotional disorders in children whose mothers use alcohol during their pregnancy; this condition is more common than the full fetal alcohol syndrome scenario.

fifth disease a disease caused by infection with human parvovirus B19, which infects only humans. It manifests as a mild rash illness that occurs most commonly in children. The ill child typically has a "slapped-cheek" rash on the face and a lacy red rash on the trunk and limbs.

first-degree relative any relative who is one meiosis away from a particular individual in a family (i.e., parent, sibling, offspring).

fluorescence in situ hybridization (FISH) an analytic technique in which a nucleic acid labeled with a fluorescent dye is hybridized to suitably prepared cells or histological sections; it is then used to look for specific transcription or localization of genes to specific chromosomes.

founder effect accumulation of random genetic changes in an isolated population as a result of its proliferation from only a few parent colonizers.

frameshift mutation an insertion or deletion involving a number of base pairs that is not a multiple of three and consequently disrupts the triplet reading frame, usually leading to the creation of a premature termination (stop) codon and resulting in a truncated protein product.

gain-of-function mutation a genetic change that increases the activity of a gene protein or increases the production of the protein.

gene a region of DNA containing genetic information, which is usually transcribed into an RNA molecule that is processed and either functions directly or is translated into a polypeptide chain; the hereditary unit.

generalized anxiety disorder a major mood disorder characterized by at least 6 months of anxious symptoms.

genetic heterogeneity the production of the same or similar phenotypes by different genetic mechanisms.

Genetic Information Nondiscrimination Act of 2008 (GINA) federal legislation that provides a baseline level of protection against genetic discrimination for all Americans.

genetic modifiers genes that influence phenotypic variation by affecting penetrance, dominance, and expressivity to alter the expression of another gene.

genetic test an analysis of human DNA, RNA, chromosomes, proteins, or metabolites that is intended to detect genotypes, mutations, or chromosomal changes.

genocopy a genotype that determines a phenotype that closely resembles the phenotype determined by a different genotype.

genomics systematic study of an organism's genome using large-scale DNA sequencing, gene-expression analysis, or computational methods.

germinal mutation a mutation that takes place in a reproductive cell.

germline mutation a change in a gene in the body's reproductive cell (egg or sperm) that becomes incorporated into the DNA of every cell in the body of the offspring.

glioma any neoplasm derived from one of the various types of cells that form the interstitial tissue of the brain, spinal cord, pineal gland, posterior pituitary gland, and retina.

granulocyte a mature granular leukocyte, including any of the neutrophilic, acidophilic, and basophilic types of polymorphonuclear leukocytes (e.g., neutrophils, eosinophils, and basophils).

hamartoma a focal malformation that resembles a neoplasm, grossly and even microscopically, but results from faulty development in an organ.

head and neck squamous cell carcinoma cancer originating from the mucosal lining (epithelium) of the head and neck.

hemarthroses bleeding into joints.

hematoma bleeding into soft tissue, such as muscle or visceral organs.

hemizygous describes an individual who has only one member of a chromosome pair or chromosome segment rather than the usual two; refers in particular to X-linked genes in males who, under usual circumstances, have only one X chromosome.

hemoglobin C disease a type of hemoglobin-related disease characterized by episodes of abdominal and joint pain, an enlarged spleen, and mild jaundice, but no severe crises. This disease occurs mostly in African Americans, who may show few symptoms of its presence.

hemoglobin SC disease a type of hemoglobin-related disease that occurs in people who have one copy of the gene for sickle cell disease and one copy of the gene for hemoglobin C disease.

hemophilia a bleeding disorder in which a specific clotting factor protein—namely, factor VIII or IX—is missing or does not function normally.

hemophilia A a deficiency or absence of factor VIII; also called "classic" hemophilia. It is the most common severe bleeding disorder.

hemophilia B a deficiency or absence of factor IX; also called "Christmas disease" after the first family identified with the condition.

hemophilia B Leyden a rare variant of hemophilia B inherited in an X-linked pattern.

hemophilia C a deficiency or absence of factor XI; more commonly known as plasma thromboplastin antecedent deficiency.

hemophilia treatment centers a group of federally funded hospitals that specialize in treating patients with coagulation disorders.

hemostasis the process by which the body stops bleeding.

hepatic ultrasound an imaging study of the liver used to detect the presence of tissue changes such as tumors, abscesses, and cysts.

hepatitis inflammation of the liver causing impaired function as a result of toxins (e.g., alcohol, iron, drugs), autoimmune disorders, or infectious agents (viruses).

hepatoma the most common type of nonmetastatic liver cancer; also known as primary hepatocellular carcinoma.

hepatomegaly enlargement of the liver.

hepatotoxic relating to an agent that damages the liver.

hereditary hemochromatosis an autosomal recessive disorder usually caused by a single mutation in the HFE gene, which causes increased intestinal absorption of iron and results in increased iron storage in body tissues.

hereditary nonpolyposis colorectal cancer (HNPCC) an inherited colorectal cancer syndrome in which only a small number of polyps are present or not present at all. Also known as Lynch syndrome.

herpes simplex virus any of a class of double-stranded DNA viruses that infect a particular cell type, specifically the neurons.

heterozygote advantage a mutated allele at the same locus as a normal allele that confers the advantage of protection against a disease and increases survival.

heterozygous carrying dissimilar alleles of one or more genes; not homozygous.

homozygous having the same allele of a gene in homologous chromosomes.

human leukocyte antigen (HLA) system designation for the gene products of at least four linked loci (A, B, C, and D) and a number of subloci on the sixth human chromosome that have been shown to have a strong influence on human allotransplantation, transfusions in refractory patients, and certain disease associations. More than 50 alleles are recognized, most of which are found at loci HLA-A and HLA-B; they are passed on through autosomal dominant inheritance.

huntingtin the product of the Huntington's disease gene on chromosome 4.

hydrocephalus a condition marked by an excessive accumulation of cerebrospinal fluid, resulting in dilation of the cerebral ventricles and raised intracranial pressure; it may also result in enlargement of the cranium and atrophy of the brain.

hypertrichosis growth of hair in excess of the normal.

hypomania a state of elevated or irritable mood that is abnormal but does not impair one's ability to function.

inborn error of metabolism a genetically determined biochemical disorder, usually in the form of an enzyme defect that produces a metabolic block.

information gathering interviewing the patients and family members to ascertain their family history and developing a three generational pedigree from that information.

information giving the process in which patients are provided with information regarding the genetic condition, including, as appropriate, inheritance patterns and risks of occurrence or reoccurrence.

inner cell mass (ICM) the cells at the embryonic pole of the blastocyst, which are concerned with formation of the body of the embryo.

insertion a chromosome abnormality in which material from one chromosome is inserted into another nonhomologous chromosome; a mutation in which a segment of DNA is inserted into a gene or other segment of DNA, potentially disrupting the coding sequence.

interleukins white blood cell cytokine.

international normalized ratio (INR) a system established by the World Health Organization and the International Committee on Thrombosis and Hemostasis for reporting the results of blood coagulation (clotting) tests. All results are standardized using the international sensitivity index for the particular thromboplastin reagent and instrument combination used to perform the test. Regardless of which laboratory checks the prothrombin time, the result should be the same even if different thromboplastins and instruments are used.

inversion   a structural aberration in a chromosome in which the order of several genes is reversed from the normal order.

investigators   genetic counselors who decipher medical and family histories to identify possible genetic etiologies and access the most current literature and research to ensure that patients receive the most up-to-date information and options.

iris flocculi   an ocular abnormality found in persons with familial thoracic aortic aneurysms and dissections that is highly associated with ACTA2 mutations.

karyotype   the chromosome complement of a cell or organism; often represented by an arrangement of metaphase chromosomes according to their lengths and the positions of their centromeres.

kindred   an aggregate of genetically related persons.

Klinefelter syndrome   a disorder that occurs when an ovum with an extra X chromosome is fertilized by a sperm with a Y chromosome. This results in an XXY genotype male who is sterile.

left ventricular hypertrophy (LVH)   enlargement of the muscle tissue in the wall of the left ventricle, often involving the intraventricular septum.

lentivirus   a type of complex retrovirus that can enter nondividing cells through pores in the nuclear membrane. Human immunodeficiency virus is an example.

Li-Fraumeni syndrome   caused by a mutation in the *TP53* gene (a tumor suppressor gene), this syndrome is associated with an increased risk for breast cancer, osteosarcoma, and soft tissue sarcomas, as well as leukemias and adrenal carcinoma.

liposome   an artificial lipid sphere with an aqueous core.

Lisch nodule   iris hamartomas, typically seen in type 1 neurofibromatosis.

livedo reticularis   a purplish skin discoloration in a lacy pattern caused by constriction of deep dermal capillaries.

locus   the site or position of a particular gene on a chromosome.

loss-of-function mutation   a genetic change that reduces the activity of a gene protein or decreases the production of the protein.

low-density lipoprotein   the type of lipoprotein responsible for transport of cholesterol to extrahepatic tissues.

lymph node mapping   a procedure in which a radioactive substance or blue dye is injected near the tumor, then flows through lymph ducts to the first lymph node or nodes where cancer cells are likely to have spread. Lymph nodes that are marked with the dye are then surgically removed and examined microscopically by a pathologist for evidence of cancer cells.

magnetic resonance imaging (MRI)   a procedure that uses a magnet, radio waves, and a computer to make a series of detailed images of areas inside the body.

major depressive disorder   a major mood disorder characterized by depressed mood for at least 2 weeks.

major mood disorder   a family of behavioral health disorders that affect a large portion of society.

Marfan syndrome   a connective tissue, multisystemic disorder characterized by skeletal changes (arachnodactyly, long limbs, joint laxity), cardiovascular defects (aortic aneurysm that may dissect, mitral valve prolapse), and ectopia lentis. It is passed on through autosomal dominant inheritance of a mutation in the fibrillin-1 gene on chromosome 15.

meconium ileus obstruction of the intestines due to retention of a dark green waste product (meconium) that is normally passed shortly after a child's birth.

melanomagenesis the formation of melanoma.

Mendelian genetics the mechanism of inheritance in which the statistical relations between the distribution of traits in successive generations result from three factors: (1) particulate hereditary determinants (genes), (2) random union of gametes, and (3) segregation of unchanged hereditary determinants in the reproductive cells.

menorrhagia excessive bleeding during the time of menses, in terms of duration, volume, or both.

merlin a tumor suppressor gene encoded on chromosome 22 (*NF2* gene). Mutation of this gene disrupts tumor suppressor activity and leads to the formation of schwannomas associated with type 2 neurofibromatosis.

mesoderm the middle of the three primary germ layers of the embryo (the others being ectoderm and endoderm). The mesoderm is the origin of connective tissues, myoblasts, blood, the cardiovascular and lymphatic systems, most of the urogenital system, and the lining of the pericardial, pleural, and peritoneal cavities.

messenger ribonucleic acid (mRNA) an RNA molecule that is transcribed from a DNA sequence and translated into the amino acid sequence of a polypeptide.

microcephaly abnormal smallness of the head; a term applied to a skull with a capacity of less than 1,350 mL. Microcephaly is usually associated with mental retardation.

microfibrils Here, structural molecules found in load-bearing tissues.

microsatellite instability a change that occurs in the DNA of certain cells (e.g., tumor cells) in which the number of repeats of microsatellites (short, repeated sequences of DNA) is different than the number of repeats that appeared in the DNA when it was inherited. The cause of microsatellite instability may be a defect in the ability to repair mistakes made when DNA is copied in the cell.

mild hemophilia a categorical term used to describe someone with a factor VIII or IX level ranging between 5% and 25% of normal blood levels.

missense mutation a mutation in which a base change or substitution results in a codon that causes insertion of a different amino acid into the growing polypeptide chain, giving rise to an altered protein.

mitochondrial chromosome a small circular chromosome found in each mitochondrion that encodes tRNA, rRNA, and proteins that are involved in oxidative phosphorylation and ATP generation.

moderate hemophilia a categorical term used to describe someone with a factor VIII or IX level ranging between 1% and 5% of normal blood levels.

monogenic of, relating to, or controlled by a single gene, especially by either of an allelic pair.

monosomy a condition in an otherwise diploid organism in which one member of a pair of chromosomes is missing.

morning-after pill a form of emergency birth control used to prevent a woman from becoming pregnant after she has engaged in unprotected vaginal intercourse.

morula the earliest stage of embryo after cell division, consisting of a ball of identical cells.

MTX Methotrexate.

multifactorial multiple factors.

mutation heritable alteration in a gene or chromosome; also, the process by which such an alteration happens.

myelofibrosis fibrosis of the bone marrow associated with myeloid metaplasia of the spleen and other organs.

myocardial infarction death of the heart muscle, caused by occlusion of the coronary vessels.

myocardium the heart muscle cells responsible for contractility of the heart.

neoplastic related to the pathologic process that results in the formation and growth of a neoplasm or abnormal tissue that may be either benign or malignant.

nephrotoxic   relating to an agent that damages renal cells.

neurofibroma   a benign, encapsulated tumor resulting from proliferation of Schwann cells that are of ectodermal (neural crest) origin and that form a continuous envelope around each nerve fiber of peripheral nerves.

neurofibromin   a tumor suppressor gene encoded on chromosome 17 (*NF-1* gene). Loss of tumor suppression due to a mutation in this gene leads to the formation of neurofibromas associated with type 1 neurofibromatosis.

nondisjunction   failure of chromosomes to separate (disjoin) and move to opposite poles of the division spindle; the result is loss or gain of a chromosome.

nonsense mutation   a single base-pair substitution that prematurely codes for a stop in amino acid translation (stop codon).

novel property mutation   a mutation that confers a new property on the protein product.

NSAIDs   Nonsteroidal anti-inflammatory drugs.

oligoarthritis   arthritis affecting two to four joints during the first 6 months of disease.

oligonucleotide   a DNA sequence consisting of a small number of nucleotide bases.

oncogene   any of a family of genes that, under normal circumstances, code for proteins involved in cell growth or regulation (e.g., protein kinases) but that may foster malignant processes if mutated or overexpressed.

organogenesis   formation of organs during development.

osteogenesis imperfecta (OI)   comes from the increasing likelihood of fracture, often from seemingly minor injuries, or in some cases, from no apparent cause at all.

osteopenia   a condition in which bone mineral density is lower than normal.

osteoporosis   is a condition of fragile bone with an increased susceptibility to fracture.

packaging cells   cells in which replication-deficient viruses are placed so that the replication machinery of the packaging cell can produce viral copies.

pannus   scar tissue.

paracrines   a group of chemical messengers that communicate with neighboring cells by simple diffusion.

parturition   the process of birth.

pedigree analysis   a diagram representing the familial relationships among relatives.

penetrance   the proportion of organisms having a particular genotype that actually express the corresponding phenotype. If the phenotype is always expressed, penetrance is complete; otherwise, it is incomplete.

Peutz-Jeghers syndrome (PJS)   caused by a mutation in the *STK11* gene (a tumor suppressor gene), this syndrome is associated with growths of hamartomas in the stomach and intestine; dark freckling in the axilla, perioral area, and buccal mucosa; and an increased risk for developing pancreatic, gastrointestinal, ovarian, and breast cancers.

pharmacogenetics   the study of the interrelation of hereditary constitution and response to drugs.

pharmacogenomics   the study of the combination of pharmacology and genomics; the aim is to develop effective and safe medications to compensate for genetic differences in patients that cause varied responses to a single therapeutic regimen.

phenylalanine hydroxylase (PAH)   the enzyme that converts phenylalanine to tyrosine and that is defective in phenylketonuria.

phenylketonuria (PKU)   a hereditary human condition resulting from inability to convert phenylalanine into tyrosine. It causes severe intellectual disability unless treated in infancy and childhood by a low-phenylalanine diet.

Philadelphia chromosome   an abnormal chromosome formed by a rearrangement of chromosomes 9 and 22 that is associated with chronic myelogenous leukemia.

phocomelia defective development of arms, legs, or both so that the hands and feet are attached close to the body, resembling the flippers of a seal.

phototype a classification system based on a person's sensitivity to sunlight as measured by the ability to tan.

placenta a structure consisting of maternal and fetal tissues that allows for exchange of gases, nutrients, and wastes between the mother's circulatory system and the circulatory system of the fetus.

point mutation the alteration of a single nucleotide to a different nucleotide.

polycythemia vera a chronic form of polycythemia of unknown cause characterized by bone marrow hyperplasia, an increase in both blood volume and the number of red cells, redness or cyanosis of the skin, and splenomegaly.

polygenic genetic disorder resulting from the combined action of alleles of more than one gene.

polymerase chain reaction (PCR) repeated cycles of DNA denaturation, renaturation with primer oligonucleotide sequences, and replication, resulting in exponential growth in the number of copies of the DNA sequence located between the primers.

polymorphisms natural variations in a gene, DNA sequence, or chromosome that have no adverse effects on the individual and occur with fairly high frequency in the general population.

polyp a usually nonmalignant growth or tumor protruding from the mucous lining of an organ such as the nose, bladder, or intestine, often causing obstruction.

polysomy condition of a diploid cell or organism that has three or more copies of a particular chromosome.

porencephaly the occurrence of cavities in the brain substance, communicating usually with the lateral ventricles.

portal hypertension elevation of pressure in the hepatic portal circulation due to cirrhosis or other changes in liver tissue. When pressure exceeds 10 mm Hg, collateral circulation may develop to maintain venous return from structures drained by the portal vein; engorgement of collateral veins can lead to esophageal varices and, less often, caput medusae.

positron emission tomography (PET) scan an imaging procedure used to locate malignant tumor cells in the body by identifying areas of tissue with greatest glucose utilization.

proband an affected person as identified in a family pedigree.

probe a labeled DNA or RNA molecule used in DNA-RNA or DNA-DNA hybridization assays.

proctocolectomy a surgical procedure involving the excision of the colon and rectum and the formation of an ileoanal reservoir or pouch.

prodrug a class of drugs in which the pharmacologic action results from conversion by metabolic processes within the body.

prothrombin time a clotting test done to test the integrity of part of the clotting scheme, which is commonly used as a method of monitoring the accuracy of blood thinning treatment (anticoagulation) with warfarin. The test measures the time needed for clot formation after thromboplastin (plus calcium) has been added to plasma.

proto-oncogene a gene in the normal human genome that appears to have a role in normal cellular physiology and is involved in regulation of normal cell growth or proliferation; as a result of somatic mutations, these genes may become oncogenic.

pseudohypertrophy increase in size of an organ or a part that is not due to an increase in size or number of the specific functional elements, but to that of some other tissue, fatty or fibrous.

psychosocial support the support provided by genetic counselors which may include incorporating empathy and compassion into their sessions and making sure individuals and families have access to appropriate health and educational interventions.

PTEN hamartoma tumor syndrome (PHTS) a spectrum of disorders caused by mutations of the *PTEN tumor* suppressor gene in egg or sperm cells (germline).

recessive refers to an allele, or the corresponding phenotypic trait, that is expressed only in homozygotes.

recurrent melanoma cancer that has returned, either to the original site or in other areas of the body, after it has been treated.

renal cell carcinoma a type of kidney cancer in which the cancerous cells are found in the lining of very small tubes (tubules) in the kidney.

residual risk the risk that an individual carries an abnormal gene after a negative (normal) screening test result.

rhizomelia a disproportion in the length of the proximal limb, creating a shorter than normal limb.

ribosomal RNA (rRNA) a type of RNA molecule that is a component of the ribosomal subunits.

ribozymes RNA molecules with enzyme activity that can cleave messenger RNA.

risk assessment identifying possible genetic diagnoses and hereditary patterns for both rare genetic conditions and common diseases based on the pedigree and medical history/characteristics of the proband.

robertsonian translocation a structural rearrangement involving one or more of the acrocentric chromosomes (chromosomes 13, 14, 15, 21, or 22).

sarcomere the simplest unit of muscle tissue that allows the muscle to contract.

satellite moles new moles that grow in a pattern around existing moles.

schwannoma a benign, encapsulated neoplasm in which the fundamental component is structurally identical to a syncytium of Schwann cells. The neoplasm may originate from a peripheral or sympathetic nerve or from various cranial nerves, particularly the eighth nerve.

senescence Age deterioration.

sentinel node the first lymph node to receive lymphatic drainage from a tumor.

serum ferritin levels a measure that estimates the amount of iron stored in the body.

serum iron levels a measure of the amount of unbound iron that has been transported to the blood.

severe combined immune deficiency any of a group of rare, sometimes fatal, congenital disorders characterized by little or no immune response.

severe hemophilia a categorical term used to describe someone with a factor VIII or IX level that is less than 1% of normal blood levels.

sex chromosome a chromosome, such as the human X or Y, that plays a role in the determination of sex.

sex-influenced phenotype a phenotype expressed in both males and females but with different frequencies in the two sexes.

sibling (sib) a brother or sister, each having the same parents.

sickle cell trait the heterozygous state of the gene for hemoglobin S in sickle cell anemia.

somatic mutation a mutation arising in a somatic cell.

spontaneous bleeding heavy bleeding without history of trauma.

steatorrhea excretion of excess fat in the feces.

synergistic hepatotoxic effects toxic effects that work together such that the total toxic effect is greater than the sum of the two (or more) single effects.

target cell an erythrocyte with a dark center surrounded by a light band that is encircled by a darker ring; thus, it resembles a shooting target.

thalassemia any of a group of inherited disorders of hemoglobin metabolism in which there is impaired synthesis of one or more of the polypeptide chains of globin.

therapeutic phlebotomy removal of a portion of the blood volume to alleviate symptoms.

thoracic aortic aneurysm widening or bulging of the upper portion of the aorta that may occur in the descending thoracic aorta, the ascending aorta, or the aortic arch.

thrombocythemia a primary form of thrombocytopenia, in contrast to secondary forms that are associated with metastatic neoplasms, tuberculosis, and leukemia involving the bone marrow, or occurring as the result of direct suppression of bone marrow by the use of chemical agents.

thrombocytopenia a condition in which an abnormally small number of platelets appear in the circulating blood.

tolerance no longer responding to the substance in the same way as initially responded, and a larger dose is required to achieve the initial effect.

total iron-binding capacity (TIBC) a measure of all proteins available to bind iron and an indirect measure of transferrin levels.

transcription the process by which the information contained in a template strand of DNA is copied into a single-stranded RNA molecule of complementary base sequence.

transduction transfer of genetic material (and its phenotypic expression) from one cell to another by viral infection.

transfer ribonucleic acids (tRNA) a small RNA molecule that translates a codon into an amino acid in protein synthesis; it has a three-base sequence, called the anticodon, complementary to a specific codon in mRNA, and a site to which a specific amino acid is bound.

transferrin the globulin protein that transports iron to the bone marrow.

transferrin saturation levels the portion of transferrin bound to iron. This value is found by dividing the serum iron by the total iron-binding capacity.

translation the process by which the amino acid sequence of a polypeptide is synthesized on a ribosome according to the nucleotide sequence of an mRNA molecule.

translocation a mutation that results from an exchange of parts of two chromosomes.

triplet repeat expansion a condition in which the number of repeating triplet units in a gene is so great that it interferes with gene expression and causes more severe disease.

trisomy a disorder in which a normally diploid organism has an extra copy of one of the chromosomes.

trophoblast the cell layer covering the blastocyst that erodes the uterine mucosa and through which the embryo receives nourishment from the mother. The cells do not enter into the formation of the embryo itself, but rather contribute to the formation of the placenta.

truncated protein a protein that does not achieve its full length or its proper form and thus is missing some of the amino acid residues that are present in a normal protein. A truncated protein generally cannot perform the function for which it was intended because its structure is incapable of doing so.

tumor suppressor gene a gene that encodes a protein involved in controlling cellular growth; inactivation of this type of gene leads to deregulated cellular proliferation, as in cancer.

tumorigenesis production of a new growth or growths.

Turner syndrome a monosomy syndrome that results when an ovum lacking the X chromosome is fertilized by a sperm that contains an X chromosome. It may also occur when a genetically normal ovum is fertilized by a sperm lacking an X or Y chromosome. The result is an offspring with 22 pairs of autosomes and a single, unmatched X chromosome.

unifactorial one factor.

variable expressivity variation in which the disease symptoms are present.

varices an enlarged and tortuous vein, artery, or lymphatic vessel.

vector the vehicle used to carry a DNA insert (e.g., a virus).

von Willebrand's disease a bleeding disorder in which von Willebrand factor, a blood protein, is either missing or does not function properly. It is the most common congenital bleeding disorder in the United States.

wide local excision a surgical procedure to remove some of the normal tissue surrounding the area where melanoma was found to check for cancer cells not visible on gross examination.

Wolff-Parkinson-White syndrome an electrocardiographic pattern sometimes associated with paroxysmal tachycardia; it consists of a short P-R interval (usually 0.1 second or less, occasionally normal) together with a prolonged QRS complex with a slurred initial component (delta wave).

xanthomas a cutaneous manifestation of lipid accumulation in the large foam cells that presents clinically as small eruptions with distinct morphologies along tendons such as the Achilles tendon.

xanthelasmata sharply demarcated yellowish collections of cholesterol in foam cells observed underneath the skin, and especially on the eyelids.

X-linked recessive recessive inheritance pattern of alleles at loci on the X chromosome that do not undergo crossing over during male meiosis.

yolk sac the sac of extraembryonic membrane that is located ventral to the embryonic disk and, after formation of the gut tube, is connected to the midgut; by the second month of development, this connection has become the narrow yolk stalk. The yolk sac is the first hematopoietic organ of the embryo.

zygote fertilized ovum before cleavage begins.

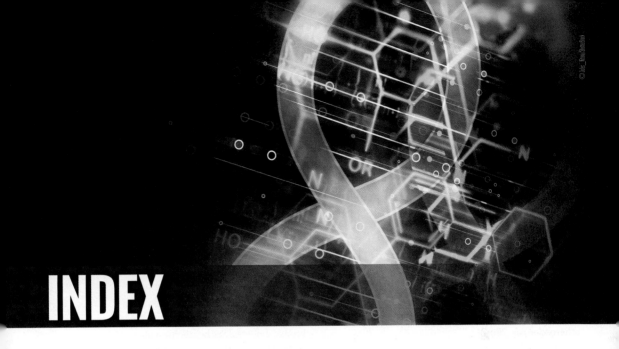

INDEX